110 PUZZLING CASES OF EPILEPSY

T0373679

The cover artwork, 'Barbican Fair', is the Plymouth Barbican where the Pilgrims departed for New England. The artist, Simon Powell, is an English artist with epilepsy.

110 PUZZLING CASES OF EPILEPSY

Edited by

Dieter Schmidt

Emeritus Professor of Neurology
Free University of Berlin;
Managing Editor of Epilepsy Research
Epilepsy Research Group
Goethestr. 5
D-14163 Berlin
Germany

Steven C Schachter

Medical Director, Office of Clinical
Trials and Research;
Director of Clinical Research
Comprehensive Epilepsy Center
Beth Israel Deaconess Medical Center
Associate Professor of Neurology
Harvard Medical School
Boston MA, USA

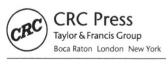 **CRC Press**
Taylor & Francis Group
Boca Raton London New York

CRC Press is an imprint of the
Taylor & Francis Group, an **informa** business

CRC Press
Taylor & Francis Group
6000 Broken Sound Parkway NW, Suite 300
Boca Raton, FL 33487-2742

First issued in paperback 2019

© 2002 by Taylor & Francis Group, LLC
CRC Press is an imprint of Taylor & Francis Group, an Informa business

No claim to original U.S. Government works

ISBN-13: 978-0-367-39659-6

**Visit the Taylor & Francis Web site at
http://www.taylorandfrancis.com**

**and the CRC Press Web site at
http://www.crcpress.com**

Contents

vi

Contributors

Christine Adam MD
UEROS, Soisy sur Seine, France.

Claude Adam MD
Department of Neurology 1,
EEG video
Hopital de la Pitié-Salpêtrière, Paris,
France.

Albert P Aldenkamp MD
Professor and Head, Department of
Behavioural Science and Psychological
Services
Epilepsiecentrum Kempenhaeghe,
Heeze, The Netherlands.

Taoufik Alsaadi MD
Assistant Professor of Clinical
Neurology, Co-director,
Comprehensive Epilepsy Program,
Department of Neurology, Sacramento
CA, USA.

Jørgen Alving MD
Department of Clinical
Neurophysiology, Dianalund Epilepsy
Hospital, Dianalund, Denmark.

Eva Andermann MD PhD FCCMG
Neurogeneticist, Montreal
Neurological Hospital, Montreal PQ,
Canada.

Frederick Andermann MD FRCPC
Neurologist, Montreal Neurological
Hospital, Montreal PQ, Canada.

Jesus Andres MD PhD
Assistant of Pediatrics, Hospital Rio
Carrion, Palencia, Spain.

Mary R Andriola MD
Professor of Neurology and Pediatrics,
Director, Divisions of Clinical
Neurophysiology and Child
Neurology, Department of Neurology,
School of Medicine, State University of
New York at Stony Brook Health
Sciences Center, Stony Brook NY,
USA.

Richard E Appleton MBBS DCH
MA(Oxon) FRCP FRCPCH
Consultant Paediatric Neurologist and
Honorary Clinical Lecturer in Child
Health, The Roald Dahl EEG Unit,
Alder Hey Children's Hospital,
Liverpool, UK.

Julio Ardura MD PhD
Professor of Pediatrics, Head of
Pediatrics, Hospital University,
Valladolid, Spain.

Johan Arends MD PhD
Head, Department of Clinical
Neurophysiology, Epilepsiecentrum
Kempenhaeghe, Heeze, The
Netherlands.

Santiago Arroyo MD PhD
Unidad Epilepsia, Hospital Clínico de
Barcelona, Barcelona, Spain.

Gus A Baker PhD FBPsS
Senior Lecturer in Clinical
Neurophysiology, The Walton Centre
for Neurology & Neurosurgery,
Liverpool, UK.

Hoan Linh Banh MD
Toronto, Ontario, Canada.

Claudio Bassetti MD
Abteilung für Neuropsychologische
Rehabilitation, Neurologische Klinik,
Inselspital Bern, Bern, Switzerland.

Gerhard Bauer MD
University Hospital for Neurology,
Innsbruck, Austria.

Jürgen Bauer MD
Neurologist, Klinik für Epileptologie,
Universität Bonn, Bonn, Germany.

Michel Baulac MD
Professor and Head of Epileptology
Hopital Pitié-Salpêtrière, Paris,
France.

Christoph Baumgartner MD
Head, Epilepsy Monitoring Unit,
Universitätsklinik für Neurologie,
Vienna, Austria.

Carl W Bazil MD
Assistant Professor of Neurology,
Columbia University College of
Physicians and Surgeons; Director,
Clinical Anticonvulsant Drug Trials,
Columbia Comprehensive Epilepsy
Center, New York-Presbyterian
Hospital, New York NY, USA.

Mark D Bej MD
Section of Epilepsy and Sleep
Disorders, Section of Neurological
Computing, Department of
Neurology, Cleveland Clinic
Foundation, Cleveland OH, USA.

Elinor Ben-Menachem MD
Department of Clinical Neuroscience,
Sahlgrenska University Hospital,
Göteborg University, Göteborg,
Sweden.

**Roy G Beran MD FRACP
FRACGP FAFPHM**
Neurologist, Chatswood NSW,
Australia.

David Berry PhD LRIC
Principal Biochemist, Medical
Toxicology Unit, Guy's Hospital,
London, UK.

Edward H Bertram III MD
Associate Professor, FE Dreifuss
Comprehensive Epilepsy Program,
Department of Neurology, University
of Virginia, Charlottesville VA, USA.

Frank M C Besag MD FRCPsych FRCPCH
Consultant Neuropsychiatrist, Learning Disabilities Service, Bedfordshire and Luton Community NHS Trust, Specialist Medical Department, Twinwoods Health Resource Centre, Clapham, Beds, UK.

David B Bettis MD
Paediatric Neurology of Idaho, Children's Specialty Center, Boise ID, USA.

Tim Betts FRCPsych
Reader in Neuropsychiatry, University of Birmingham, Honorary Consultant Neuropsychiatrist, South Birmingham Mental Health Trust, Birmingham, UK.

Ahmad Beydoun MD
Associate Professor of Neurology; Director, Epilepsy Program and Clinical Neurophysiology Laboratories, University of Michigan, Ann Arbor MI, USA.

Nadir E Bharucha MD
Chief, Department of Neuroepidemiology, Medical Research Centre, Mumbai, India.

Christian G Bien MD
Department of Epileptology, University of Bonn, Bonn, Germany.

Warren T Blume MD FRCP(C)
Professor, Department of Clinical Neurological Sciences, Epilepsy and Clinical Neurophysiology, London Health Sciences Center, London ON, Canada.

Jane Boggs MD
Associate Professor of Neurology, Director, EpiCenter USA, University of South Alabama, Mobile AL, USA.

Kirsten A Bracht MD
Co-Medical Director, CNI Epilepsy Center, Colorado Neurological Institute, Englewood CO, USA.

Martin J Brodie MD FRCP
Professor of Medicine and Clinical Pharmacology; Director, Epilepsy Unit, University of Glasgow, Glasgow, Scotland.

Edward B Bromfield MD
Chief, Division of Epilepsy and EEG, Department of Neurology, Brigham and Women's Hospital, Boston MA, USA.

Daniel J Brotman MD
Associate Staff, Department of Internal Medicine, The Cleveland Clinic Foundation, Cleveland OH, USA.

Carol S Camfield MD FRCP(C)
Professor of Pediatrics, Dalhousie University Medical School, IWK Health Centre, Halifax NS, Canada.

Peter R Camfield MS FRCP(C)
Professor and Chair of the Department
of Pediatrics, Dalhousie University
Medical School, IWK Health Centre,
Halifax NS, Canada.

Enrique J Carrazana MD
Executive Director, Neurosciences
Scientific Operations, Novartis
Pharmaceuticals Corporation, East
Hanover NJ, USA.

Catherine Chiron MD PhD
Neuropediatrician and Specialist in
Childhood Epilepsy, Neuropediatric
Department, Hopital St Vincent de
Paul, Paris, France.

Cesare Maria Cornaggia MD
UO Handicap Psicorganico Adulto,
Bergamo, Italy.

**Paulo Rogério M de Bittencourt
MD**
Director, Unidade de Neurologia
Clinica, Curitiba, Brazil.

Orrin Devinsky MD
Professor of Neurology, Neurosurgery
& Psychiatry, NYU School of
Medicine; Director NYU–Mount Sinai
Epilepsy Center; Director, St Barnabus
Institute of Neurology, New York NY,
USA.

Joost P H Drenth MD
Department of Endocrinology,
University Medical Center St
Radboud, Nijmegen, The Netherlands.

François Dubeau MD FRCPC
Neurologist, Montreal Neurological
Hospital, Montreal PQ, Canada.

P Barton Duell MD
Associate Professor of Medicine,
Division of Endocrinology, Diabetes,
and Clinical Medicine; Director,
Metabolic Disorders Clinic, Oregon
Health Sciences University, Portland
OR, USA.

Olivier Dulac MD
Professor of Pediatrics
Université René Descartes, Paris;
Hôpital Saint-Vincent-de-Paul, Service
de Neuropédiatrie, Paris, France.

Keith R Edwards MD
Director, Neurological Research
Center Inc, Bennington VT, USA.

Manuel Eglau MD
Department of Neurology–Center for
Epilepsy, University of
Erlangen–Nürnberg, Erlangen,
Germany.

Christian E Elger MD PhD FRCP
Professor and Chairman, Department
of Epileptology, University of Bonn,
Bonn, Germany.

Maurizio Elia MD
Department of Neurology, Oasi
Institute for Research on Mental
Retardation and Brain Aging, Troina,
Italy.

Eloy Elices MD
Unidad Epilepsia, Hospital Clínico de
Barcelona, Barcelona, Spain.

Alan B Ettinger MD
Associate Professor of Clinical
Neurology, Albert Einstein College of
Medicine; Director, LIJ
Comprehensive Epilepsy Center and
Huntington Hospital Seizure
Monitoring Program; Chief, Division
of EEG and Epilepsy, EEG Laboratory,
Long Island Jewish Medical Center,
New Hyde Park NY, USA.

Edward Faught MD
Professor and Interim Chairman,
Department of Neurology, University
of Alabama School of Medicine,
Birmingham AL, USA.

Natalio Fejerman MD
Chief, Servicio de Neurologia,
Hospital Nacional de Pediatria 'Juan P
Garrahan', Buenos Aires, Argentina;
and Secretary General of the
International League Against Epilepsy.

Robert S Fisher MD PhD
Director, Stanford Comprehensive
Epilepsy Center; Professor of
Neurology and Neurological Sciences,
Department of Neurology, Stanford
University Medical Center, Stanford
CA, USA.

Majid Fotuhi
Instructor in Neurology, and Fellow in
Neurophysiology, Department of
Neurology, Massachusetts General
Hospital, Harvard Medical School,
Boston MA, USA.

Jacqueline A French MD
Professor of Neurology, Associate
Director, Penn Epilepsy Center,
University of Pennsylvania,
Philadelphia PA, USA.

Lucia Fusco MD
Neurologist, Division of Neurology,
Bambino Gesù Hospital, Rome, Italy.

John R Gates MD
President, Minnesota Epilepsy Group,
PA, St Paul, MN; Clinical Professor,
Department of Neurology, University
of Minnesota, Minneapolis MN, USA.

Giuseppe Gobbi MD
UO Handicap Psicorganico Adulto,
Bergamo, Italy.

James Santiago Grisolia MD
Chairman, Advocacy Committee,
Epilepsy Foundation National
Professional Advisory Board, Scripps
Mercy Hospital; Associate Clinical
Professor of Neurosciences, UCSD
School of Medicine, San Diego CA,
USA.

Donald W Gross MD FRCPC
Neurologist, Montreal Neurological
Hospital, Montreal PQ, Canada.

Thomas Grunwald MD PhD
Senior Neurologist, Department of
Epileptology, University of Bonn,
Bonn, Germany.

Marilisa M Guerreiro
Assistant Professor of Child Neurology,
Department of Neurology, University
of Campinas (UNICAMP) Campinas,
São Paulo, Brazil.

Hajo M Hamer MD
Department of Neurology, University
of Marburg, Marburg. Germany.

Cynthia L Harden MD
Associate Professor of Neurology and
Neuroscience, Comprehensive
Epilepsy Center, Weill Cornell
Medical Center, New York
Presbyterian Hospital, New York NY,
USA.

Ad R M M Hermus MD
Department of Endocrinology,
University Medical Center St
Radboud, Nijmegen, The Netherlands.

Christian W Hess MD
Abteilung für Neuropsychologische
Rehabilitation, Neurologische Klinik,
Inselspital Bern, Bern, Switzerland.

Peter Höllinger MD
Abteilung für Neuropsychologische
Rehabilitation, Neurologische Klinik,
Inselspital Bern, Bern, Switzerland.

Peter Hopp MD
Department of Neurology–Center for
Epilepsy, University of
Erlangen–Nürnberg, Erlangen,
Germany.

Kazuie Iinuma MD PhD
Department of Pediatrics, Tohoku
University School of Medicine, Sendai,
Japan.

Yushi Inoue MD
Head, Clinical Division, National
Epilepsy Center, Shizuoka Medical
Institute for Neurological Disorders,
Shizuoka, Japan.

Jouko Isojärvi MD
Department of Neurology, University
of Oulu, Oulu, Finland.

Satish Jain MD DM
Professor in Neurology, Neurosciences
Centre, All India Institute of Medical
Sciences, New Delhi, India.

Isabelle Jambaqué MD
Hopital Saint-Vincent-de-Paul, Service
de Neuropédiatrie, Paris, France.

Reetta Kälviäinen MD
Department of Neurology, University
of Kupio, Kupio, Finland.

Sunao Kaneko MD PhD
Professor and Chairman, Department
of Neuropsychiatry, Hirosaki
University Hospital, Hirosaki, Japan.

Andres M Kanner MD
Associate Professor of Neurological
Sciences and Psychiatry; Director,
Laboratory of Electroencephalography
and Video-EEG Telemetry, Rush-
Presbyterian St Luke's Medical
Center, Chicago IL, USA.

Jaideep Kapur MD PhD
Associate Professor, FE Dreifuss
Comprehensive Epilepsy Program,
Department of Neurology, University
of Virginia, Charlottesville VA, USA.

Dorotheé GA Kasteleijn-Nolst Trenité MD PhD MPH
Department of Neurology, Medical Center Alkmaar, Alkmaar, The Netherlands.

Pavel Klein MB BChir
Department of Neurology, Georgetown University Medical Center, Washington DC, USA.

Susanne Knake MD
Department of Neurology, University of Marburg, Marburg. Germany.

Sookyong Koh MD PhD
Assistant in Neurology, Children's Hospital; Instructor, Harvard Medical School, Boston MA, USA.

Ronald E Kramer MD
Co-Medical Director, CNI Epilepsy Center, Colorado Neurological Institute, Englewood CO, USA.

Gregory L Krauss MD
Assistant Professor of Neurology, Johns Hopkins University Hospital, Baltimore MD, USA.

Ennapadam S Krishnamoorthy MD
Assistant Director, Research Faculty, National Neuroscience Institute, Singapore.

Kaarkuzhali Babu Krishnamurthy MD
Director, Women's Health in Epilepsy, Comprehensive Medical Center, Beth Israel Deaconess Medical Center, Boston MA, USA.

Martin Kurthen MD
Senior Neurologist, Department of Epileptology, University of Bonn, Bonn, Germany.

Thomas Kuruvilla MD
Research Associate, Department of Neuroepidemiology, Medical Research Centre, Bombay Hospital, Mumbai, India.

Ekrem Kutluay MD
Epilepsy Program and Clinical Neurophysiology Laboratories, University of Michigan, Ann Arbor MI, USA.

David M Labiner MD
Associate Professor of Neurology and Pharmacy Practice and Science; Associate Department Head and Director of Residency Training, Department of Neurology; Director, Arizona Comprehensive Epilepsy Program, the University of Arizona, Colleges of Medicine and Pharmacy, Tucson AZ, USA.

Paul M Levisohn MD
Assistant Professor of Pediatrics and Neurology, University of Colorado Health Sciences Center; Medical Director, Children's Epilepsy Program, The Children's Hospital, Denver CO, USA.

Dick Lindhout MD PhD
Professor of Medical Genetics, Chairman, Department of Medical Genetics, University Medical Center Utrecht, Utrecht, The Netherlands.

xix

Susan M Lippmann MD
Neurologist/Epileptologist, The
Comprehensive Epilepsy Care Center
for Children and Adults PC,
Chesterfield, Chesterfield MO, USA.

Brian Litt MD
Assistant Professor of Neurology and
Bioengineering, Penn Epilepsy Center,
Department of Neurology, University
of Pennsylvania School of Medicine,
Hospital of the University of
Pennsylvania, Philadelphia PA, USA.

Cesare T Lombroso MD PhD
Professor of Neurology, Harvard
Medical School (Emeritus); Director of
Clinical Neurophysiology Division and
of Seizure Unit (Emeritus), Children's
Hospital, Boston MA; Adjunct
Professor in Neurology, Department
of Neurology, University of Rochester
Medical School, Rochester NY, USA.

Gerhard Luef MD
Division of EEG and Seizure
Disorders, Department of Neurology,
University Hospital Innsbruck,
Innsbruck, Germany; First Secretary of
the Austrian Chapter of the ILAE
(1996–2000).

Vijay Maggio MD
Assistant Professor of Neurology;
Adult Epileptologist, Texas
Comprehensive Epilepsy Program,
University of Texas at Houston,
Houston TX, USA.

Alessandra Mascarini
Department of Clinical Psychiatry
University of Milano Bicocca, San
Gerardo Hospital, Monza, Italy.

Fumisuke Matsuo MD
Professor of Neurology, University of
Utah School of Medicine, Salt Lake
City UT, USA.

Cassandra I Matteo MD
New York Medical College
Department of Neurology
Munger Pavilion, Valhalla NY, USA.

Heinz-Joachim Meencke MD
Professor, Epilepsy Center Berlin,
Evangelisches Krankenhaus Königin
Elisabeth Herzberge, Teaching
Hospital of Humboldt University,
Berlin, Germany.

Jens Carsten Möller MD
Department of Neurology, University
of Marburg, Marburg, Germany.

Martha J Morrell MD
Director, Department of Epilepsy, The
Neurological Institute, New York-
Presbyterian Hospital, New York NY,
USA.

George Lee Morris III MD
Medical College of Wisconsin,
Milwaukee WI, USA.

Lisa Nashef MB FRCP
Consultant Neurologist and Honorary
Senior Lecturer, Kent and Canterbury
Hospital, Canterbury, and Kings
College Hospital, London, UK.

Wolfgang H Oertel MD
Director, Department of Neurology,
University of Marburg, Marburg.
Germany.

Christa Pachatz MD
Resident in Neurology, Division of
Neurology, Bambino Gesù Hospital,
Rome, Italy.

Erasmo A Passaro MD
Assistant Professor of Neurology;
Director, Adult Epilepsy Laboratory,
University of Michigan, Ann Arbor
MI, USA.

Marie-José Penniello MD
Hopital Saint-Vincent-de-Paul, Service
de Neuropédiatrie, Paris, France.

Gerlach F F M Pieters MD
Department of Endocrinology,
University Medical Center St
Radboud, Nijmegen, The Netherlands.

Perrine Plouin MD
Hopital Saint-Vincent-de-Paul, Service
de Neuropédiatrie, Paris, France.

Mark Quigg MD MS
Assistant Professor, FE Dreifuss
Comprehensive Epilepsy Program,
Department of Neurology, University
of Virginia, Charlottesville VA, USA.

R Eugene Ramsay MD
International Center for Epilepsy,
Department of Neurology, University
of Miami, School of Medicine, Miami
FL, USA.

Willy O Renier MD PhD
Professor of Epileptology, University
Medical Center, University of
Nijmegen, Nijmegen, The
Netherlands.

David C Reutens MD FRACP
Neurologist, Austin and Repatriation
Center, Melbourne, Australia.

William E Rosenfeld MD
Director, The Comprehensive
Epilepsy Care Center for Children and
Adults PC, Chesterfield, Chesterfield
MO, USA.

Felix Rosenow MD
Professor, Department of Neurology,
University of Marburg, Marburg,
Germany.

A James Rowan MD
Professor and Vice Chairman,
Department of Neurology, Mount Sinai
School of Medicine, Neurology Faculty
Associates, New York NY, USA.

Rajesh C Sachdeo MD
UMDNJ Robert Wood Johnson
Medical Center, New Brunswick NJ,
USA.

Steven C Schachter MD
Medical Director, Office of Clinical
Trials and Research, Director of
Clinical Research, Comprehensive
Epilepsy Center, Beth Israel Deaconess
Medical Center, and Associate
Professor of Neurology, Harvard
Medical School, Boston MA, USA.

**Ingrid E Scheffer MBBS PhD
FRCAP**
Paediatric Neurologist, Senior
Lecturer, Epilepsy Research Institute,
University of Melbourne, Austin and
Repatriation Medical Centre, Royal
Children's Hospital and Monash
Medical Centre, Melbourne, Australia.

Dieter Schmidt MD
Emeritus Professor of Neurology, Free University of Berlin; Managing Editor, Epilepsy Research, Epilepsy Research Group, Berlin, Germany.

Bettina Schmitz MD PhD
Epilepsy Research Group, Department of Neurology, Charité, Campus Virchow-Klinikum, Humboldt University, Berlin, Germany.

Donald L Schomer MD
Director, Comprehensive Epilepsy Center, Department of Neurology, Beth Israel Deaconess Medical Center, Boston MA, USA.

Masakazu Seino MD
Honorary President, National Epilepsy Center, Shizuoka Medical Institute for Neurological Disorders, Shizuoka, Japan.

Matti Sillanpää MD PhD
Professor Emeritus and Senior Researcher, Departments of Child Neurology and Public Health, University of Turku, Turku, Finland.

Joseph I Sirven MD
Director, EEG and Epilepsy, Mayo Clinic Scottsdale; Assistant Professor of Neurology, Mayo Medical School, Department of Neurology, Mayo Clinic, Rochester MN, USA.

Brien J Smith MD
Senior Staff Neurologist; Director, Epilepsy Monitoring Unit, Henry Ford Health System, Detroit MI, USA.

Michael R Sperling MD
Baldwin Keyes Professor of Neurology, Thomas Jefferson University; Director, Jefferson Comprehensive Epilepsy Center, and Director, Clinical Neurophysiology Laboratory, Thomas Jefferson University Hospital, Philadelphia PA, USA.

Carl E Stafstrom MD PhD
Associate Professor of Neurology and Pediatrics, University of Wisconsin, Madison WI, USA.

Hermann Stefan MD
Professor of Neurology/Epileptology, Department of Neurology–Center for Epilepsy, University of Erlangen–Nürnberg, Erlangen, Germany.

Paolo Tinuper MD
Research Fellow, Epilepsy Center, Neurological Institute, University of Bologna, Bologna, Italy.

Torbjörn Tomson MD PhD
Associate Professor, Department of Clinical Neuroscience, Division of Neurology, Karolinska Institute; Consultant Neurology, Department of Neurology, Karolinska Hospital, Stockholm, Sweden.

Alan R Towne MD
Professor and Chair, Department of Neurology, Virginia Commonwealth University MCV Campus, Richmond VA, USA.

xxii

Edwin Trevathan MD
Associate Professor of Neurology and
Pediatrics, Director, Neurology and
Pediatrics, Pediatric Epilepsy Center,
Washington University School of
Medicine, St Louis Children's
Hospital, St Louis MO, USA

Michael R Trimble MD
Professor of Behavioural Neurology,
Institute of Neurology, London, UK.

Eugen Trinka MD
Epilepsiemonitoring-Einheit,
Universitätsklinik für Neurologie,
Innsbruck, Austria.

**Jing-Jane Tsai MD Dr.Med
(Germany)**
Associate Professor in Neurology,
Chief, Division of Epileptology,
Department of Neurology, National
Heng Kung University Hospital,
Tainan, Taiwan.

Peter Uldall PhD
Child Neurologist and Consultant,
Rigshospitalet, Children's
Department, Juliane Marie Center,
Copenhagen, and Dianalund Epilepsy
Hospital, Dianalund, Denmark.

Walter van Emde Boas MD
Instituut voor Epilepsiebestrijding,
'Meer en Bosch' / 'De
Cruquiushoeve' Heemstede, The
Netherlands.

Federico Vigevano MD
Chief of the Neurological Division,
Bambino Gesù Hospital, Rome, Italy.

Nathalie Villenueve MD
Neuropediatrician and Specialist in
Childhood Epilepsy, Epilepsy Center,
Hopital St Paul, Marseille, France.

Biene Weber MD
Child Neurologist, Department of
Neurology, University Hospital of
Maastricht, Maastricht; Programme for
Child Neurology and Learning
Disabilities, Epilepsiecentrum
Kempenhaeghe, Heeze, The
Netherlands.

James W Wheless MD
Professor of Neurology and Pediatrics;
Director, Epilepsy Monitoring Unit;
Director, Texas Comprehensive
Epilepsy Program, University of Texas
at Houston, Houston TX, USA.

Andrew N Wilner MD FACP
Newport RI, USA.

Kazuichi Yagi MD
Director, National Epilepsy Center,
Shizuoka Medical Institute of
Neurological Disorders, Shizouka,
Japan.

Hiroyuki Yokoyama MD
Department of Pediatrics, Tohoku
University School of Medicine, Sendai,
Japan.

PREFACE

'In the system of the universe, what happens every day deserves the most attention'.

Cabanis: *Rapports du physique et du moral du homme*, 1802.

In the field of epilepsy, original observations are often the key to diagnosis and successful treatment. Indeed, the acumen to recognize the unexpected or unusual case distinguishes astute physicians. Further, case observations may prompt and stimulate basic science experiments and well-controlled clinical research. Yet illustrative reports and vignettes seem to have lost their appeal and are increasingly viewed with disdain as evidence-free medicine.

We believe that original observations are fine examples of human curiosity and the quintessence of medical science, especially in epilepsy. For this reason, we asked eminent colleagues from around the world to each contribute a case study, one that taught the clinician an important lesson and influenced the way they approached the care of their patients.

If you are curious to learn how experts are intrigued and informed by individual cases, or what clues patients may hold to the mysteries of epilepsy, this book may be of interest to you. Its purpose is to remind us that original observations still have a role by benefiting the practicing physician as well as inspiring the clinical scientist dedicated to solving today's unanswered questions in epilepsy.

Dieter Schmidt, Berlin
Steven C Schachter, Boston

I

Diagnostic Puzzles

Case 1

A YOUNG WOMAN WITH MOUTH JERKING PROVOKED BY READING

Taoufik Alsaadi

History

A 20-year-old left-handed junior college student (who has a family history of left-handedness) reports episodes of jerking of her mouth that have been present since the age of 16 years. She was born at full term after a normal pregnancy and delivery. She experienced her first febrile convulsion at the age of 18 months. Convulsions persisted until she went to kindergarten. She then remained free of seizures until the episodes of mouth jerking that began when she was 16. Both her grandfather and her paternal great-aunt had seizures in adulthood.

These episodes of mouth jerking were mostly provoked by reading, especially reading aloud but also by reading silently; rarely, they were triggered by conversational speech. Singing never triggered them. Spontaneous attacks did not occur. She has suffered a total of three of these convulsions since their onset. One of theses occurred while she was hospitalized for video-EEG monitoring.

The jerks responded poorly to carbamazepine, although generalized convulsions were prevented. Topiramate monotherapy of 100 mg twice a day controlled both the jerks and the convulsions.

Examination and investigations

Neurological examination, including mental status and language assessment, was normal. Her evaluation has already included admission for video-EEG monitoring. Several of her typical spells of mouth-jerking were recorded: one attack progressed to a secondarily generalized seizure. This attack was associated with rhythmic spikes arising from the left central region (Fig. 1.1).

Magnetic resonance imaging (MRI) scan of the brain with surface coils did not show any abnormalities.

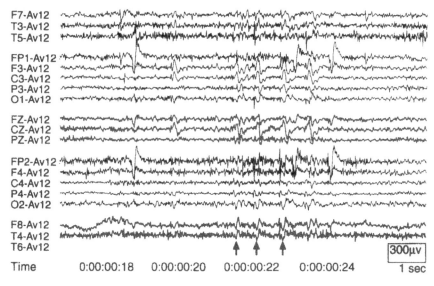

Figure 1.1 *Ictal EEG recording showing left central spikes (arrows) during the patient's typical 'click'.*

Diagnosis

Primary (inherited) reading epilepsy.

Treatment and outcome

Treatment with topiramate 100 mg twice a day was able to control her spells almost completely. She can now read well enough without having jerks. She has had no convulsions while talking.

The patient is currently engaged to be married and is planning to start a family in the near future. She was able to complete her college studies successfully and has now started to study to be a dental assistant.

Commentary

Why did I choose this case?

First, this case and other cases of reflex epilepsy have long fascinated me. They are rare and offer tantalizing glimpses into the mechanism of epileptogenesis and the organization of cognitive function.

3

Second, reading epilepsy can go unrecognized for years since it can be easily mistaken for tics or hysterical fits or for a primary language disorder if convulsions do not occur. Consequently, these patients may suffer psychosocial consequences for a long time before an accurate diagnosis is made.

Third, failure to recognize reading epilepsy may result in unnecessary investigations and delay in initiating the appropriate treatment, since it can be successfully treated in most cases with anticonvulsants, especially valproate or clonazepam.[7,8]

What did I learn from this case?

This patient's reading epilepsy was an inherited form of localization-related epilepsy that first manifests in early adolescence with mouth jerking or 'clicking' that is provoked by reading for some time, but not by writing or thinking. Convulsions may occur if reading persists for a longer time.[1-4] This disorder should by distinguished from the secondary (symptomatic) form of reading epilepsy by:

- the lack of interictal EEG abnormalities;
- the lack of spontaneous seizures;
- a normal neurological examination; and
- a normal MRI study.

A positive family history of seizures or primary reading epilepsy, or both, is another common feature of this disorder.[5-6] In some cases, but not all, jerks are associated with spikes, sharpened elements and paroxysmal rhythmical delta activity over the dominant temporoparietal region.

Although spontaneous remission is unlikely, these cases respond well to anticonvulsant treatment, as suggested by previous studies in the literature.[7,8] In most cases, life-long treatment is required.

References

1. Login IS, Kolakovich TM. Successful treatment of primary reading epilepsy with clonazepam. *Ann Neurol* 1978;4:155–6.

2. Vanerzant C, Fitz R, Holmes G, *et al*. Treatment of primary reading epilepsy with valproic acid. *Arch Neurol* 1982;39:452–3.

3. Valenti MP, Tinuper P, Cerullo A, Carcangiu R, Marini C. Reading epilepsy in a patient with previous idiopathic focal epilepsy with centrotemporal spikes. *Epileptic Disord* 1999;1:167–71.

4. Pegna AJ, Picard F, Martory MD, *et al*. Semantically-triggered reading epilepsy: an experimental case study. *Cortex* 1999;35:101–11.

4

5.   Yalcin AD, Forta H. Primary reading epilepsy. *Seizure* 1998;**7**:325–7.

6.   Wolf P, Mayer T, Reker M. Reading epilepsy: report of five new cases and further considerations on the pathophysiology. *Seizure* 1998;**7**:271–9.

7.   Saenz-Lope E, Herranz-Tannaro FJ, Masdeu JC. Primary reading epilepsy. *Epilepsia* 1985;**26**:649–56.

8.   Daly RF, Forster FM. Inheritance of reading epilepsy. *Neurology* 1975;**25**:1051–4.

Case 2

JERKY EYE MOVEMENTS IN A 2-YEAR-OLD-BOY WITH EPILEPTIC SEIZURES

Richard E Appleton

History

A 10-year-old boy initially presented at the age of 29 months after one generalized tonic–clonic seizure and one partial seizure. His birth, perinatal history and early development were normal. The patient's father had idiopathic generalized epilepsy; three siblings were all well. His parents were unrelated to each other.

An initial EEG at 30 months of age showed infrequent focal spike and slow waves over the left temporal region and photosensitivity. He was started on valproate but continued to experience infrequent tonic–clonic and simple partial motor seizures. Five months after presentation he developed atonic and myoclonic seizures, the latter up to 15–20 times a day. His development continued to progress although his mother felt that he had become clumsy and unsteady. His behaviour deteriorated and he became irritable and aggressive.

Examination and investigations

A paediatric neurologist subsequently saw the patient when he was 3½ years old. The patient's general physical examination was normal. Fundoscopy was normal – there was no optic atrophy or abnormal retinal pigmentation. Neurological examination showed no abnormalities of speech, hearing or vision. His gait was mildly ataxic and his fine motor skills were delayed to that of a child aged between 18 and 20 months. Cranial nerve examination was normal. There was no nystagmus, but his eye movements were jerky. Muscle tone was increased in his lower limbs and muscle stretch reflexes were brisk with extensor plantar responses. Frequent, brief myoclonic seizures affecting his head and body were observed.

A repeat EEG at 3½ years of age showed frequent paroxysms of high amplitude, irregular polyspike and spike–wave discharges against a normal background. Grade 3 and 4 photoparoxysmal responses were observed   intermittent photic

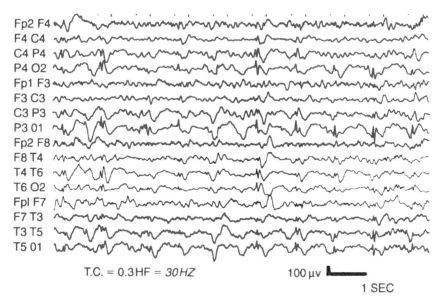

Fp2 F4
F4 C4
C4 P4
P4 O2
Fp1 F3
F3 C3
C3 P3
P3 O1
Fp2 F8
F8 T4
T4 T6
T6 O2
Fpl F7
F7 T3
T3 T5
T5 O1

T.C. = 0.3HF = 30HZ   100 μv
1 SEC

Figure 2.1: *A repeat EEG at 3½ years of age showed frequent paroxysms of high-amplitude, irregular polyspike and spike–wave discharges on a normal background and persisting photosensitivity with grade 3 and 4 photoparoxysmal responses. Intermittent photic stimulation (IPS) using single flashes at a frequency of 1 Hz demonstrated high-amplitude (>160 μV), bioccipital spike discharges, which appeared to be time-locked with each flash.*

stimulation using single flashes at a frequency of 1 Hz demonstrated high-amplitude (>160 μV), bioccipital spike discharges that appeared to be time-locked with each flash (Fig. 2.1); some of these discharges were associated with a whole-body myoclonic seizure.

Cranial magnetic resonance imaging showed enlarged lateral and third ventricles and generous extraventricular cerebrospinal fluid spaces, suggesting cerebral atrophy. Visual evoked potentials were markedly increased (>150 μV) and the electroretinogram was absent. Electron microscopy of the skin and rectum showed the presence of numerous curvilinear bodies and abnormal storage material.

Diagnosis

Late infantile neuronal ceroid lipofuscinosis (NCL2), also known as Batten–Bielschowsky–Jansky disease.

7

Treatment and outcome

The most effective treatment has been a combination of valproate (35 mg/kg per day), clonazepam (0.25 mg/kg per day) and benzhexol (3 mg/kg per day). Piracetam (up to a maximum dose of 600 mg/kg per day) was very effective in controlling this patient's non-epileptic myoclonus when he was 7–9 years of age. Lamotrigine was thought to have exacerbated his epileptic and non-epileptic myoclonus.

The patient is currently aged 11 years. He has severe spastic quadriplegia and cortical blindness. He has a feeding gastrostomy tube and requires 24-hour nursing care. He experiences daily myoclonic seizures and tonic–clonic seizures every 6–8 weeks. The patient also shows very frequent non-epileptic myoclonus that is largely spontaneous, but also stimulus-sensitive, as well as other involuntary (predominantly choreiform) movements.

Commentary

This child presented at 2½ years of age with two seizures. He was otherwise normal. The subsequent development of frequent myoclonic seizures, mild ataxia and behaviour changes, together with photosensitivity on the EEG, clearly raised a possible diagnosis of a form of progressive myoclonic epilepsy and an underlying neurodegenerative disorder.

The occurrence of photosensitivity is an unusual finding at this age (3 years), but in itself is not pathognomonic or diagnostic of any one specific neurodegenerative disorder. However, when attempting to identify photosensitivity, IPS should always include a flash frequency of 1 Hz. The occurrence of high-amplitude discharges that appear to be time-locked to each flash is virtually pathognomonic of late infantile NCL. The failure to use single flashes during IPS may contribute to a delay in the diagnosis of this disorder. Early diagnosis is important both for genetic counselling (including the possible prenatal identification of affected fetuses) and for the detection of younger, asymptomatic affected siblings.

What did I learn from this case?

The initial diagnosis was simply 'epilepsy.' 'Epilepsy' in itself is not an adequate diagnosis; any child with epileptic seizures must be ascribed, or classified into, a specific syndrome whenever possible and an underlying cause must then be considered (and often actively sought).

In addition to the important issues outlined above, this case also reinforces the role and importance of the EEG not only in helping to classify an epilepsy syndrome but also in providing valuable clues as to the underlying cause.

How did this case alter my approach to the care and treatment of my epilepsy patients?

When teaching medical and EEG technical staff, I routinely use this patient's history and evolution to illustrate the importance of the 'four-level' diagnostic approach in the assessment of every child who presents with possible epilepsy:

* are the child's episodes epileptic or non-epileptic?
* what is (are) the type (or types) of epileptic seizure(s)?
* what is the epilepsy syndrome?
* what is the cause of this child's epilepsy?

Further reading

Brett E. Progressive neurometabolic brain disease. In: Brett E, ed. *Paediatric Neurology* 3rd ed. London: Churchill–Livingstone, 1997:149–50.

Lyon G, Adams RD, Kolodny EH. Late infantile progressive genetic encephalopathies (metabolic encephalopathies of the second year of life). In: Lyon G, Adams RD, Kolodny EH, eds. *Neurology of Hereditary Metabolic Diseases of Children* 2nd ed. New York: McGraw–Hill, 1996:148–50.

Mole S, Gardiner M. Molecular genetics of the neuronal ceroid lipofuscinoses. *Epilepsia* 1999;**40(suppl 3)**:29–32.

Naqvi SZ, Beach RL, Armao DM, Greenwood RS. Photoparoxysmal response in late infantile neuronal ceroid lipofuscinosis. *Ped Neurol* 1998;**19**:395–8.

Acknowledgement

The author is grateful to Margaret Beirne, Chief EEG technician, for her assistance with the neurophysiological investigations in this patient.

Case 3

A PATIENT WHO WOULD NOT LEAVE HIS APARTMENT FOR HOURS EVERY THREE DAYS

Jürgen Bauer

History

The patient was a 52-year-old man who developed epilepsy at the age of 45 years. The only type of seizure he experienced was non-convulsive status epilepticus of focal temporal onset. Over the course of the preceding 7 years, the seizure frequency had increased to one seizure every 3 days. In between seizures, the patient was able to care for himself. However, during the seizures the patient stayed in his flat until the seizure activity ceased. There was incomplete amnesia for the period of the seizure.

Phenytoin (serum concentration >20 μg/ml) as monotherapy and combined with clobazam (20 mg/day) were without effect.

Examination and investigations

The interictal neurological and psychiatric examinations were normal. Similarly, the interictal EEG showed neither focal or generalized slowing nor epileptic discharges (Fig. 3.1). A magnetic resonance imaging scan of the brain was normal.

During a prolonged seizure, the patient's behaviour changed. In particular, his memory and speech fluency were impaired. EEG monitoring showed that his seizures lasted for several hours up to 1 day and that normalization occurred within a short time. During his seizures, bitemporal rhythmic theta-wave activity was documented on EEG (Fig. 3.2).

Diagnosis

Cryptogenic epilepsy characterized by focal non-convulsive status epilepticus.

10

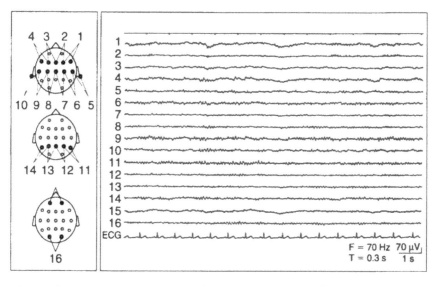

Figure 3.1: Interictal EEG without focal slowing or epileptiform activity.

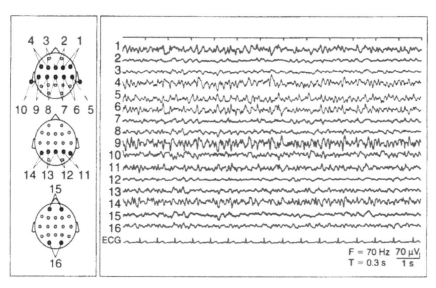

Figure 3.2: Ictal EEG showing bitemporal rhythmic theta-wave activity.

11

Treatment and outcome

Lamotrigine was added to the phenytoin and increased to 800 mg/day. At the time of the patient's last visit, his seizure frequency had decreased from one seizure every 3 days to one every 2 weeks.

Commentary

Non-convulsive status epilepticus, such as absence status epilepticus, is a rare event in patients suffering from epilepsy, but this patient demonstrates an even rarer form of epilepsy in which the sole manifestation is non-convulsive status epilepticus of focal (temporal) onset.[1,2]

Non-convulsive status epilepticus is usually treated acutely with benzodiazepines, phenytoin (for focal non-convulsive status epilepticus) or valproate (for absence status epilepticus). In patients with repetitive non-convulsive status epilepticus, however, acute therapy will not prevent further episodes. In such patients, chronic antiepileptic drug therapy is necessary. Interestingly, lamotrigine has proven to be an effective drug for the prevention of non-convulsive status epilepticus.[3]

In patients with epilepsy, non-convulsive status epilepticus may occur as a consequence of antiepileptic drug therapy. For example, carbamazepine and phenytoin may provoke absences in patients with idiopathic generalized epilepsy,[4] and tiagabine has been implicated as a cause of focal non-convulsive status epilepticus or atypical absence status in patients with focal epilepsy.[5] There was no evidence for an iatrogenic cause in this patient.

Epileptic non-convulsive status epilepticus may be mimicked by psychogenic seizures, which can last for hours or days.[6] Unlike in this case, an ictal EEG will not exhibit any abnormal findings related to the event. Similarly, endocrine disorders may also be mistaken for non-convulsive status epilepticus. I investigated a 30-year-old woman suffering from daily episodes of delayed responsiveness that had been classified as non-convulsive status epilepticus. The episodes of altered behaviour occurred after waking and lasted until breakfast. On investigation, it was determined that her serum glucose concentrations decreased to less than 28 mg/100ml during the night. Not surprisingly, carbamazepine had no influence on the frequency of her 'seizures'.

References

1.   Shorvon S. *Status Epilepticus*. Cambridge: Cambridge University Press; 1994.

2.   Bauer J, Helmstaedter C, Elger CE. Nonconvulsive status epilepticus with generalized 'fast' activity. *Seizure* 1997;6:67–70.

3. Bauer J, Wagner G, Elger CE. Sturzanfälle und Status nonkonvulsiver Anfälle als besondere Behandlungsindikation von Lamotrigin: Ergebnisse einer add-on Studie bei 46 Patienten mit pharmakoresistenten epileptischen Anfällen. *Aktuel Neurol* 1995;**22**:51–4.

4. Bauer J. Seizure-inducing effects of antiepileptic drugs: a review. *Acta Neurol Scand* 1996;**94**:367–77.

5. Ettinger AB, Bernal OG, Andriola MR, *et al.* Two cases of nonconvulsive status epilepticus in association with tiagabine therapy. *Epilepsia* 1999;**40**:1159–62.

6. Flügel D, Bauer J, Elger CE. Kriterien zur Differenzierung epileptischer und psychogener Fugue-Zustände. *Epilepsieblätter* 1995;**8**:39–41.

13

Cases 4 and 5

Two Adult Patients With Infantile Spasms

Carol S Camfield and Peter R Camfield

History

The first patient is currently an 18-year-old woman who is moderately mentally handicapped and has two predominant seizure types – partial complex seizures and persistent infantile spasms.

She was born after a normal pregnancy to healthy, non-related parents with no family history of neurological problems. At 6 months of age she had a 4-day history of myoclonic seizures and flexor spasms occurring in clusters. Neurologic examination and development were normal for age. A routine EEG showed typical hypsarrhythmia without focal features. and a computed tomography (CT) scan was normal. A diagnosis of West syndrome was made and she was treated with adrenocorticotropic hormone (ACTH) (40 units intramuscularly) and nitrazepam (0.2 mg/kg twice daily) with an immediate, marked decrease in spasms and a normalization of the EEG over 3 weeks. However, occasional spasms continued for the next 6 weeks and ACTH was increased to 60 units/day for an additional 6 weeks. ACTH was discontinued at 8 months of age and nitrazepam at 10 months of age.

At the age of 21 months the patient's development was normal, however, she had 'six strings of four to five spasms'. With each spasm, her arms 'shot up' and her head dropped forward for 2–5 seconds. She could remain standing during the spasms. Nitrazepam was restarted but was ineffective despite an increase in the dose to clinical toxicity. Valproate was added 2 weeks later. The runs of spasms decreased but did not stop.

About the same time she developed brief staring spells several times a day that were associated with speech interruption, odd facial expression, a small grunt and occasional eye deviation to the right with clonic arm movements. ACTH 60 units/day was given for 5 weeks with a major decrease in the frequency of the spasms. The EEG was normal. Valproate was stopped and nitrazepam was continued. Over the next 5 months, strings of spasms recurred. Her development still seemed normal.

14

When the patient was 4 years old, Professor Jean Aicardi paid a memorable visit to Halifax and felt that the patient had an 'excellent' prognosis for intellectual development with an emerging partial complex seizure disorder. Even the great ones are not always correct!

Starting at the age of 4½ years, carbamazepine was added for her complex partial seizures and her spasms continued with one 'string' a day despite nitrazepam. She appeared disoriented during a string of spasms and briefly afterwards. Sadly, her development plateaued, especially her speech.

The spasms continued, and at the age of 15 years, her complex partial seizures became more severe she would wander aimlessly for up to 5 minutes during a complex partial seizure, which was obviously dangerous for her. A magnetic resonance imaging (MRI) scan was normal. Clobazam was ineffective and vigabatrin was of transient benefit. At the age of 18 years, vigabatrin was replaced with lamotrigine. Her spasms recurred with a remarkable string of spasms that lasted for 45 minutes. She continues treatment with vigabatrin plus carbamazepine.

The second patient (case 5) is a 21-year-old woman who is mildly to moderately mentally handicapped with tuberous sclerosis. On the second day of life she had right-sided clonic seizures that were treated with phenobarbital. Her neurologic and skin examinations were normal. The EEG showed a left central focal spike discharge.

Seizures persisted and were resistant to phenobarbital, carbamazepine and phenytoin. At 6 months of age, she had a 1-week history of somnolence and loss of eye contact associated with the onset of typical infantile spasms. Spasms consisted of raising both arms and upward eye deviation for 1–2 seconds, with spasms repeating every 10–20 seconds for 5 10 minutes.

Her sibling and parents did not have a history of seizures or skin or retinal abnormalities.

The EEG showed a burst suppression pattern and hypsarrhythmia. For the first time, the typical hypopigmented macules of tuberous sclerosis were noted, but a CT scan (her first) was normal.

A diagnosis of West syndrome was made and she was treated with prednisone for 8 weeks, resulting in a more than 90 % decrease in both the spasms and the brief right-sided focal seizures. Subsequently the spasms disappeared, but the partial seizures gradually evolved into partial complex seizures and her EEG showed multifocal spike discharges.

At the age of 8 years, she began to have spasms again, and these have continued. She has 20–30 spasms in a series with one or two strings of spasms nearly every day. She is often incontinent during the string of spasms, which causes major restrictions in her social life. At the age of 18 years, she had her first and only generalized tonic–clonic seizure, which frightened her family more than any previous experience.

15

Over the years, treatment of her partial seizures and spasms has been ineffective; it has included phenobarbital, phenytoin, carbamazepine, prednisone, clonazepam, valproate, nitrazepam, the ketogenic diet, clobazam, felbamate (which produced a partial response with severe anorexia), vigabatrin and lamotrigine.

Now, at the age of 21 years, her spasms occur daily with urination during the attacks. Her skin examination shows typical hypopigmented macules and adenoma sebaceum. Her CT scan shows multiple calcified tubers, but ultrasound of her kidneys is normal. Her EEG continues to show a multifocal spike pattern.

She works happily in a sheltered workshop and functions at the mild to moderate mentally handicapped level. Through Special Olympics she goes bowling and skating regularly.

Commentary

Both patients illustrate that symptomatic and cryptogenic infantile spasms can persist into adulthood, apparently indefinitely. Experts in several recently published textbooks suggest that West syndrome is a disorder of infants only, which is true if persistent hypsarrhythmia is required for the diagnosis. Dulac, Plouin and Schlumberger note that 'hypsarrhythmia and therefore West syndrome is self-limited'.[1] Indeed, the hypsarrhythmia stops but they do note that when West syndrome is followed by Lennox–Gastaut syndrome, 'clusters of spasms persist in addition to the more characteristic seizures of Lennox–Gastaut.' Jeavons and Livet do not mention persistence of spasms in their chapter on West syndrome in an authoritative book.[2]

What did we learn from these cases?

First, infantile spasms may reappear in adult life. Adults with spasms must be rare and we do not think that spasms begin *de novo* in adulthood – they always start before the age of 4 years. In both of these patients, the spasms began in the first year of life, stopped completely for several years during early childhood but then later returned. Both patients had persistent partial complex seizures; however, the parents immediately recognized when the spasms returned, although the EEG did not revert to hypsarrhythmia. When the spasms returned they were completely unresponsive to current treatment. At first glance, the spasms seem relatively trivial; however, the first patient was transiently confused after a string of spasms and the second patient was incontinent. These problems have serious consequences as to whether patients can be free from supervision, and an effective treatment would be welcome.

We conclude that our patients no longer continue to fulfill the criteria for

West syndrome because of the evolution of the EEG; however, their problem is persistent spasms and it is a real problem. Spasms are not strictly age-related.

The most effective treatment for infantile spasms is ACTH. The first patient had an excellent response to the first course of ACTH but at the age of 2 years she had only a transient reduction in spasms. We have seen several other patients with spasms persisting into adulthood who also did not respond to repeated courses of ACTH.

Secondly, tuberous sclerosis may be difficult to diagnose in infants. The second patient had persistent partial seizures in the newborn period. We were very aware of the possibility of tuberous sclerosis and searched carefully for skin lesions, but there weren't any. She was born in 1978 when CT scanning of the newborn was just beginning. The electromagnetic interference scan of the day was normal but did not have the resolution of our current spiral CT scans. Presumably an MRI scan would have shown tubers. However, we had to wait until the onset of spasms at 6 months of age before the typical depigmented ash-leaf spots of tuberous sclerosis were first seen.

Since then we have seen another newborn with partial seizures whose mother has definite tuberous sclerosis. Two child neurologists and a dermatologist searched with and without a Wood's lamp and could not find any skin lesions. When the patient was aged 12 months they suddenly 'popped up'! The lesson is to keep looking if you suspect tuberous sclerosis.

How did these cases alter our approach to the care and treatment of our epilepsy patients?

In the follow-up of infantile spasms, we continue to ask about their re-emergence. The spasms are relatively easily misdiagnosed in older people. The recognition of their intractability is depressing but an important reality. Since our experience with these two cases, we are now aware of four other patients in our center and several more in other centers.

References

1.   Dulac O, Plouin P, Schlumberger E. Infantile spasms. In: Wyllie E, ed. *The treatment of epilepsy: principles and practice* 2nd ed. Baltimore: Williams and Wilkins; 1996:540–72.

2.   Jeavons PM, Livet MO. West syndrome: infantile spasms. In: Roger J, Bureau M, Dravet C, Dreiffus FE, Perret A, Wolf P, eds. *Epileptic syndromes in infancy, childhood and adolescence* 2nd ed. John Libbey; 1992:53–65.

Case 6

AN INFANT WITH PARTIAL SEIZURES AND INFANTILE SPASMS

Catherine Chiron and Nathalie Villeneuve

History

A baby girl experienced infantile spasms with hypsarrhythmia at 6 months of age. Her pregnancy and psychomotor development were normal. Spasms were stopped by vigabatrin monotherapy and the hypsarrhythmia disappeared, but a right temporal focus of spikes persisted. A magnetic resonance imaging (MRI) scan was normal.

The child continued to develop satisfactorily until spasms recurred on vigabatrin at 12 months of age; these spasms were associated with partial seizures. The spasms were again rapidly controlled using hydrocortisone, but partial seizures persisted. They were stereotyped in semiology: the child hid her eyes with her right arm and cried for about 30 seconds, and then she recovered immediately. Ictal EEG showed paroxysmal activity over the right hemisphere, but the onset could not be localized more precisely. The seizures were refractory to antiepileptic drugs (carbamazepine, valproate, benzodiazepines, phenytoin, lamotrigine and stiripentol) and to the ketogenic diet. She had between five and 10 seizures a day until she was 2½ years of age.

Examination and investigations

Neurological examination was normal except for moderate global mental retardation with predominant language dysfunction and hyperkinesia. A second MRI scan at age 2½ years was said to be normal. Ictal single photon emission computed tomography (SPECT) scanning imaged a 20-second seizure with the semiology described above; this scan showed a focus of hyperperfusion in the right temporal pole, in contrast to right temporal hypoperfusion seen interictally (Fig. 6.1). Further review of the MRI and comparison with subtraction interictal–ictal SPECT scans co-registered with MRI (see Fig. 6.1) discovered an abnormal gyrus in the right temporal pole with a focal cortical dysplasia.

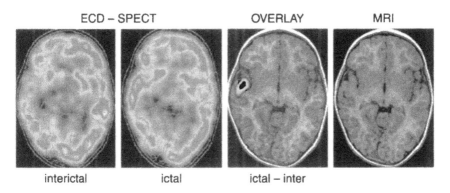

ECD – SPECT		OVERLAY	MRI
interictal	ictal	ictal – inter	

Figure 6.1: From left to right, interictal SPECT showing a right temporal hypoperfusion, ictal SPECT showing a right temporal hyperperfusion, subtraction image locating the ictal onset focus, and MRI showing a subtle cortical abnormality in the right temporal pole, in a 2½-year-old girl presenting with refractory partial seizures. This focus corresponds to a dysplastic lesion, which has been discovered on MRI after analysis of the ictal SPECT (MRI had previously been interpreted as normal). After right temporal lobectomy limited to the pole, the child became seizure-free.

Diagnosis

Infantile spasms (West Syndrome) and right temporal lobe epilepsy with a focal cortical dysplasia.

Treatment and outcome

The child underwent surgical resection of the right temporal pole without intracranial EEG recording. She has been seizure-free for 3 years and without antiepileptic drugs for 2 years. Language and behaviour improved when she was aged 5, though she continues to have mild mental retardation.

Commentary

Why did we choose this case?

We chose this case for three reasons. First, it shows that children with a focal lesion may have a generalized epilepsy. During the first year of life, infantile spasms with generalized seizures (epileptic spasms) and generalized EEG features between

19

spasms (hypsarrhythmia) can be associated with partial seizures. This combination is quite frequent – a focal lesion is found in more than 50 % of infantile spasms.

Secondly, such a lesion, although actively searched for on MRI, is often missed before the age of 2 years, owing to myelin immaturity. Among the cause of infantile spasms, focal cortical dysplasia may present with subtle MRI features limited to a lack of delineation of grey and white matter. These signs may not be present until myelin is mature. MRI should be repeated at least once after the age of 2 years using new sequences such as FLAIR, which appear to increase MRI sensitivity in infants.

Thirdly, focal surgical resection can be successfully performed in very young children. Whereas spasms are usually easily controlled in focal cortical dysplasia, partial seizures are known to be highly refractory to medical treatment. Presurgical investigations in young children should involve the same procedures as in adults, namely video–EEG monitoring of seizures, MRI, neuropsychological evaluation and functional imaging, if possible. In the present case, ictal SPECT had a great impact on our decision to proceed with surgery. The excellent concordance between ictal semiology, ictal SPECT and the lesion on MRI allowed us to perform the resection without the need for additional ictal recordings with intracranial EEG, as it is often done in adults.

What did we learn from this case and how did it alter our approach to the care and treatment of our epilepsy patients?

Two particular aspects of this case impressed us and have modified our approach to our patients. First, the interictal EEG focus – right temporal spikes – was noticed from the beginning of the story and proved to be a key point. It represented the only focal sign and was present for many months. In retrospect, this finding was highly relevant. We have to be aware of such subtle and peculiar features.

Secondly, ictal SPECT was a crucial component of the presurgical examination, although the patient's seizures were short and we had some difficulty identifying them clinically. Because the parents were able to recognize the onset of every seizure, their presence when ictal SPECT was performed was the most important reason for the success of this examination.

Further reading

Chugani HT, Shields WD, Shewmon DA, Olson DM, Phelps ME, Peacock WJ. Infantile spasms: I. PET identifies focal cortical dysgenesis in cryptogenic cases for surgical treatment. *Ann Neurol* 1990;**27**:406–13.

Dulac O, Chugani H, Dalla-Bernadina B, eds. *Infantile spasms and West syndrome*. London: WB Saunders; 1994.

Chiron C, Vera P, Kaminska A, *et al*. Single-photon emission computed tomography: ictal perfusion in childhood epilepsies. *Brain Dev* 1999;**100**:1–3.

Case 7

Epilepsia Partialis Continua Versus Non-Epileptic Seizures

Alan B Ettinger

History

A 42-year-old right-handed male was evaluated for episodes of twitching movements of the right hand that began 2 weeks earlier. He had a 3-year history of bipolar disorder, which was well controlled on valproate 1500 mg/day. He was moderately overweight and had a history of sleep apnea treated with continuous positive air pressure (CPAP).

The episodes were stereotypic, beginning with numbness of the left hand and arm and a flushed feeling in his face. This was followed by uncontrollable twitching movements of the right hand. The episodes lasted from 10 minutes to 4 hours and occurred an average of four times a week. Lorazepam 2 mg/kg intravenously had been administered at another hospital during a prolonged episode but had no effect. All episodes occurred while the patient was awake and there were no precipitants such as sleep deprivation.

Previous diagnostic testing included normal magnetic resonance imaging, EEG, complete blood count and blood chemistry as well as a negative Lyme titre.

Examination and investigations

Video-EEG monitoring revealed stereotyped sensorimotor episodes beginning with a sensation of numbness in the left hand and in the neck and face. Subsequently, right-sided flexion—extension movements occurred. These movements involved the second, third, fourth and fifth digits at the metacarpophalyngeal joints or the entire hand. The movements were usually arrhythmic but were sometimes rhythmic at 1–3 Hz. Movements would intermittently stop for several seconds. The episodes lasted 7–10 minutes and did not occur during sleep.

The episodes stopped briefly when the patient's attention was diverted while performing a left upper extremity task. There was no weakness during or between episodes. The patient appeared to be in no emotional distress during the

21

episodes and would speak calmly to examiners. One episode that began 6 hours before a second admission to our unit was terminated immediately with a placebo 'antidote' administered intravenously. During the episodes, there was no change on EEG. An ictal single-photon emission computed tomography (SPECT) scan revealed no perfusion abnormalities.

Diagnosis

Psychogenic non-epileptic seizures.

Treatment and outcome

The patient initially accepted the diagnosis of non-epileptic seizures but subsequently expressed skepticism and sought a second opinion because of persistent episodes.

Commentary

Epilepsia partialis continua (EPC) is a relatively rare form of seizures that is characterized by localized, prolonged myoclonic jerking.[1] This disorder can affect most muscle groups, especially in the distal limbs.[2] Among different cases of EPC, motor activity varies in distribution, rate, rhythm and intensity.[2,3] EPC may lack a visually detectable scalp EEG correlate.[2,4]

Psychogenic non-epileptic seizures resemble epileptic seizures but result from psychological factors, not from central nervous system dysfunction.[5,6] Although the medical literature usually focuses on cases with bilateral motor activity and unresponsiveness,[7,9] non-epileptic seizures are also associated with focal muscle activity and preserved responsiveness. In such cases, differentiating partial motor seizures from non-epileptic seizures can be very challenging.

What did I learn from this case?

This case demonstrated to me the difficulties in distinguishing non-epileptic seizures with prolonged focal motor activity from EPC, as well as the potential hazards of misdiagnosis.

Several features helped distinguish this case from true EPC. The appearance of the movements suggested a potential psychogenic origin. Movements varied between episodes, on one occasion with flexion–extension movements at the metacarpophalangeal joints and at other times with flexion–extension movements at the wrist.

22

A psychogenic mechanism was further supported by the transient abolition of movements when the face or contralateral extremity was engaged in an effortful task. This probably occurred because of the patient's inability to co-ordinate simultaneous movements on a functional basis. A similar finding has emerged in studies of posthypnotic suggestion. Task interference occurs when subjects receive a posthypnotic suggestion to search for one number and are asked to search for another number in a series of digits.[10] Thus, although posthypnotic suggestion and conversion symptoms are executed without conscious awareness, they tap the same attentional networks that are used to execute conscious tasks. Although inhibition or activation of movements related to EPC may occur with voluntary motor tasks or sensory stimulation of the affected limb,[11,12] this patient and two others I have seen demonstrated abolition of activity when they performed tasks using other parts of the body. Eliciting and abolishing typical episodes with normal saline and suggestion provide very strong support for the diagnosis of non-epileptic seizures.

Most patients with EPC demonstrate varying degrees of peri-ictal muscle weakness. This patient had no paresis immediately before, during or between episodes.[1,2,12 14] Furthermore, his calm demeanor – he appeared undisturbed by the events – also suggested non-epileptic seizure, although this was a less definitive sign.

The failure to see hyperperfusion on ictal SPECT scan also suggests non-epileptic seizure. Although the sensitivity of ictal SPECT scanning in EPC is unknown, several reports suggest that SPECT scanning is sensitive and can reveal hyperperfusion even in the absence of EEG changes.[15,16]

Our patient had no demonstrable etiology for EPC despite vigorous blood testing and neuroimaging. Although the number of idiopathic cases of EPC is unknown, most reports of EPC describe readily identified causes such as metabolic,[17] inflammatory,[18] infectious,[19 21] vascular,[2] neoplastic[13] and other structural[22] etiologies. Although one of my patients had a history of seizures, the other two showed no evidence of neurological or metabolic disturbance.

A number of features demonstrated in this case were not helpful in distinguishing non-epileptic seizure from EPC. For example, the arrhythmic movements did not prove their functional nature, since EPC movements are often arrhythmic.[2] The failure to demonstrate episodes during sleep does not exclude EPC since it can diminish or stop during sleep.[2] A previous psychiatric history was also not helpful since psychiatric disturbances, including depression[23 26] and anxiety,[27,28] are common in epilepsy.[29] Finally, the failure of these episodes to respond to antiepileptic drugs did not exclude EPC, since the response to antiepileptic drugs, including intravenous benzodiazepines, is often poor in EPC.[2]

Other techniques can help distinguish EPC from non-epileptic seizure. Supplemental scalp electrodes near the sensory–motor strip may enhance the identification of changes on EEG during the episodes. Other electrophysiological techniques, including demonstration of giant somatosensory evoked potentials[30,31] and isolated spikes preceding myoclonic jerks on back-averaged EEG,[4,31] can also help to diagnose EPC.

How did this case alter my approach to the care and treatment of my patients with epilepsy?

I have learned to recognize the possibility of non-epileptic events resembling EPC by the presence of the following features:

- variability in the areas of motor activity in the same patient;
- distribution and spread of motor activity without a neuroanatomic basis;
- transient abolition of movements with distraction (e.g. when other body parts are engaged in effortful tasks);
- eliciting and abolishing typical episodes with suggestive techniques;
- absence of motor weakness during or in between episodes;
- absence of EEG correlate of motor activity; and
- absence of hyperperfusion on ictal SPECT scan.

References

1. Watanabe K, Kuroiwa Y, Toyokura Y. Epilepsia partialis continua. Epileptogenic focus in motor cortex and its participation in transcortical reflexes. *Arch Neurol* 1984;**41**:1040–4.

2. Thomas JE, Reagan TJ, Klass DW. Epilepsia partialis continua. *Arch Neurol* 1977;**34**:266–75.

3. Schomer DL. Focal status epilepticus and epilepsia partialis continua in adults and children. *Epilepsia* 1993;**34(suppl 1)**:S29–S36.

4. Hallett M, Chadwick D, Marsden CD. Cortical reflex myoclonus. *Neurology* 1979;**29**:309–18.

5. Ozkara C, Dreifuss FE. Differential diagnosis in pseudoepileptic seizures. *Epilepsia* 1993;**34**:294–8.

6. Bazil CW, Kothari M, Luciano D, *et al.* Provocation of nonepileptic seizures by suggestion in a general seizure population. *Epilepsia* 1994;**34**:768–70.

7. Gulick TA, Spinks IP, King DW. Pseudoseizures: ictal phenomena. *Neurology* 1982;**32**:24–30.

8. Gumnit RJ, Gates JR. Psychogenic seizures. *Epilepsia* 1986;**27**:S124–S129.

9. Gates JR, Ramani V, Whalen S, *et al.* Ictal characteristics of pseudoseizures. *Arch Neurol* 1985;**42**:1183–7.

10. Kihlstrom JF. The cognitive unconscious. *Science* 1987;**237**:1445–52.

11. Wieser HG, Graf HP, Bernoulli C, Siegfried J. Quantitative analysis of intracerebral recordings in epilepsia partialis continua. *Electroencephalogr Clin Neurophysiol* 1977;**44**:14–22.

12. Hefter H, Witte OW, Reiners K, Niedermeyer E, Freund HJ. High frequency bursting during rapid finger movements in an unusual case of epilepsia partialis continua. *Electromyogr Clin Neurophysiol* 1994;**34**:95–103.

13. Botez MI, Brossard L. Epilepsia partialis continua with well-defined subcortical frontal tumor. *Epilepsia* 1974;**15**:39–43.

14. Juul-Jension P, Denny-Brown D. Epilepsia partialis continua. *Arch Neurol* 1966;15:563–78.

15. Katz A, Bose A, Lind S, Spencer S. SPECT in patients with epilepsia partialis continua. *Neurology* 1990;**40**:1848–50.

16. Sztriha L, Pavics L, Ambrus E. Epilepsia partialis continua: follow-up with 99mTc-HMPAO-SPECT. *Neuropediatrics* 1994;**25**:250–4.

17. Singh BM, Strobos RJ. Epilepsia partialis continua associated with nonketotic hyperglycemia: clinical and biochemical profile of 21 patients. *Ann Neurol* 1980;**8**:155–60.

18. Gray F, Serdaru M, Baron H. Chronic localized encephalitis (Rasmussen's) in an adult with epilepsia partialis continua. *J Neurol Neurosurg Psychiatry* 1987;**50**:747–51.

19. Komsuoglu SS, Liman O, Gurkan H. Epilepsia partialis continua following pertussis infection. *Clin Electroencephalogr* 1985;**16**:45–7.

20. Piatt JH, Hwang PA, Armstrong DC. Chronic focal encephalitis (Rasmussen syndrome): six cases. *Epilepsia* 1988;**29**:268–79.

21. Chalk CH, McManis PG, Cascino GD. Cryptococcal meningitis manifesting as epilepsia partialis continua of the abdomen. *Mayo Clin Proc* 1991;**66**:926–9.

22. Andermann F. Epilepsia partialis continua and other seizures arising from the precentral gyrus: high incidence in patients with Rasmussen syndrome and neuronal migration disorders. *Brain Dev* 1992;**14**:338–9.

23. Ettinger AB, Krupp LB, Jandorf L. Fatigue and depression in epilepsy. *Epilepsia* 1994;**35 (suppl 8)**:79.

24. Victoroff JI, Benson DF, Engel J Jr, Grafton S, Mazziotta JC. Interictal depression in patients with medically intractable complex partial seizures: electroencephalography and cerebral metabolic correlates. *Ann Neurol* 1990;**28**:221.

25. Robertson MM. Depression in patients with epilepsy: an overview and clinical study. In: Trimble MR, ed. *The psychopharmacology of epilepsy*. Chichester, UK: John Wiley; 1985.

25

26. Mendez MF, Cummings JL, Benson DF. Depression in epilepsy. *Arch Neurol* 1986;**43**:766–70.

27. Francis S, Weisbrot DM, Jandorf L, Krupp LB, Ettinger AB. Anxiety in epilepsy (abstract). *Epilepsia* 1996;**37(suppl 5)**:3.

28. Altshuler LL, Devinsky O, Post RM, Theodore W. Depression, anxiety, and temporal lobe epilepsy. *Arch Neurol* 1990;**47**:284–8.

29. Perrine K, Congett S. Neurobehavioral problems in epilepsy. In: Devinsky O, ed. *Neurologic clinics.* Philadelphia: WB Saunders: 1994:129–52.

30. Chauvel P, Liegeois-Chauvel C, Marquis P, Bancaud J. Distinction between the myoclonus-related potential and the epileptic spike in epilepsia partialis continua. *Electroencephalogr Clin Neurophysiol* 1986;**64**:304–7.

31. Cowan JMA, Rothwell JC, Wise RJS, Marsden CD. Electrophysiological and positron emission studies in a patient with cortical myoclonus, epilepsia partialis continua and motor epilepsy. *J Neurol Neurosurg Psychiatry* 1986;**49**:796–807.

Case 8

VOMITING IN AN 8-YEAR-OLD GIRL WITH STATUS EPILEPTICUS

Natalio Fejerman

History

This patient is an 8-year-old girl who was born to healthy parents. Her neurological and psychiatric development was normal. Her brother had a simple febrile convulsion at the age of 3 years.

Her first seizure occurred during sleep at the age of 5 years. She woke up with vomiting and head and eye deviation to the right. Consciousness became clouded, and right-sided tonic–clonic contractions started and then became secondarily generalized. The whole episode lasted almost 1 hour and was followed by right hemiparesis for 4 hours. One year later, she had a second brief seizure, also during sleep, with vomiting and ocular deviation to the right.

Examination and investigations

Neurological examination after recovery from the prolonged seizure was normal. Routine laboratory examinations were normal. The EEG obtained the next morning showed left occipital high-amplitude spikes that were non-reactive to eye opening. The frequency of the spikes increased during sleep (Fig. 8.1). Computed tomography and magnetic resonance imaging scans of the brain were normal.

Diagnosis

Idiopathic partial epilepsy with occipital spikes (Panayiotopoulos type).

Treatment and outcome

Treatment with carbamazepine 15 mg/kg/day was started after the first episode.

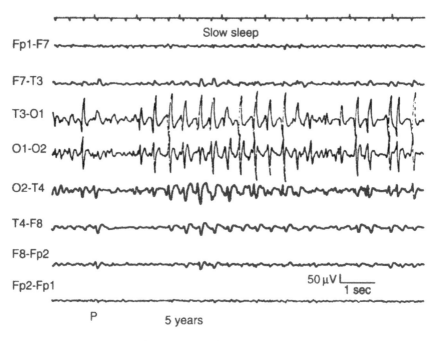

Figure 8.1: EEG with left occipital high-amplitude spikes during sleep.

The patient has remained seizure-free since then, and has been without medication during the last year.

Commentary

The way in which this patient presented might have suggested a severe cerebral insult. However, it is known that a significant number of patients with this benign form of epilepsy present with prolonged seizures, and yet the prognosis is good. On the other hand, vomiting in children has not usually been recognized as an initial ictal manifestation.

In my experience, this epileptic syndrome is about three or four times less common than benign partial epilepsy with centrotemporal spikes, but three or four times more common than the Gastaut type of childhood epilepsy with occipital paroxysms. I have suggested that this new syndrome be included in the International League Against Epilepsy's next classification of epileptic syndromes.

What did I learn from this case?

This was the first case in my series of 66 cases with the Panayiotopoulos type of childhood epilepsy with occipital paroxysms. In addition I learnt that:

- good clinical observation and judgement is essential to diagnosis of epilepsy syndrome;
- benign idiopathic partial epilepsy may present as an apparently grave condition;
- recognition of specific epileptic syndromes is of paramount importance for making treatment decisions and establishing the prognosis.

Further reading

Caraballo R, Cersosimo R, Medina C, Fejerman N. Panayiotopoulos-type benign childhood occipital epilepsy. *Neurology* 2000;**55**:1096–100.

Caraballo R, Cersosimo R, Medina C, Tenembaum S, Fejerman N. Epilepsias parciales idiopaticas con paroxismos occipitales. *Rev Neurol* 1997;**25**:1052–8.

Commission on Classification and Terminology of the International League Against Epilepsy. Proposal for revised classification of epilepsies and epileptic syndromes. *Epilepsia* 1989;**30**:389–99.

Fejerman N. New idiopathic partial epilepsies. *Epilepsia* 1997;**38(suppl 7)**:26.

Kivity S, Ephraim T, Weitz R, Tamir A. Childhood epilepsy with occipital paroxysms: Clinical variants in 134 patients. *Epilepsia* 2000;**41**:1522–33.

Oguni H, Hayashi K, Imai K, Muto K, Osawa M. Study on the early-onset variant of benign childhood epilepsy with occipital paroxysms otherwise described as early-onset benign occipital seizure susceptibility syndrome. *Epilepsia* 1999;**40**:1020–30.

Panayiotopoulos CP. Benign nocturnal childhood occipital epilepsy: a new syndrome with nocturnal seizures, tonic deviation of the eyes, and vomiting. *J Child Neurol* 1989;**4**:43–9.

Panayiotopoulos CP. *Benign childhood partial seizures and related epileptic syndromes.* London: John Libbey; 1999.

Panayiotopoulos CP. Early-onset benign childhood occipital seizure susceptibility syndrome: a syndrome to recognize. *Epilepsia* 1999;**40**:621–30.

Vigevano F, Ricci S. Benign occipital epilepsy of childhood with prolonged seizures and autonomic symptoms. In: Andermann F, Beaumanoir A, Mira L, Roger J, Tassinari CA, eds. *Occipital seizures and epilepsies in children.* London: John Libbey; 1993;133–40.

Case 9

PANIC ATTACKS IN A WOMAN WITH FRONTAL LOBE EPILEPSY

Thomas Grunwald, Martin Kurthen and Christian E Elger

History

A 32-year-old woman presented with frequent simple and complex partial
seizures since the age of 22. Often she would suffer from attacks of intense panic,
which were frequently followed by *déjà-vu* experiences or by a poorly localized
tingling sensation in the body. During these episodes she would normally tremble
and utter short phrases such as, 'Oh, no' or 'Oh, God'. These symptoms
sometimes preceded a partial or complete loss of consciousness during which the
patient would verbalize recurring syllables ('a ta ta ta ta'). She then would display
perseverative movements that resembled body-rocking or complex actions that
sometimes had an aggressive quality. For instance, we recorded seizures during
which she tore off the electrode cap and pulled the mattress off her bed.

These seizures had never been controlled despite treatment with
carbamazepine, phenytoin, lamotrigine and clonazepam in monotherapy and in
combination. The patient had graduated from extended elementary school and
had begun training to be a nurse. However, she had to abandon her plans because
of frequent seizures. When she was admitted for presurgical evaluation she was
unemployed and single.

Examination and investigation

On admission, the patient's neurological and psychiatric examinations were
normal. Neuropsychological tests revealed prominent non-verbal memory
deficits. Scalp EEG recordings showed an interictal right temporal sharp wave
focus. Ictal recordings, which were initially obscured by muscle artifacts, were
characterized by theta-wave activity over the right temporal lobe. Magnetic
resonance imaging (MRI) scans were negative but positron emission tomography
demonstrated right temporal hypometabolism consistent with the localization of
hyperperfusion during an ictal single photon emission computed tomography
examination.

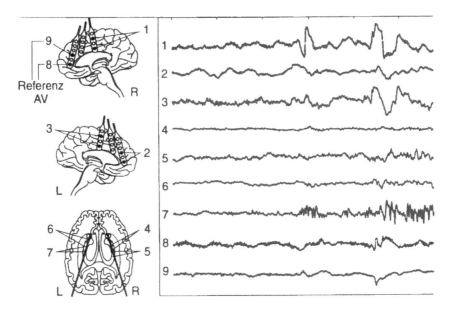

Figure 9.1: *Intracranial recording of the initial part of a complex partial seizure. Channel 8 shows low-amplitude fast activity in the anterior cingulate gyrus before and during a fast spread of seizure activity to the left hippocampus (channel 7) and right hippocampus (channel 5).*

Four seizures were recorded invasively using bilateral basal and lateral temporal as well as interhemispheric subdural strip and hippocampal depth electrodes. All seizures started with characteristic low amplitude fast activity within the right anterior cingulate gyrus (Fig. 9.1).

Diagnosis

Cryptogenic frontal lobe epilepsy with simple and complex partial cingulate seizures.

Treatment and outcome

An anterior mesial frontal resection, which included the anterior half of the right superior frontal gyrus and the right anterior cingulate gyrus, was performed. This procedure resulted in complete seizure control. Postoperative histopathological examinations revealed a glioneural hamartoma within the anterior cingulate gyrus.

31

Because the patient has now been seizure-free for 24 months, we have started to taper her carbamazepine and lamotrigine.

Commentary

This case demonstrates the importance of seizure semiology. During the presurgical evaluation of our patient, the results from non-invasive electrophysiological and functional imaging studies all pointed to the seizures originating within the right temporal lobe. In addition, our patient experienced auras with fear and *déjà-vu* and exhibited non-verbal memory deficits. These symptoms can also be associated with right-sided temporal lobe epilepsy. The only clue that the seizures arose from the anterior cingulate gyrus was the motor and hypermotor (complex movement) signs, which had a somewhat aggressive quality. This single clinical observation necessitated the use of interhemispheric subdural strip electrodes and, eventually, permitted the localization of the primary epileptogenic area.

Secondly, this case shows that morphological lesions causing symptomatic focal epilepsy can remain undetected by MRI scans. This is important because the correlation between structural lesions and the prognosis of epilepsy surgery is well known, especially in patients with seizures of extratemporal origin. Although 60–80 % of patients with lesional focal epilepsy become seizure-free postoperatively, outcome in non-lesional patients is often less successful. Our case indicates, however, that clearly localizing signs and findings may be related to a minor lesion that can be demonstrated histopathologically but that may have been too small to be detected by MRI. In such cases, invasive recordings are warranted and necessary to prove the localization of focal seizure onset. On the other hand, if localizing signs and findings cannot be obtained, it seems advisable to postpone further invasive studies until improved imaging techniques may justify the implantation of electrodes.

What did we learn from this case?

The anterior cingulate gyrus maintains massive interconnections, both with the limbic system and with the frontal, temporal and parietal neocortex. Therefore, cingulate seizures can have different possible propagation pathways, which may be responsible for the variability of their expression as seizures. Thus patients suffering from cingulate epilepsy can present with findings that are normally associated with epileptogenic foci in different areas of the brain. Ictal symptoms may include, for instance, somatosensory feelings, absence-like arrest, fear, vocalizations and verbalizations as well as complex (hypermotor) movements. Moreover, electrostimulation of this area in humans can elicit both movements and feelings of anxiety while in non-human primates it can also elicit vocalizations indicative of alarm or separation anxiety. Thus, the anterior cingulate gyrus may subserve the association of complex behavior with adequate emotional qualities and vice versa. However, its pathological activation can also elicit one without the other because cingulate gelastic seizures are characterized by laughter without the subjective feeling of mirth. Because this structure seems to be capable of mediating neocortical and limbic functions, it is an important target of neuropsychological research on cognitive processes in both healthy volunteers and patients with psychopathological disorders.

This case suggests that there may be other patients with cingulate epilepsy in whom all the findings point to a temporal lobe origin. Therefore, if results from non-invasive examinations are consistent with temporal lobe epilepsy but are not backed by MRI studies, the search for another possible seizure focus should continue and should always include the anterior cingulate gyrus.

Further reading

Devinsky O, Morrell M, Vogt BA. Contributions of anterior cingulate gyrus to behavior. *Brain* 1995;118:279–306.

Grunwald Th, Kurthen M, Elger CE. Predicting surgical outcome in epilepsy: how good are we? In: Schmidt D, Schachter SC, eds. *Epilepsy: Problem Solving in Clinical Practice*. London, Martin Dunitz; 2000:399–410.

Jurgens U. Vocal communications in primates. In: Kesner RP, Olton DS, eds. *Neurobiology of Comparative Cognition*. New Jersey: Erlbaum; 1990.

Mazars G. Criteria for identifying cingulate epilepsies. *Epilepsia* 1970;11:41–7.

So KN. Mesial frontal epilepsy. *Epilepsia* 1998;**39(suppl 4)**:49–61.

von Cramon D, Jurgens U. The anterior cingulate cortex and the phonatory control in monkey and man. *Neurosci Biobehav Rev* 1983;7:423–5.

Williamson PD, Spencer DD, Spencer SS, Novelly RA, Mattson RH. Complex partial seizures of frontal lobe origin. *Ann Neurol* 1985;18:497 504.

Case 10

MISDIAGNOSED EPILEPSY IN A YOUNG GIRL

Satish Jain

History

A young girl presented in 1992 with a history of four generalized tonic–clonic seizures that had begun at the age of 13 years. She had no history of febrile convulsions, absences or myoclonic jerks. A scalp EEG showed occasional generalized sharp waves, and a brain computed tomography (CT) scan was normal. She was started on carbamazepine 500 mg/day.

She continued to have occasional generalized tonic–clonic seizures during wakefulness and the dose of carbamazepine was gradually increased to 800 mg/day. She had another 10–12 generalized tonic–clonic seizures, and acetazolamide was added. She continued to have recurrent generalized tonic–clonic seizures and was admitted to the hospital for video-EEG recording. Some of the seizures recorded during the video-EEG were interpreted as pseudoseizures, and fluoxetine was added to the carbamazepine (which was increased to 1000 mg/day) and acetazolamide.

Two years later, recurrent seizures resulted in falls to the ground and tongue biting. Serum carbamazepine concentration was within the therapeutic range and a magnetic resonance imaging (MRI) scan of the brain was normal. She continued to have generalized tonic–clonic seizures, and phenobarbital (60 mg/day) was added without any beneficial effect. Phenobarbital was stopped and carbamazepine was increased to 1200 mg/day with minimal benefit.

In June 1996, she reported that she was not being allowed to go outside the house because of her frequent seizures. She was very depressed and emotionally upset.

Her entire clinical history was reviewed. For the first time, she admitted that she had occasional myoclonic jerks dating back a couple years. The jerks were not precipitated by sleep deprivation, would occur at any time during the day and would frequently result in her dropping objects. There was no family history of seizures or epilepsy.

34

Examination and investigations

Her examination was normal. She had gained about 30 kg weight over the last 8 years. Her brain imaging (both CT and MRI scans) was normal. An EEG done while she was on carbamazepine revealed generalized sharp waves, slow waves and isolated generalized spike–wave discharges. There was no photoparoxysmal response. The serum carbamazepine level was 12.6 μg/ml.

Diagnosis

Juvenile myoclonic epilepsy.

Treatment and outcome

The patient was started on valproate and carbamazepine was gradually tapered off. Currently she is on valproate (1000 mg/day) and has had no generalized tonic–clonic seizures or myoclonic jerks since valproate was begun. She is no longer depressed but gets emotionally upset because her friends and relatives still say that she gets seizures. When last seen in the outpatient clinic, she was very happy and was looking forward to starting a business and becoming independent.

Commentary

This patient's seizures had never responded to carbamazepine, despite good compliance. In fact, she often had flurries of seizures while on carbamazepine alone or in combination with acetazolamide and phenobarbital. Her seizures were finally controlled with valproate alone. Her weight gain was partly due to the growth process and the fact that she was confined to home, but it could also have been due to long-term intake of carbamazepine and valproate. Her emotional disturbance was certainly related to the poorly controlled seizures and her family's attitude towards her epilepsy.

I chose this case for several reasons. First, it is a classical example of juvenile myoclonic epilepsy being misdiagnosed. There was a delay of almost 4 years before a correct diagnosis was reached.

Secondly, this case exemplifies the importance of using a syndromic approach when classifying patients with epilepsy. If one uses the International League Against Epilepsy classification of epilepsies and epileptic syndromes proposed in 1989,[1] the approach to management of patients with epilepsy can be totally

35

different. Classifying patients by epilepsy syndrome will result in the choice of proper antiepileptic drugs and can even avoid unnecessary imaging procedures.

Thirdly, seizures in certain epilepsy syndromes such as juvenile myoclonic epilepsy can be refractory to inappropriate antiepileptic drugs or can be made more frequent, as in this case. Carbamazepine is a commonly used drug to initiate treatment in young people with generalized tonic–clonic seizures but it can exacerbate seizures in patients with juvenile myoclonic epilepsy.

What did I learn from this case?

My clinical approach towards classifying epilepsy patients into different epilepsy syndromes was reinforced by my experience with this patient and other similar patients. I have learned with experience that young people who present with generalized tonic–clonic seizures that are not controlled with routine antiepileptic drugs (carbamazepine, diphenylhydantoin and phenobarbital) should be re-evaluated. If the EEG shows generalized spike–wave discharges and brain imaging (CT and MRI scans) is normal, then a common epilepsy syndrome such as juvenile myoclonic epilepsy should be considered.

The history from the patient was crucial in making a correct diagnosis. Every patient should be asked specifically whether myoclonic jerks have occurred and should be encouraged to demonstrate the jerks if the answer is yes. Special attention must be paid to eliciting a history of mild and transient events like myoclonic jerks, because they are often inconspicuous and therefore missed.

How did this case alter my approach to the care and treatment of my patients with epilepsy?

Juvenile myoclonic epilepsy is a common age-related idiopathic generalized epileptic syndrome with fairly well-defined clinical and EEG features. It has been reported to account for about 10 % of all epilepsy cases seen in different centres all over the world. In large series, seizures respond to valproate in nearly 90 % of cases.

In all young patients who present with onset of generalized tonic–clonic seizures during early adolescence, I always ask for a history of myoclonic jerks and absences. This is even more important when seizures have not responded to antiepileptic drugs such as carbamazepine or phenytoin and EEGs show generalized spike–wave discharges. In such situations, I use valproate for seizure prophylaxis. Valproate is a broad spectrum antiepileptic drug that successfully controls generalized tonic–clonic seizures, myoclonic jerks and absences in the majority of patients with idiopathic generalized epilepsy syndromes. I now routinely use the International Classification of Epileptic Syndromes for classifying epilepsies in all my patients.

References

1.   Commission on Classification and Terminology of the International League Against Epilepsy. Proposal for classification of epilepsies and epileptic syndromes. *Epilepsia* 1989;**30**:389–99.

Further reading

Janz D. Epilepsy with impulsive petit mal (juvenile myoclonic epilepsy). *Acta Neurol Scand* 1985;**72**:449–59.

Jain S, Padma MV, Puri A, Maheshwari MC. Juvenile myoclonic epilepsy: disease expression among Indian families. *Acta Neurol Scand* 1998;**97**:1–7.

Jain S, Padma MV, Maheshwari MC. The syndrome of juvenile myoclonic epilepsy: AIIMS experience. *Ann Indian Acad Neurol* 1999;**2**:9–14.

Jain S, Padma MV, Narula A, Maheshwari MC. EEG photosensitivity and response to valproate segregate together in Indians with juvenile myoclonic epilepsy. *Neurol J Southeast Asia* 1999;**4**:61–6.

Case 11

THE VALUE OF DIAGNOSTIC PERSISTENCE

Gregory L Krauss

History

The patient is a 26-year-old right-handed woman with a history of complex partial seizures beginning at approximately 1 year of age. She typically had one or two complex partial or secondary generalized seizures every morning with as many as 50–60 seizures in one day. She became aware of her seizures at the age of 5, describing 'weird feelings in her head' followed by a scared look, and then her head and eyes would roll back with stiffening and shaking.

Several routine EEGs were normal. Her seizures failed to respond to all available antiepileptic drugs. During video-EEG monitoring at the age of 16, she had diffuse anterior hemispheric seizure onset, maximal on the left, as well as numerous psychic sensations that were unaccompanied by EEG changes. She was thought to have a mixed disorder with seizures and pseudoseizures or some seizures that did not project to the surface. Magnetic resonance imaging (MRI) scanning was normal. She failed additional treatment with methsuximide, vigabatrin and clorazepate maximized to 18.75 mg/day. She had an occipital hemorrhage as a result of a seizure-related head injury at the age of 26. She had a positive antinuclear antibody secondary to phenytoin. She had ovarian cysts, possibly associated with her antiepileptic drugs. She also had an episode of serial seizures that required several days of barbiturate coma therapy with airway intubation.

Examination and investigations

The patient's neurological and general examinations were normal. At the age of 21, additional video-EEG monitoring was performed. Interictally there were frequent spike and sharp waves that were widely distributed over the anterior midline and frontal regions bilaterally. Spikes were sometimes slightly maximum on the left. She had 22 seizures during 4 days of monitoring, including two secondary generalized seizures. These secondary generalized seizures began with eye opening and then staring and chewing followed by fast hyperventilation with

38

pursed lips. These seizures were poorly localized with widely distributed bilateral frontal spikes, maximal over the midline, followed by generalized slowing. Four seizures that occurred after medication withdrawal showed an anterior midline spike pattern followed by generalized electrodecremental pattern and then generalized slowing.

Several months later, the patient underwent depth electrode seizure recording. She had electrode tresses placed bilaterally superiorly in the frontal lobes, with additional electrodes projecting into amygdala and hippocampus. During her seizures there were no ictal patterns recorded on the depth electrodes.

The patient was offered several options: vagal nerve stimulation, anterior callosal sectioning to stop secondary generalized seizures and lateralize her seizures, experimental medications and additional intracranial monitoring.

She received investigational treatment with felbamate, but continued to have several seizures a day. Three years after her unsuccessful depth electrode monitoring, the patient had additional intracranial seizure monitoring. She had subdural strips placed bilaterally, with four 1×8 cm strips placed over each anterior frontal lobe. She also had a 2×8 cm electrode grid placed over the saggital midline with bilateral electrodes. These electrodes covered the anterior medial frontal lobe, including the cingulate cortex. The patient had nine complex partial seizures, of which seven were secondarily generalized. Six of these seizures were well localized to the right medial frontal and right anterior lateral frontal lobe with an anterior cingulate seizure maximum. She also had two clinically atypical partial seizures beginning from the left frontal lobe.

Diagnosis

Right anterior cingulate and anterior lateral frontal lobe seizures.

Treatment and outcome

The patient tolerated resective surgery well. Preoperatively she had between two and four complex partial and secondary generalized seizures a day. Since surgery she has been free of seizures for the past 6 years. Because she had two clincally atypical seizures originating from the left anterior frontal lobe during intracranial recording, she has continued on carbamazepine 600 mg four times daily. Before surgery she had been a very pleasant but insecure young woman who, despite her uncontrolled epilepsy, walked to work several miles each day and frequently had seizures on the roadside. She is now able to be employed full time and is engaged to be married.

39

Commentary

The patient had extremely difficult-to-control complex partial and secondary generalized seizures that were life-long and not associated with MRI changes. She attempted to work despite daily seizures. She was very shy, lacked confidence and was socially impaired as a result of her episodes. Over the years it was felt that some of her episodes could have been pseudoseizures, but in fact these were partial seizures beginning in the frontal lobe. The patient had poorly localized seizures on initial scalp video-EEG recording and had several additional years of additional medication trials with no benefit before her surgery.

The patient then had scalp monitoring with extra recording electrodes and had a large number of seizures that showed a frontal midline seizure onset. This detailed scalp recording allowed effective intracranial mapping using subdural electrode strips to be performed.

The majority of patients with extratemporal epilepsy and no structural lesions are reported to do poorly with epilepsy surgery. This patient, however, became seizure-free after right anterior cingulate and lateral frontal resection.

What did I learn from this case?

This case illustrates the difficulty of localizing seizures in extratemporal neocortex. It also highlights the possibility that some patients with uncontrolled but stereotyped seizures may have focal ictal zones and may benefit from surgical treatment.

How did this case alter my approach to the care and treatment of my epilepsy patients?

Patients whose seizures fail to respond to several standard antiepileptic drugs at high doses are unlikely to become seizure-free on newer drugs. In this patient, surgery had a remarkably beneficial effect on her life.

Patients with non-lesional extratemporal epilepsy are reported to be poor candidates for surgery. This case demonstrates, however, that some patients with frontal lobe seizures, particularly if the seizures are localized to medial frontal areas, may be good candidates for surgery. Patients with frontal lobe seizures often have diffuse ictal EEG patterns, owing to rapid seizure propagation and sometimes to large areas of cortex being involved. This patient, however, had a diffuse anterior seizure onset with a midline maximum and, in fact, turned out to have anterior cingulate involvement on intracranial mapping. Her case illustrates the importance of effective sampling using intracranial electrodes. The patient had no seizures localized with depth electrodes placed through the superior lateral frontal lobes but had discrete seizure localization with bilateral subdural electrode strips and grids.

Further reading

Williamson PD. Frontal lobe seizures: problems of diagnosis and classification. In: Chauvel P, Delgado-Escueta AV, Halgren E, Bancand J. Frontal lobe seizures and epilepsy. *Advances in neurology*, vol 57. New York: Raven; 1992.

Case 12

FREQUENT NIGHT TERRORS*

Cesare T Lombroso

History

A 6-year-old boy was referred because of nightly events thought to be nightmares. These events had started when he was 4 years old and had progressively increased until they happened several times a night. They adversely affected his daytime performance and caused stress in the family.

No benefit had been obtained from benzodiazepines or counseling with a behavioral therapist familiar with sleep disorders. His past medical history was unremarkable. There was some relevant family background: a sibling, an aunt and a cousin had suffered from febrile convulsions, the cousin later developing non-febrile seizures.

Examination and investigations

The patient had normal general and neurological examinations. Metabolic screening and scalp EEGs were normal. He was admitted for scalp video-EEG long-term monitoring (LTM). Several stereotypical events were captured, all occurring at night. He would awaken from quiet, non-rapid eye movements (non-REM) sleep, sit up looking frightened and seeking and grabbing his mother, and fleetingly exhibit dystonic posturing of his flexed left arm. There were also several bouts of a dry cough without drooling. The events lasted less then 1 minute, after which he quickly returned to sleep. Similar episodes recurred between four and eight times during the night. In the morning he had some vague recollection of the events and specifically stated that he had awoken because of 'fear and a feeling in my throat'.

The accompanying ictal EEG showed an arousal pattern out of non-REM sleep and, amidst muscle artifacts, some bilateral frontal low-voltage theta activity. An ictal single-photon emission computed tomography scan demonstrated an area of hyperperfusion within the left frontotemporal lobes. A magnetic resonance imaging scan was normal.

*Case published in part (*Epilepsia* 2000; 41:1221 26).

Another trial with clonazepam did not help. Carbamazepine at top blood levels reduced the frequency of the episodes by about 30–40 %. Trials with lamotrigine and gabapentin caused skin rashes.

At this point, clinical and imaging data had increased the suspicion of an epileptic disorder but routine EEGs and the scalp LTM had failed to demonstrate interictal or ictal discharges that might localize a presumed epileptogenic focus. Therefore, an invasive LTM was performed (Fig. 12.1) because the parents insisted that 'all be done' to help their child.

On invasive LTM, all seizures began with low-voltage spikes originating focally within the left rolandic cortex (identified by electrical stimulation and evoked potentials). The discharge soon spread to the left superior parietal and to the first temporal lobe gyrus.

Diagnosis

Medically refractory partial seizures arising from the left primary motor cortex.

Treatment and outcome

Based on the invasive recordings, resective surgery was recommended. At surgery, electrocorticography recorded vigorous spiking in a restricted zone, which was again confirmed to lie within the primary motor cortex. Multiple subpial slicings were performed in this area. There were no postsurgical motor or language deficits.

The nocturnal episodes have been 90 % controlled on 5-year follow up. The child still receives a small dose of carbamazepine.

Commentary

Paroxysmal behaviors during sleep in children are classified as either sleep-induced epileptic seizures or as parasomnias.[1][3] The most common parasomnias are night terrors, followed by confusional arousals or sleep walking. The great majority of night terrors are parasomnias caused by a benign developmental disorder of arousal.[1-3] However, studies of paroxysmal events occurring during sleep have shown that some events that are considered to be parasomnias are actually ictal events, as in this case.[4,5]

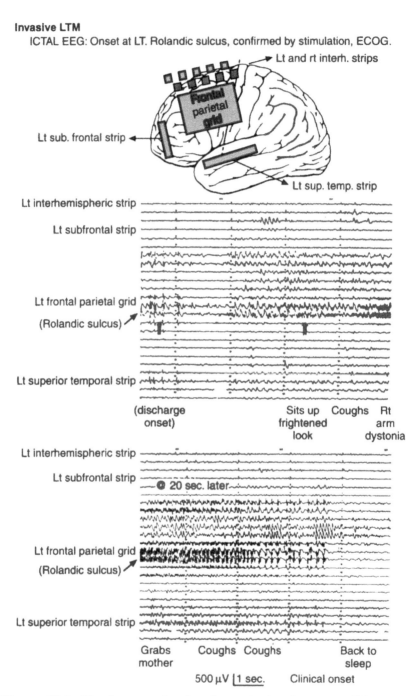

Figure 12.1: *The placement of grids and strips (top) and a portion of the many ictal EEGs accompanying the events (bottom) recorded on invasive long-term monitoring.*

What did I learn from this case and how did it alter my approach to the care and treatment of my epilepsy patients?

My evaluation of this patient and investigations of several other children with atypical, frequent night terrors show that it is reasonable to consider epileptic events in the differential diagnosis. The main features that suggest an ictal origin for episodes mimicking the common night terrors or confusional arousals are listed in Table 12.1. Perhaps one important clue is the dystonic or tonic posturing of one or more limbs, although this may occur only fleetingly. Subtle posturing might suggest other types of frontal lobe epilepsy, such as those arising from the supplementary motor areas[6-8] or so-called nocturnal paroxysmal

Table 12.1 Main features suggesting an ictal origin for episodes mimicking the common night terrors or confusional arousals.

	N.T.	C.A.	E.N.T.
FAMILIAL INCIDENCE	Yes	± Yes	?
NREM ONSET	Yes Early	Yes Anytime	Yes
NIGHTLY EVENTS	Usually Once	Usually Once	Several
INTENSE FEAR	Yes	No	Yes
STEREOTYPY	No	No	Yes
HALLUCINATIONS	Probably	No	No
DURATION	> 4–5 mins	Variable 1–5 mins	< 2 mins
RESPONSIVENESS	No	±	Yes
DYSTONIA	No	No	Yes
AUTONOMIC SIGNS	No	No	Yes
AMNESIA	Yes	±	No

N.T. = Night Terrors; C.A. = Confusional Arousals; E.N.T. = Epileptic Night Terrors

45

dystonia, also once considered to be a parasomnia.[1,4,5] These seizures, and some other types of partial epilepsy arising from frontal lobe cortex, differ significantly from the ictal nocturnal events described in children who are thought to suffer from night terrors.[5,6–10]

How frequently are 'night terrors' actually seizures? From my study alone it is impossible to estimate the frequency of ictal events masquerading as parasomnias and, specifically, the frequency of those mimicking night terrors or confusional arousals. My referred population is evidently strongly biased towards those children who do not respond favorably to the use of benzodiazepines or behavioral counseling and who exhibit multiple episodes during their sleep. It is very probable that the great majority of the common night terrors are not epileptic in origin. The few that are seizures can be suspected only from careful histories, adequate LTM investigation and the other parameters listed in Table 12.1, and they represent another example of the kaleidoscopic group of distinct clinical phenotypes from epileptogenic foci within the frontal lobes.

References

1. Thorpy MJ. Classification and nomenclature of the sleep disorders. In: Thorpy MJ, ed. *Sleep disorders*. New York: Marcel Dekker; 1990:155–78.

2. Broughton RJ. Sleep disorders: disorders of arousal? *Science* 1968;**159**: 1070–8.

3. Guilleminault C, Silvestri R. Disorders of arousal and epilepsy following sleep. In: Sterman MB, Shouse MN, Passuants P, eds. *Sleep and epilepsy*. New York: Academy Press; 1982:513–31.

4. Lugaresi E, Cirignotta F, Montagna P. Nocturnal paroxysmal dystonia. *J Neurol Neurosurg Psychiatry* 1986;**49**:375–80.

5. Lombroso CT. Nocturnal paroxysmal dystonia due to a subfrontal cortical dysplasia. *Epileptic Disord* 2000;**2**:15–20.

6. Penfield W, Welch K. The supplementary motor area of the cerebral cortex. *Arch Neurol Psychiatr* 1951;**66**:289–317.

7. Wieser HG, Swartz BC, Delgado-Escueta AV, *et al*. Differentiating frontal lobe seizures from temporal lobe seizures. In: Chauvel P, Delgado-Escueta AV, *et al*, eds. *Advances in neurology*, vol 57. Raven: New York; 1992:272–4.

8. Williamson PD, Van Hess PC, Wieser HG. Surgically remediable extratemporal syndromes. In: Engel J Jr, ed. *Surgical treatment of the epilepsies*, 2nd ed. Raven: New York; 1993:68–73.

9. Vigevano F, Fusco L. Hypnic tonic postural seizures in healthy children provide evidence for a partial epileptic syndrome of frontal lobe origin. *Epilepsia* 1993;**39**:110–9.

10. Scheffer IE, Bhatia KP, Lopes-Cendes I, *et al.* Autosomal dominant nocturnal frontal lobe epilepsy: a distinctive clinical disorder. *Brain* 1995;**118**:61 73.

Case 13

GENERALIZED EPILEPSY WITH FEBRILE SEIZURES PLUS

Ingrid E Scheffer

History

A 5½-year-old girl presented in January 2001 with recent onset of generalized tonic–clonic, absence and atonic seizures. Her first afebrile generalized tonic–clonic seizure occurred in September 2000 and lasted 90 seconds. There was neither apparent aura nor any focal features. She had three further brief afebrile generalized tonic–clonic seizures over the ensuing 4 months.

Atonic drop attacks began at the end of October 2000. Her eyelids fluttered briefly, she crumpled forwards or backwards and lost awareness for only a second. She sustained facial injuries with these attacks. Brief absence seizures also occurred on two occasions. These consisted of staring for 1–5 seconds without eyelid fluttering or automatisms.

She has not had myoclonus, tonic seizures or febrile seizures. Perinatal history and developmental history were normal. She is right-handed and developmentally normal.

The family history is significant (Fig. 13.1). The patient is the elder of two daughters to unrelated Australian parents. There is no family history of epilepsy on the mother's side but there is an extensive family history of seizures on the father's side, although the father himself has not had seizures.

Examination and investigations

General and neurological examinations were normal. There were no neurocutaneous stigmata or dysmorphic features.

Routine EEG showed three irregular generalized polyspike–wave discharges during hyperventilation. Intermittent photic stimulation did not evoke epileptiform abnormalities. Neuroimaging has not been performed.

Molecular genetic analysis was performed and showed the same SSCA band shift as the c.387C→G mutation in the β-1 subunit gene of the neuronal sodium channel (SCN1B) in the wider family – sequencing of other family members had confirmed this band shift as c.387C→G.

48

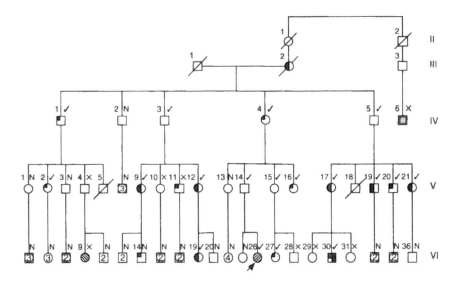

Figure 13.1 *Pedigree of an Australian GEFS⁺ family showing the presence of the C121W mutation in SCN1B. The arrow denotes the patient described here.*

✓ = SCN1B(C121W) mutation; ✗ = negative for mutation; N = not tested. ▣ febrile seizures (FS); ◧ febrile seizures plus (FS⁺); ▣ FS and partial epilepsy; ⧖ neonatal, febrile and partial seizures; ◩ GTCS; ▨ GTCS, absences and atonic seizures; ⊘ deceased; □ unaffected male; ○ unaffected female; ▢ mixed gender; II-IV denotes generations.

Diagnosis

Generalized epilepsy with febrile seizures-plus (GEFS-plus) with the patient's phenotype comprising generalized tonic–clonic seizures, atonic seizures and absence seizures.

Treatment and outcome

The patient was commenced on valproate but her attacks were not fully controlled on 38 mg/kg per day. She had a further cluster of seizures in December 2000, including unusual attacks with bilateral facial clonic activity with limp limbs; these attacks required rectal diazepam after 5 minutes. Higher doses of valproate will be tried, and if this does not produce full seizure control, lamotrigine will be introduced in combination with valproate.

Commentary

This is one of the more severe epilepsy phenotypes in the spectrum of GEFS-plus, which we originally described in 1997.[1] GEFS-plus is a genetic epilepsy syndrome with phenotypic heterogeneity. The mildest end of the spectrum includes febrile seizures and febrile seizures-plus. In febrile seizures-plus, the child either has febrile seizures that extend past the usual accepted maximum age limit of 6 years or has afebrile generalized tonic–clonic seizures in early to mid-childhood. The more severe phenotypes include febrile seizures or febrile seizures-plus with other types of generalized seizures such as atonic, myoclonic or absence seizures, and also myoclonic–astatic epilepsy.[2] The absence seizures differ from those typically seen in childhood absence epilepsy[3] because in GEFS-plus, absence seizures tend to be infrequent. By contrast, in childhood absence epilepsy, absence seizures typically occur 20 or more times a day. Many patients with GEFS-plus have normal routine EEG studies but some have generalized spike and wave activity. The phenotypic spectrum of GEFS-plus has expanded with further family studies[4,5] to include some patients with partial seizures and, more recently, severe myoclonic epilepsy of infancy.[6]

Molecular genetic studies of GEFS-plus have shown mutations of three different neuronal sodium channel subunits. Initially a mutation was found in *SCN1B* in a large Tasmanian family.[7] Subsequently, mutations have been found in the α-1 subunit gene (*SCN1A*), with different mutations found in different families.[8,9] Very recently, mutations in the alpha 2 subunit gene of the sodium channel (SCN2A) and the gamma 2 subunit gene of the GABA-A receptor (GABRG2) have been reported in families with GEFS-plus.[9,10] To date, only two further families with GEFS-plus have been found with *SCN1B* mutations.[12,13]

This patient's family is the second family in which a *SCN1B* mutation has been demonstrated.[12] The extended family contained 19 members with seizures, including 16 with typical GEFS-plus phenotypes. The mutation (c.387C$\rightarrow$G) in *SCN1B*, found in this family and in the original Tasmanian family, changes a conserved cysteine residue (C121W), disrupting a putative disulphide bridge that maintains an extracellular immunoglobulin-like fold.[7,12] Functional studies of the brain sodium channel comprising a mutant β-1 subunit with a wild type alpha subunit in *Xenopus* oocytes found a loss-of-function effect.

The patient and her father both carry this mutation and the patient's phenotype can be regarded as one of the moderately severe phenotypes of the GEFS-plus spectrum. More severe phenotypes include myoclonic–astatic epilepsy[2] and severe myoclonic epilepsy of infancy.[6,14] The patient's course is difficult to predict – the majority of patients with GEFS-plus have a good prognosis but some continue to have refractory epilepsy.

Why did I choose this case?

I chose this case because it demonstrates the clinical relevance of GEFS-plus. This patient shows that the clinical diagnosis can be made on the basis of the electroclinical presentation in the setting of a significant family history. A key to making the diagnosis lies in obtaining further details about the family history so that the genetic context of the patient's epilepsy can be understood.

This case is important in demonstrating the spectrum of the more severe phenotypes of GEFS-plus. This patient may have evolving myoclonic-astatic epilepsy presenting without febrile seizures and her epilepsy may prove difficult to control.

What did I learn from this case?

This case once again emphasizes how genetic epilepsies that follow autosomal-dominant inheritance, as GEFS-plus does in this patient's family, result in further family members becoming affected over time. Genetic epilepsies are not always benign and easily controlled, nor do they always resolve spontaneously.

Many cases of GEFS-plus follow complex inheritance (where multiple genes and environmental factors play a part), so that the family history will not always be as striking as in this child. Nevertheless, the nature of seizure disorders in a few other family members may be a valuable clue to the aetiology and diagnosis. Importantly, bilineal inheritance of seizure disorders is not uncommon and suggests that the patient is at risk of inheriting more than one epilepsy gene.

References

1. Scheffer IE, Berkovic SF. Generalized epilepsy with febrile seizures plus. A genetic disorder with heterogeneous clinical phenotypes. *Brain* 1997;**120**:479–90.

2. Doose H, *et al*. Centrencephalic myoclonic–astatic petit mal. *Neuropediatrics* 1970;**2**:59–78.

3. Commission on Classification and Terminology of the International League Against Epilepsy: proposal for revised classification of epilepsies and epileptic syndromes. *Epilepsia* 1989;**30**:389–99.

4. Singh R, *et al*. Generalised epilepsy with febrile seizures plus (GEFS$^+$): a common, childhood onset, genetic epilepsy syndrome. *Ann Neurol* 1999;**45**:75–81.

5. Baulac S, *et al*. A second locus for familial generalized epilepsy with febrile seizures plus maps to chromosome 2q21-q33. *Am J Hum Genetics* 1999;**65**:1078–85.

6. Singh R, *et al*. Severe myoclonic epilepsy of infancy: extended spectrum of GEFS$^+$? *Epilepsia* 2001;**42**:837–44.

51

7. Wallace RH, *et al.* Febrile seizures and generalized epilepsy associated with a mutation in the Na⁺-channel β1 subunit gene SCN1B. *Nat Genetics* 1998;**19**:366–70.

8. Escayg A, *et al.* Mutations of SCN1A, encoding a neuronal sodium channel, in two families with GEFS⁺². *Nat Genetics* 2000;**24**:343–5.

9. Wallace RH, *et al.* Neuronal sodium channel α1 subunit (SCN1A) mutations in generalised epilepsy with febrile seizures plus. *Am J Hum Genetics* 2001;**68**:859–65.

10. Sugawara T, Tsurubuchi Y, Agarwala K, *et al.* A missense mutation of the Na⁺ Channel alpha II subunit gene Na(v)1.2 in a patient with febrile and afebrile seizures causes channel dysfunction. *Prod Nat Acad Sci USA* 2001;**98**:6384–9.

11. Baulac S, Huberfeld G, Gourfinkel-An I, *et al.* First genetic evidence of GABAA receptor dysfunction in epilepsy: mutation in the gamma 2-subunit gene. *Nat Genet* 2001;**28**:46–8.

12. Wallace R, *et al.* Generalised epilepsy with febrile seizures plus: mutation of the sodium channel sub-unit SCN1B and evidence for a founder effect. *Neurology*; under review.

13. Scheffer IE, *et al.* Temporal lobe epilepsy and febrile seizures associated with a sodium channel β1 subunit (SCN1B) mutation. *Epilepsia* 2000;**41**:71.

14. Dravet C. Les epilepsies graves de l'enfant. *Vie Med* 1978;**8**:543–8.

Acknowledgements

The author is indebted to the patient, her family and Dr Robyn Wallace for performing the molecular studies on this patient and her family.

Case 14

A Visit To The Borderland Of Neurology And Psychiatry

Donald L Schomer

History

Mrs N was 52 years old in 1980 when I first met her. She was referred by her psychiatrist for an opinion about her behavior.

In 1963 she was admitted to a psychiatric facility for profound depression after the birth of her fifth child. She had a previous history of depression but was now thought to be acutely psychotic. She failed to respond to multiple antidepressants but subsequently responded to electroconvulsive therapy. She required long-term use of both antidepressants and antipsychotics.

In 1974 she was riding in a car that was involved in an accident, and she struck her head on the windshield. Between 6 and 8 months later she began experiencing complex visual hallucinations. She would suddenly see six German soldiers stacked in a triangular formation one on top of two on top of three. They wore Kaiser Willhelm helmets reminiscent of World War I and occasionally spoke to her in muffled tones telling her to harm herself. These were interpreted as command hallucinations. She was committed to a locked psychiatric unit for several years.

In 1977 she was struck in the head by another inpatient and rendered unconscious for several days. She suffered a subarachnoid hemorrhage. A few months later, she began having a second type of complex visual hallucination. This time the image was of an elderly woman sitting in a rocking chair that reminded her of a painting by Grandma Moses. She felt that this woman was a premonition of her own future. The woman rocked back and forth while several small rat-like animals chewed at her fingers, which were dangling to the side of the chair. Mrs N would get comfort only by cutting herself with a sharp object when these hallucinations were present. The frequency of their occurrence steadily increased over the years to the point where they happened several times daily.

The referring psychiatrist had first met Mrs N in 1979. The history that he had obtained revealed that the patient saw these images only in her left visual field. An EEG was performed (the first EEG in her now long medical–psychiatric history), and this showed frequent right parietal and temporal interictal spikes. He treated her initially with phenytoin, but she developed a rash after 1 day. She was switched to carbamazepine, which she tolerated. She remained without hallucinations for the next 6 months, the longest symptom-free period in 5 years. The hallucinations then started to recur, prompting the referral to me.

Examination and investigations

My examination revealed a pleasant, engaging woman who was knowledgeable about current events and told me several humorous stories about her interactions with her congressman, which I was later able to confirm as being accurate. She had mild left arm drift and posturing, slight left-sided hyper-reflexia and absent Babinski responses. Of note, she had normal visual fields and intact higher-level cognitive sensory functions. She was found to have a small nodular contrast-enhancing abnormality in the right parietotemporo-occipital junction on computed tomography scanning. Her EEG confirmed the previously described abnormalities.

Diagnosis

Recurrent simple partial seizures coming from the right parietotemporal region, secondary to a probable arteriovenous malformation.

Treatment and outcome

My initial treatment was with medication. First, the carbamazepine was raised to maximum tolerated levels, which produced some improvement. Phenytoin was re-introduced and she tolerated it without developing a rash. She went for many years with very few seizures. Her evaluation for the 'lesion' revealed a probable old arteriovenous malformation that had been obliterated by the hemorrhage that followed the physical attack she had suffered several years earlier.

After about 7 years of good seizure control, the seizures again gradually increased in frequency until she was experiencing them every 1–2 days. There had been no significant change in other medication except that conjugated estrogen had been added about 4 years earlier to treat menopausal symptoms.

She then underwent a surgical approach. Intraoperatively, with electrodes over the exposed right lateral temporoparietofrontal neocortex and with acute depth electrodes in the right anterior hippocampus and amygdala, she experienced a seizure. Co-incident with the appearance of the German soldiers, she had sustained seizure activity posterior to a scarred-appearing area at the junction of the right posterior superior temporal gyrus and the inferior parietal junction. She felt fear and the desire to injure herself at the same time that the discharge spread to the deeper structures in the temporal lobe. The pathology revealed an old occluded arteriovenous malformation on the surface, as well as hippocampal sclerosis.

Postoperatively, she did well for a number of years until she slipped on the ice and suffered an acute intracerebral hemorrhage that left her with a left hemiparesis and hemianopia. Several years later, she developed acute leukemia and died of its complications in 1997.

Commentary

This unfortunate woman had symptoms of partial epilepsy of a neocortical onset that went unrecognized for many years. She was treated with multiple drugs that were targeted at alleviating symptoms without really treating the underlying disorder. She underwent numerous electroconvulsive therapy sessions that may have contributed to her overall state of intractability. All the while she harbored an undiagnosed arteriovenous malformation that declared itself following an assault.[1]

What did I learn from this case?

The following lessons were evident to me:

- The history is perhaps the most important clinical tool that we have available.[2] When in doubt, retake the history. There were many clues in this case that the events were convulsive in origin. The symptoms were paroxysmal in origin, not related to environmental triggers. Their appearances were stereotypic. Her interpersonal skills were normal, not typical of a psychotic person. The EEG and clinical responses to antiseizure medication supported the diagnosis.
- Partial seizures may have a progressive pattern without evidence for an underlying progressive lesion.[3] In her case, perhaps the use of unopposed estrogen played a role in the progressive nature of her epilepsy.[4,5]
- The appearance of a rash following the initiation of high doses of phenytoin does not always preclude its potential long-term use.[6,7]
- Epilepsy surgery is not the exclusive domain of the young – Mrs N responded well to the surgical approach until she was injured in an accident. If she had been diagnosed earlier and treated aggressively, I am convinced she would have had a more benign course.[8]
- Dual pathology may play a significant role in the development of

55

intractability.[9] Improved brain imaging allows us to diagnose dual pathology earlier and should be considered whenever neocortical-onset seizures that later take on a clinical picture of temporolimbic epilepsy are recognized.

- Did her years of exposure to a variety of antidepressants, antipsychotics and AEDs predispose her to her final illness – acute leukemia?[10]

How did this case alter my approach to the care and treatment of my epilepsy patients?

For the reasons noted above, I teach the importance of the history to my residents and fellows. I am cautious about the use of unopposed estrogen when there is the history of symptom progression after the introduction of estrogen therapy. I weigh the pros and cons of aggressive medical–surgical treatment in all my patients. Finally, my group uses newer non-invasive technology at an early stage in an attempt to improve our understanding of the pathological basis for epilepsy.

References

1. LeBlanc R, Feindel W, Ethier R. Epilepsy from cerebral arteriovenous malformations. *Can J Neurol Sci* 1983;**10**: 91–5.

2. Schomer DL, O'Connor M, Spiers P, Seeck M, Bear D, Mesulam MM. Temporal limbic epilepsy and behavior. In: Mesulam MM, ed. *Behavioral neurology*. London: Oxford University Press; 2000:373–405.

3. Elwes RDC, Johnson AL, Reynolds EH. The course of untreated epilepsy. *Lancet* 1988;**297**:948–50.

4. Logothitis J, Harner R, Morrell F, Torres F. The role of estrogens in catamenial exacerbation of epilepsy. *Neurology* 1959;**9**:352–60.

5. Herzog A, Seibel MM, Schomer DL, Vaitukaitis JL, Geschwind N. Reproductive endocrine disorders in women with partial seizures of temporal lobe origin. *Arch Neurol* 1986;**43**:341–6.

6. Kimball OP, Horan TN. The use of Dilantin in the treatment of epilepsy. *Ann Intern Med* 1939;**13**:787–93.

7. Wilson JT, Hojer B, Tomson G. High incidence of concentration dependent skin reactions in children treated with phenytoin. *BMJ* 1978;**1**:1583–6.

8. Elwes RDC, Reynolds EH. First seizure in adult life. *Lancet* 1988;**ii**:36.

9. Levesque MF, Nakasoto N, Vinters HV, Babb TL. Surgical treatment of limbic epilepsy associated with extra hippocampal lesions: the problem of dual pathology. *J Neurosurg* 1991;**75**:354–70.

10. White S, McLean A, Howland C. Anticonvulsant drugs and cancer: a cohort study in patients with severe epilepsy. *Lancet* 1979;**ii**:458–61.

Case 15

A Case Of Complex Partial Status Epilepticus

Alan R Towne

History

The patient is a 56-year-old man who was admitted to the hospital for bizarre behavior. He had a history of hypertension and hypercholesterolemia, which had been diagnosed approximately 15 years ago. Six years before admission he experienced a cerebral infarct in the distribution of the left middle cerebral artery distribution, and he had mild residual right hemiparesis. Approximately 1 year after this he was noted to have episodes of staring followed by confusion that lasted for approximately 15 minutes. A neurological evaluation at that time demonstrated left temporal spike discharges emanating maximally from the T3 electrode, with minimal temporal slowing. A diagnosis of complex partial seizures was made and the patient was started on carbamazepine and had no further seizures after attaining a dose of 1200 mg/day.

On the day of admission the patient was found wandering in the street by another pedestrian. He was taken to the closest emergency department.

Examination and investigations

In the emergency department, the patient was found to be confused and unable to answer simple questions. He was slightly lethargic and oriented to name only. One-step commands were performed with difficulty. General physical examination, including vital signs, was unremarkable. Neurological examination revealed right hemiparesis. Laboratory tests including complete blood count, serum electrolytes, magnesium and toxicology screen were normal. Computed tomography (CT) scanning of the head revealed an old left middle cerebral artery infarct without acute changes. The carbamazepine level was 3 µg/ml.

The patient was kept in the emergency department for continued observation. He was noted to have changes in mentation ranging from mild impairment of consciousness to almost complete unresponsiveness, during which he would not respond to simple questions. Past medical history was unobtainable and the

57

patient had no identification on his person. Because no previous medical information was available, the working diagnosis by the emergency room staff was drug or toxin exposure or a psychiatric, encephalopathic or cerebrovascular etiology.

Neurological and psychiatric consultations were obtained. As part of his work-up, the neurology consultant ordered an EEG, which demonstrated rhythmic left posterior temporal sharp activity with intermittent spread to the right hemisphere. This activity was continuous with the frequency of the ictal discharges ranging from 0.5 to 6 Hz.

Diagnosis

Complex partial status epilepticus (CPSE) associated with low carbamazepine levels.

Treatment and outcome

On the basis of the EEG findings, the patient was given 5 mg lorazepam by slow intravenous push followed by 1000 mg of fosphenytoin.

Fifteen minutes after the injection of lorazepam the patient was noted to be slightly lethargic but able to follow simple one-step commands. The EEG demonstrated cessation of the continuous seizure activity. However, the left hemispheric slowing remained. The patient was able to give his full name and the fact that he had discontinued taking his carbamazepine approximately 3 days before admission.

The importance of compliance with antiepileptic medication was stressed to the patient, and he has had no further seizures. He was told not to make any changes to his regimen unless this was discussed with his neurologist.

Commentary

This case illustrates some important points pertinent to the diagnosis and management of CPSE. As in this patient, 30–50 % of patients with CPSE have a history of seizures before developing CPSE.[1] In those adult patients who develop CPSE without an antecedent history, CPSE occurs most commonly in association with symptomatic neurological disease such as herpes simplex encephalitis or cerebral infarction. In patients with a history of epilepsy, precipitating factors include recent infection and inadequate anticonvulsant levels. A possible precipitant of status epilepticus in this patient may have been the low carbamazepine level. CPSE has also been reported after cerebral angiography and can be associated with thrombotic thrombocytopenic purpura. Other precipitants include alcohol withdrawal, drug overdose, myelography, tumor and certain medications (e.g. cephalosporins).

The incidence of CPSE is difficult to assess because the paucity of clinical symptoms may not raise a suspicion of possible status epilepticus and because there are few population-based studies. A population-based study carried out in Richmond, Virginia, USA, revealed that CPSE represented approximately 5 % of the total number of convulsive and non-convulsive episodes and 35 % of non-convulsive episodes.[2] Other studies have demonstrated that CPSE accounts for 10–40 % of all cases of non-convulsive status epilepticus (SE).[1,3]

CPSE is defined as 30 minutes or more of discrete or continuous partial seizures without full recovery of consciousness. The characteristic clinical manifestation is impairment of consciousness, which can vary from mild alteration of mentation to complete unresponsiveness. CPSE may also be characterized by a cyclic pattern in which phases of unresponsiveness alternate with partially responsive phases. During the periods of partial responsiveness, automatisms and abnormal speech patterns may be present. During the unresponsive phase, complete speech arrest usually occurs, occasionally accompanied by stereotyped automatisms.[4,5]

The clinical manifestations of CPSE are varied and may be difficult to differentiate from generalized non-convulsive SE. The accompanying behavior can range from confusion to bizarre or psychotic-type behavior. Lateralizing or localizing neurological deficits (e.g. aphasia, ictal paresis) may also be seen. Although the duration of CPSE is usually between 30 minutes and several hours, recent reports have described examples of CPSE lasting for months, indicating that prolonged fugue states can be caused by CPSE.

CPSE should be suspected in any patient who is being evaluated for confusion or unresponsiveness. Other conditions that may be confused with CPSE include absence status epilepticus, prolonged post ictal states, psychiatric syndromes (such as somatoform disorder and psychosis) and cerebral circulation disorders, including transient ischemic attacks and stroke with delirium. Other conditions such as encephalopathies, migraine and transient global amnesia also need to be considered in the differential diagnosis.

To prevent serious morbidity and mortality, CPSE must be promptly diagnosed and treated. Among patients with convulsive SE, mortality ranges from 10 to 40 % depending on the etiology, the duration of SE and the response to treatment. Recent studies have indicated that CPSE is also associated with increased morbidity and mortality.[6] Identification of CPSE may be delayed in patients who are comatose or who do not present with clinical manifestations that suggest ongoing seizure activity. Thus, EEG confirmation is mandatory to make the diagnosis for this condition. Recent studies of SE in comatose patients reveal that approximately 10 % of these patients are in electrographic SE despite the fact that the patient may not demonstrate obvious clinical activity or may demonstrate only subtle clinical manifestations. Thus, patients who have persistent alterations of mental status should be evaluated immediately by EEG.[6,7]

Diagnostic evaluation of patients with CPSE should also include studies to identify the etiology of the event. These studies include laboratory tests to investigate the possibility of metabolic disorders, infections, toxic exposure and withdrawal conditions. Neuroimaging studies such as CT or magnetic resonance imaging scanning can reveal abnormalities that may be diagnostic. Although not usually performed, ictal single-photon emission CT scanning can also provide information about the localization of the seizure, especially in atypical cases.

The treatment of CPSE is similar to that of generalized convulsive SE.[8] However, since the patient may not be obtunded during the seizures, the physician may not want to use large quantities of sedating anticonvulsants. Benzodiazepines, such as diazepam, lorazepam or midazolam, are usually used as first-line choices. A benzodiazepine is generally followed by intravenous fosphenytoin or other intravenous anticonvulsants.

What did I learn from this case?

This case illustrates that the diagnosis of complex partial seizures is not always obvious. In cases such as this, patients may not be able to give an adequate history, and previous records may not be readily available. This condition may be mistaken for a drug-related disorder or a psychiatric disorder. I realized that I would have missed this diagnosis if the patient had not undergone EEG monitoring to document the presence of ongoing seizure activity.

How did this case alter my approach to the care and treatment of my epilepsy patients?

I have become more sensitized in entertaining the diagnosis of NCSE in patients who are comatose. This applies both to patients in the emergency department and to patients in the intensive care unit. EEG seizure activity may be present even in the absence of any obvious clinical seizure activity.

References

1.   Towne AR, Waterhouse EJ. Rational diagnosis of subtle and non-convulsive status epilepticus. In: Schmidt D, Schachter SC, eds. *Epilepsy: problem solving in clinical practice*. London: Martin Dunitz; 2000:79–93.

2.   DeLorenzo RJ, Hauser WA, Towne AR, *et al*. A prospective population-based epidemiologic study of status epilepticus in Richmond Virginia. *Neurology* 1996;**46**:1029–35.

3.   Krumholz A, Sung GY, Fisher RS, Barry E, Bergey GK, Grattan LM. Complex partial status epilepticus accompanied by serious morbidity and mortality. *Neurology* 1995,**45**:1499–1504.

4.   Williamson PD. Complex partial status epilepticus. In: Engel J Jr, Pedley TA, eds. *Epilepsy: a comprehensive textbook*. Philadelphia: Lippincott–Raven; 1997:618–723.

5.   Treiman D, Delgado-Escueta A. Complex partial status epileptics. In: Delgado-Escueta A, Wasterlain C, Treiman D, *et al*, eds. *Status epilepticus*, vol 34. Raven: New York; 1983:69–81.

6.   Towne AR, Boggs JG, Smith JR, DeLorenzo RJ. Status epilepticus in patients in whom EEGs were obtained for the evaluation of coma. *Neurology* 1995;**45(suppl 4)**:A424.

7.   Towne AR, Waterhouse EJ, Boggs JG, Garnett LK, Brown AJ, DeLorenzo RJ. Prevalence of non-convulsive status epilepticus in comatose patients. *Neurology* 2000;**54**:340–5.

8.   Treiman DM. Effective treatment for status epilepticus. In: Schmidt D, Schachter SC eds. *Epilepsy: problem solving in clinical practice*. London: Martin Dunitz; 2000:253–65.

61

Case 16

AN UNUSUAL CONVULSION AT DINNER

Jing-Jane Tsai

History

A 48-year-old man was brought to the emergency service after a convulsion 15 minutes earlier. During dinner he suddenly noticed twitching in both his arms. His eyes, he told us, were forced to look upwards and to the left. He felt a tight contraction of both arms and legs in extension. At that very movement he tried to overcome the involuntary contraction of the limbs, but he failed. There was no trismus, no tongue biting, no urinary incontinence and no clouding of consciousness. The attack was over within a few minutes. After this, he felt a general weakness without impaired consciousness or confusion.

About 18 months earlier, he had the first brief episode of sudden tightness of his left limbs. There was transient weakness of the left arm and leg after the attack. The second episode happened 6 months earlier while driving a car. He suddenly felt something strange and both hands were held in a tight grasp. When the attack was over, he felt weakness in both legs.

His consciousness was clear at the beginning of all three attacks and there was possibly only a very brief lapse of consciousness, if any, during the attack.

He had arterial hypertension and a history of inferior wall myocardial infarction 7 years earlier. Coronary artery three-vessel disease had been diagnosed 3 years before this. There was no history of head injury, stroke or central nervous system infection.

Examination and investigations

The vital signs at the emergency service were a blood pressure of 180/92 mmHg, a pulse rate of 100 beats per minute and a body temperature of 37°C. Physical and neurological examinations revealed no abnormal findings. Cranial computed tomography showed a hypodense region over the right frontal lobe with negative mass effect (Fig. 16.1). Postictal EEG revealed regional slow

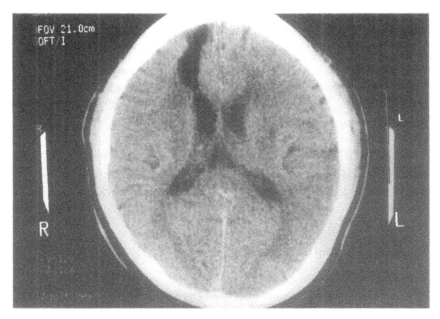

Figure 16.1: *Cranial computed tomography, revealing a longitudinal shape of encephalomalacia (2.5×1.6×3.5 cm) over the right anteriomedial frontal region. This is the lowest of the three cuts that were taken.*

waves over the right frontal area. The prolactin level during the postictal phase was 55.2 ng/ml and the follow-up prolactin level 3 days later was 11.5 ng/ml.

Diagnosis

Symptomatic frontal lobe epilepsy caused by an otherwise asymptomatic old insult with encephalomalacia of the right frontal lobe.

Treatment and outcome

The patient hesitated to start antiepileptic drugs. No attack occurred during a follow-up of 3 years.

Commentary

This case was tentatively diagnosed as a pseudoseizure by the neurological resident in the emergency room, who did not learn about the previous two attacks. The diagnostic difficulty was how to reconcile the patient's clear consciousness with the generalized tonic contractions of all four limbs and head turning to the left side. Taken together, these manifestations did not fulfill the criteria for the diagnosis of a tonic–clonic seizure or a tonic seizure. Therefore, the alternative diagnosis of a pseudoseizure was considered, although no precipitating factor for a pseudoseizure could be established in this middle aged man.

In the seizure clinic, I found out that the patient had two earlier attacks over an 18-month period. The semiology of the first two attacks correlated with his frontal lobe infarction. The motor phenomena were not identical in each attack. The clinical course was relatively benign.

What did I learn from this case?

This case demonstrated the value of measuring the prolactin level and the EEG in a patient with an unusual presentation of paroxysmal motor attacks. The unusual and inconsistent prominent motor manifestations could be the nature of the frontal lobe epilepsy. However it could also be due to the limited description of the earlier seizures. The focal signs of the first and the third attack hinted at partial seizures; however, these signs may not be diagnostically reliable. The bilateral prominent tonic motor phenomenon favored the involvement of the frontal lobe.

Further reading

Saygi S, Katz A, Marks DA, *et al*. Frontal lobe partial seizures and psychogenic seizures: comparison of clinical and ictal characteristics. *Neurology* 1992;42:1274–7.

Riggio S. Frontal lobe epilepsy: clinical syndrome and presurgical evaluation. *J Epilepsy* 1995;8:178–89.

Salanova V, Morris HH, Ness PV, *et al*. Frontal lobe seizure: electroclinical syndrome. *Epilepsia* 1995;36:16–24.

Laskowitz DT, Sperling MR, French JA, *et al*. The syndrome of frontal lobe epilepsy: characteristics and surgical management. *Neurology* 1995;45:780–7.

Case 17

A Boy With Up To 100 Partial Seizures A Day

Federico Vigevano, Christa Pachatz and Lucia Fusco

History

In August 1994, a right-handed boy aged 4 years and 9 months presented with an epileptic seizure during sleep. The seizure was characterized by awakening, moaning, vomiting and hypomotility of the left side of the body. There were no antecedents or history of head trauma. The family history was negative for epilepsy and other neurological diseases.

Twenty days later, the child started to present complex partial seizures lasting from a few seconds to 4 minutes. These seizures were characterized by psychomotor arrest, impairment of consciousness, flushing of the face, head deviation to the left or right, and motor manifestations such as palpebral jerks, deviation of the mouth to the left, and left hemiclonic jerks. Seizure frequency increased to 30 to 100 seizures a day within the first month of disease.

Two years and 7 months after the onset of epilepsy, the child showed continuous unilateral myoclonic jerks of different muscle groups on the left side, particularly the left orbicular muscle, consistent with epilepsia partialis continua.

Examination and investigations

Neurological examination was normal at epilepsy onset. One year after onset the child showed a slight left-sided faciobrachiocrural hemiparesis that deteriorated constantly during the course of the disease, with loss of ambulation at the age of 7 years and 9 months and complete loss of trunk control at the age of 8 years and 7 months. Progressive cognitive deterioration was observed, beginning 1 year after epilepsy onset.

A cerebral magnetic resonance imaging (MRI) scan revealed T2 hyperintensity in the right anterior frontal region 1 month after seizures started. Successive MRI scans showed atrophy of the right frontal lobe (at 3 months after onset), T2 hyperintensity of the right frontotemporoparietal cortex (at 10 months after onset), volumetric reduction of the right hemisphere with T2 hyperintensity in

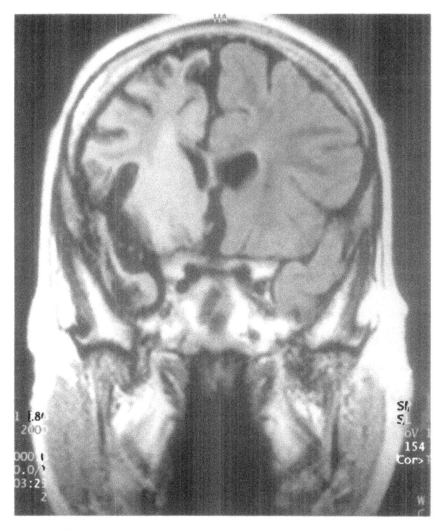

Figure 17.1: *Cerebral MRI performed 4 years and 7 months after the onset of epilepsy.*

the right frontal periventricular white matter (at 1 year and 11 months after onset) and right cerebellar atrophy (at 3 years and 11 months after onset). At 4 years and 7 months after onset, hyperintense signal of the right-sided basal ganglia and marked right frontal and temporal cortical and subcortical atrophy were diagnosed (Fig. 17.1).

The first EEG, performed 20 days after the first seizure, showed right frontotemporal theta–delta waves and spikes that evolved into right hemispheric slow and epileptiform abnormalities within the first year of the disease and, on successive EEGs, into bihemispheric synchronous and asynchronous abnormalities. Clinical and subclinical seizures originated exclusively from the right hemisphere. Marked depression of the right hemispheric cerebral activity could be documented, beginning 3 years and 10 months after seizure onset.

Diagnosis

Rasmussen's encephalitis affecting the right hemisphere.

Treatment and outcome

Antiepileptic drug treatment, including phenobarbital, phenytoin, carbamazepine, clobazam, nitrazepam, vigabatrin, valproate, felbamate and gabapentin, was ineffective. Nine months after epilepsy onset, a trial of adrenocorticotropic hormone failed. Surgical treatment was recommended, but at that time the parents did not agree to it. Further attempts with immunomodulatory therapies did not prevent continuous clinical deterioration. Eleven cycles of plasmapheresis at 1 year and 6 months after onset were unsuccessful, and combination with two cycles of cyclophosphamide decreased seizure frequency only for a few weeks. At 3 years and 4 months after epilepsy onset, the child underwent treatment with intravenous immunoglobulins without success, followed by oral corticosteroid therapy. The course of the disease was markedly aggravated by recurrent infections of the respiratory tract.

At the age of 9 years and 7 months (4 years and 10 months after epilepsy onset), the child underwent right hemispheric functional hemispherotomy, performed by Dr Olivier Delalande in Paris. Since then, the child has been seizure-free, has recovered ambulation with support and is markedly improving in cognitive functions. Permanent motor deficit consists of a left-sided faciobrachiocrural hemiparesis.

Commentary

Rasmussen's encephalitis, first described in 1958 by T Rasmussen, is an acquired chronic progressive neurological disease of unknown etiology with onset in childhood; it is characterized by severe pharmacoresistant epilepsy, cortical and subcortical atrophy of a single hemisphere, contralateral hemiparesis and progressive cognitive deterioration. Cerebral biopsy shows a characteristic inflammatory histopathology with perivascular lymphocytic cuffs throughout the cortex and, to a lesser degree, in the white matter, and microglial nodules.

67

Rasmussen's encephalitis is considered an autoimmune disease, and the role of the glutamate receptor GluR3 as the pathogenic autoantigen is discussed in the literature. Other pathogenic mechanisms, such as viral infections by cytomegalovirus or herpes virus triggering an autoimmune response, have been proposed. Furthermore, double pathologies found at pathological examination have indicated that Rasmussen's encephalitis might be a single clinical entity that occurs as a result of a variety of pathophysiological mechanisms.

What did we learn from this case?

Reports in the literature have proposed a series of immunomodulatory therapies such as corticosteroids, immunoglobulins, plasmapheresis, antiviral therapy with ganciclovir, and interferon therapy, but the clinical results remain contradictory. In our case, a large range of immunomodulatory therapies was attempted aggressively – partly because of the temporary lack of parental consent to neurosurgical treatment – but without results. Progressive deterioration of motor and cognitive functions was unavoidable and recurrent respiratory infections led to a life-threatening situation. We learnt, in concert with the literature, that neurosurgical treatment seems to be the only therapy capable of stopping the evolution of Rasmussen's encephalitis.

How did this case alter our approach to the care and treatment of our epilepsy patients?

We are convinced that surgical treatment is recommended in Rasmussen's encephalitis to prevent the inevitable progression of intellectual deterioration and incapacitating seizures. Functional hemispherotomy does not result in a further motor handicap. Cognitive functions improve markedly as a result of seizure cessation and discontinuation of treatment with antiepileptic drugs.

If we are confronted with a pharmacoresistant epilepsy in childhood and if the affected patient is a candidate for surgical treatment, we have to take care not to waste too much time and to proceed rapidly in the decision-making process.

Further reading

Asher DM, Gajdusek CD. Virologic studies in chronic encephalitis. In: Andermann F, ed. *Chronic encephalitis and epilepsy: Rasmussen's syndrome.* Boston: Butterworth–Heinemann; 1991:147–58.

Andrews PI, Dichter MA, Berkovic SF, *et al.* Plasmapheresis in Rasmussen's encephalitis. *Neurology* 1996;**46**:242–6.

Dabbagh O, Gascon G, Crowell J, *et al*. Intraventricular interferon-α stops seizures in Rasmussen's encephalitis: a case report. *Epilepsia* 1997;**38**:1045–9.

Delalande O, Pinard JM, Basdevant C, *et al*. Hemispherotomy: a new procedure for central disconnection. *Epilepsia* 1992:**33(suppl 3)**:99–100.

Freeman JM, Vining EPG, Pillas DJ, *et al*. Seizure outcome after hemispherectomy: the Johns Hopkins experience. In: Tuxhorn I, *et al*, eds. *Paediatric epilepsy syndromes and their surgical treatment*. London: John Libbey; 1997:743–8.

Hart YM, Andermann F, Robitaille Y, *et al*. Double pathology in Rasmussen's syndrome. A window on the etiology? *Neurology* 1998;**50**:731–5.

Hart YM, Cortez M, Andermann F, *et al*. Medical treatment of Rasmussen's syndrome (chronic encephalitis and epilepsy): effect of high-dose steroids or immunoglobulins in 19 patients. *Neurology* 1994;**44**:1030–6.

Krauss GL, Campbell ML, Roche KW, *et al*. Chronic steroid-responsive encephalitis without autoantibodies to glutamate receptor GluR3. *Neurology* 1996;**46**:247–9.

McLachlan RS, Levin S, Blume WT. Treatment of Rasmussen's syndrome with ganciclovir. *Neurology* 1996;**47**:925–8.

Rogers SW, Andrews I, Gahring LC, *et al*. Autoantibodies to glutamate receptor GluR3 in Rasmussen's encephalitis. *Science* 1994;**265**:648–51.

Villemure JG. Hemispherectomy techniques: a critical review. In: Tuxhorn I, *et al*, eds. *Paediatric epilepsy syndromes and their surgical treatment*. London: John Libbey; 1997:729–38.

69

Case 18

LATE-ONSET MYOCLONIC SEIZURES IN DOWN'S SYNDROME

Hajo M Hamer, Jens Carsten Möller, Susanne Knake, Wolfgang H Oertel and Felix Rosenow

History

A 55-year-old man with Down's syndrome was admitted to our hospital after a generalized myoclonic–tonic seizure. Approximately 3 years before admission, myoclonic jerks (particularly of the upper extremities) had started. These usually occurred in the morning and could be improved by administration of valproate (1800 mg/day). The dose was reduced because of daytime somnolence, and this reduction coincided with the occurrence of the first generalized myoclonic–tonic seizure, as described by a witness. Owing to aggressive behavior during the addition of lamotrigine, the medical regimen was not closely followed, and additional generalized myoclonic–tonic seizures occurred.

Examination and investigations

Apart from increased muscle tone and gait disturbance, physical examination did not reveal any significant neurological abnormalities. A mini-mental state examination yielded a score of 1 point. A computed tomography scan revealed cortical atrophy; magnetic resonance imaging was not possible because of non-compliance on the part of the patient. The clinical diagnosis of Down's syndrome was confirmed by cytogenetical analysis.

An EEG was recorded when serum valproate levels were below detection threshold; this showed generalized continuous slowing and generalized polyspike–wave complexes (Fig. 18.1). The details of the myoclonic seizures, which were preceded by generalized polyspikes on the EEG, have been described elsewhere.[1]

Diagnosis

Late-onset myoclonic epilepsy in Down's syndrome.

70

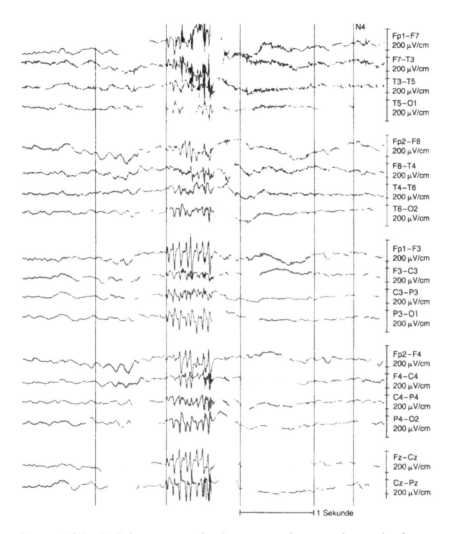

Figure 18.1: *EEG showing generalized continuous slowing and generalized polyspike–wave complexes.*

Treatment and outcome

On a low dose of valproate (900 mg/day), the patient's generalized myoclonic–tonic seizures were finally controlled but his myoclonic jerks increased over the subsequent months. Therefore, topiramate (100 mg/day) was introduced, which led to significant and sustained improvement.

Commentary

Why did we choose this case?

Epilepsy in Down's syndrome becomes more common with age, affecting more than 46 % of patients over the age of 50 years (compared with approximately 9 % of patients aged over 18 years).[2,3,4] So far, descriptions of epilepsy with onset during or after the fifth decade in Down's syndrome have been rare, but reports have included at least two patients who have myoclonic seizures as well as generalized tonic–clonic seizures.[5,6] A bimodal onset of seizures in Down's syndrome, with peaks during early childhood and in middle age, has been described by several authors.[7,8] Because the longevity of subjects with Down's syndrome is increasing, epilepsy with late onset will be encountered more frequently in the future.[9]

What did we learn from this case?

Epilepsy in Down's syndrome that is characterized by seizure onset after the fourth decade may comprise myoclonic jerks and occasional generalized tonic–clonic seizures associated with progressive dementia.[5,6,10] We therefore propose that late-onset myoclonic epilepsy in Down's syndrome (as characterized in this case) should be included in the differential diagnosis of adult-onset myoclonic epilepsies. The time-locked association of polyspike–wave complexes preceding the myoclonus in our patient[1] and in the patient reported by Genton and Paglia[5] allows it to be classified as a primary generalized epileptic myoclonus. Late-onset myoclonic epilepsy in Down's syndrome may be successfully controlled by valproate and topiramate. However, topiramate must be used with particular caution in patients with Down's syndrome since it carries a risk of cognitive side effects.

Myoclonus is also found in the majority of Alzheimer's disease patients with epilepsy.[11] Since the accumulation of β-amyloid has been found both in patients with Alzheimer's disease and in aging Down's syndrome patients with dementia,[12] a common pathogenesis of dementia and myoclonic epilepsy in elderly Down's syndrome patients and patients with Alzheimer's disease appears possible.[13]

How much did this case alter our approach to the care and treatment of our epilepsy patients?

Late-onset epilepsy in elderly, demented Downs' syndrome patients is characterized by myoclonus, occasional generalized tonic–clonic seizures or generalized myoclonic–tonic seizures, generalized epileptiform discharges on the

EEG, and slow progression. Myoclonus in this syndrome can probably be classified as primary generalized epileptic myoclonus. Late-onset myoclonic epilepsy in Down's syndrome should be included in the differential diagnosis of adult-onset myoclonic epilepsies.

References

1. Möller JC, Hamer HM, Oertel WH, Rosenow F. Late-onset myoclonic epilepsy in Down's syndrome (LOMEDS). *Seizure* 2001;**10**:303–6.

2. Veall RM. The prevalence of epilepsy among mongols related to age. *J Ment Deficiency Res* 1974;**18**:99–106.

3. Tangye SR. The EEG and incidence of epilepsy in Down's syndrome. *J Ment Deficiency Res* 1979;**23**:17–24.

4. McVicker RW, Shanks OE, McClelland RJ. Prevalence and associated features of epilepsy in adults with Down's syndrome. *Br J Psychiatry* 1994;**164**:528–32.

5. Genton P, Paglia G. Epilepsie myoclonique sénile? Myoclonies epileptiques d'apparition tardive dans le syndrome de Down. *Epilepsies* 1994;**1**:5–11.

6. Li LM, O'Donoghue MF, Sander JW. Myoclonic epilepsy of late onset in trisomy 21. *Arq Neuropsiquiatr* 1995;**53**:792–4.

7. Pueschel SM, Louis S, McKnight P. Seizure disorders in Down syndrome. *Arch Neurol* 1991;**48**:318–20.

8. Prasher VP. Epilepsy and associated effects on adaptive behaviour in Down's syndrome. *Seizure* 1995;**4**:53–6.

9. Baird PA, Sadovnick AD. Life expectancy in Down syndrome adults. *Lancet* 1988;**2**:1354–6.

10. Evenhuis HM. The natural history of dementia in Down's syndrome. *Arch Neurol* 1990;**47**:263–7.

11. Hauser WA, Morris ML, Heston LL, Anderson VE. Seizures and myoclonus in patients with Alzheimer's disease. *Neurology* 1986;**36**:1226–30.

12. Petronis A. Alzheimer's dementia and Down syndrome: from meiosis to dementia. *Exp Neurol* 1999;**158**:403–13.

13. Collacott RA. Epilepsy and associated effects on adaptive behaviour in Down's syndrome. *J Intellect Disability Res* 1993;**37**:153–60.

73

Case 19

FAINTING, FEAR AND PALLOR IN A 22-MONTH-OLD GIRL

Edwin Trevathan

History

JH, an otherwise normal 22-month-old girl, was brought to her pediatrician's office after a 'fainting spell'. JH was playing after breakfast when she ran to her mother, grabbed her mother's dress, appeared pale and then lost consciousness. After JH collapsed to the floor she slept for about 10 minutes before awaking in her usual state of health. Her examination and development were normal. The pediatrician considered a diagnosis of cardiac arrhythmia (such as paroxysmal atrial tachycardia) as well as gastroesophageal (GE) reflux, and ordered an electrocardiograph (ECG) and an esophageal pH probe, both of which were normal. The mother was reassured and the child was placed on thickened feeds for presumed gastroesophageal reflux.

Two weeks later, JH was playing with her dolls on the family kitchen floor. As JH was singing a children's song, the mother reported that she suddenly stopped singing and was noted to appear afraid and look pale before running to grab her mother's skirt and 'fainting'. The child was taken to the local emergency room, where she had a normal examination, a normal ECG, a normal chest X-ray and normal routine blood tests. As the emergency room physician was leaving the room JH had her third spell – this time witnessed by a pediatric emergency room specialist. The look of sudden panic or fear was time-locked with the sudden pale appearance and staring straight ahead and also with cessation of normal play activities. The child had subtle lip pursing movements and her hands were held at the mid-line as she 'tapped her thumbs together'. The physician noted that her pupils were dilated and that she seemed unable to respond to his questioning. Her pulse rate, previously 90 beats/minute, was noted to be 130 beats/minute and regular during the spell. After about 90 seconds (which the mother described as 'about 5 minutes'), the child fell asleep. She awoke 10 minutes later in her usual state of health. However, the emergency room physician noted that she had mild right central facial weakness upon awakening and that she did not speak for 30 minutes after waking from the spell; thereafter, she returned to her usual behavior with fluent, intact language.

Examination and investigations

I was consulted in the emergency room and noted that the patient's physical examination was normal, with the exception of a very subtle facial asymmetry – slightly less facial movement of the right face when speaking. The mother's account was reviewed in detail. All three spells were witnessed by the mother and were noted to be stereotypical. The spells were all heralded by a sudden look of fear with sudden loss of normal color of the facial skin, cessation of play, staring and subtle (but stereotypic) hand movements. An EEG performed within a few hours demonstrated left temporal theta waves, without epileptiform activity. The diagnosis of complex partial seizures of probable left temporal origin was made, and JH was started on carbamazepine (CBZ). A magnetic resonance imaging scan of the brain demonstrated thickening of the cortex within the left temporal lobe, with a significant reduction in white matter volume in the left temporal lobe compared with the same area on the right. The right hippocampus was very small, with very high signal on T2-weighted imaging.

After 7 months of freedom from seizures on CBZ, the seizures recurred. These seizures now occurred in clusters several times a week, and on rare occasions they were associated with secondary generalization. The seizures failed to respond to CBZ, phenytoin, valproate, lamotrigine, topiramate and clonazepam in maximum tolerated doses. Video–EEG monitoring demonstrated that all interictal spikes and ictal onsets came from the left temporal lobe. A modified left temporal lobectomy with complete resection of the dysplastic cortex was performed, with cessation of seizures and freedom from seizures for more than 3 years of follow-up. The pathology was consistent with focal cortical dysplasia.

Diagnosis

Left temporal lobe epilepsy.

Commentary

Both the manifestations and the pathology associated with temporal lobe seizures are different in children from adults. The semiology of JH's seizures, like other young children with temporal lobe seizures, was primarily remarkable for a look of fear, cessation of normal play activities and pallor. The typical oral and hand automatisms usually seen among adults with mesial temporal lobe epilepsy are often not seen or are so subtle in children that they are not noticed or reported by parents and non-physician observers.[1]

75

Obtaining an EEG within 24 hours of the spell[1] may increase the diagnostic yield of an EEG, but the most important diagnostic feature is the history. The manifestations of temporal lobe seizures in children are sometimes unrecognized by pediatricians and adult neurologists alike. Stereotypic spells of staring and pallor, with a look of fear or with associated clinging behaviour (or both), associated with an alteration in consciousness and sleep, are manifestations of complex partial seizures of temporal lobe origin in children.[2]

Physicians who manage children with partial seizures should realize that failure to respond to the first drug increases the likelihood that the child will develop intractable seizures. Failure to respond to three drugs used appropriately for partial seizures is predictive of intractability, and early referral to a pediatric epilepsy surgery center can improve the child's long-term outcome.[3]

References

1.   Bourgeois BF. Temporal lobe epilepsy in infants and children. *Brain Dev* 1998;20:135–41.

2.   King MA, Newton MR, Jackson GD, *et al*. Epileptology of the first-seizure presentation: a clinical, electroencephalographic, and magnetic resonance imaging study of 300 consecutive patients. *Lancet* 1998;352:1007–11.

3.   Kwan P, Brodie MJ. Early identification of refractory epilepsy. *N Engl J Med* 2000;342:314–9.

II

INTRIGUING CAUSES AND CIRCUMSTANCES

Case 20

ABNORMAL HEART RATE IN A CHILD WITH WEST SYNDROME

Julio Ardura and Jesus Andres

History

We evaluated a full-term (38 weeks of gestational age) newborn male. His mother was healthy. During prenatal monitoring, both bradycardia and late-onset decelerations were observed in the fetus. After delivery, the physical examination showed normal intrauterine growth. Apgar scores were 3/7; and cardiopulmonary resuscitation was required.

On the 3rd day of post natal life, episodes of body hyperextension and abnormal eye movements were observed. On day 11, generalized tonic-clonic convulsions occurred.

Examination and investigations

In the newborn period, the blood glucose level was 30 mg/100 ml. Blood cultures as well as a serological screening of congenital infections (toxoplasmosis, other infections, rubella, cytomegalovirus infection, herpes simplex virus infection –'TORCH') and syphilis were negative. An EEG performed 23 days after birth showed bursts of spikes in the right parietal region. A second EEG performed at the age of 3 months demonstrated a hypsarrhythmic pattern. Brain ultrasound performed on day 5 after birth showed right ventricular dilatation, and subependymal and intraventricular haemorrage. A CT scan at the 17th day of life revealed enlargement of the right lateral ventricle, and subcortical parieto-occipital atrophy.

Continuous 24-hour, polygraphic continuous recordings of heart rate were performed on days 1 (first day of life), 15, 57, 289 and 295. Data analysis was carried out using the single cosinor method, which is a statistical test for chronobiological rhythms.

Heart rate analysis disclosed no circadian rhythm at any time during this follow-up period (Table 20.1). Significant ultradian rhythms occurred within a period of 8 hours on day 1 and within a period of 4 hours on day 289.

Table 20.1 24-hour heart rate rhythm cosine parameters					
Day of life	Amplitude	SE	Achrophase	SE	Z-test
1	10.35	5.14	23:57	32	0.14
15	8.98	4.51	20:18	27	0.15
56	9.94	4.33	12:05	24	0.08
289	8.34	3.44	23:55	24	0.06
295	11.27	6.02	18:58	31	0.18

SE = Standard error
Amplitude: half the difference between the highest and lowest points in the cosine curve.
Achrophase: the timing of the highest value (hours:min)

Diagnoses

West Syndrome, birth asphyxia, cerebral hemorrhage, subcortical atrophy and seizures. Circadian disturbances of heart rate.

Treatment and outcome

Phenobarbital was initiated at a total daily dose of 60 mg (20 mg/kg). Because seizures continued, phenytoin was added (initially at a daily dose of 7 mg/kg and subsequently at 10 mg/kg). The convulsions were finally controlled with a combination of clonazepam (0.5 mg twice daily), phenytoin and phenobarbital.

When the baby was last examined at the age of 3 months, episodes of generalized flexor spasms as well as a delay in developmental milestones were noted.

Commentary

Epilepsy influences the biological rhythms of melatonin, sleep/wake and other hormones. Nevertheless, few papers have been published dealing with the study of biological rhythms in children with seizures.

We describe the patterns of circadian and ultradian heart rate rhythms during a 10-month follow-up in one case of West Syndrome. Circadian heart rate variability, which is not mature in newborn infants, usually appears at 30 days of age, continues through the 2nd and 3rd months of life, and remains throughout life. Therefore, in our patient, circadian changes of heart rate rhythm were expected to

79

occur at least by the latest recording (day 295). Nevertheless, our patient's heart rate showed no evidence of circadian rhythms during any of the recordings.

On the other hand, healthy infants have ultradian high frequency heart rate rhythms (3-hour) at birth, and low frequency rhythms at 90 days of age. In this case, the ultradian rhythms were less prevalent, and high frequency rhythms were predominant during the entire follow-up period.

What did we learn from this case?

We surmised that the absence of circadian rhythms in this patient could be accounted for by damage to his central nervous system (CNS) and speculate that this phenomenon may occur more often than is believed because it is generally not investigated in this syndrome.

In addition, we suspect that the appearance of biological rhythms in the postnatal period and during infancy may prove to be a useful indicator of normal maturation of CNS structures. On the other hand, the absence or delay of their appearance during infancy might indicate a disturbance of the CNS. Thus, circadian rhythm of heart rate might be an indirect measure of the degree of biological derangement.

How did this case alter our approach to the care and treatment of our epilepsy patients?

Based on this case, we believe that West syndrome may alter circadian rhythms permanently and modify the appearance and predominance pattern of ultradian rhythms of heart rate variability.

In our opinion, monitoring biological rhythms could be helpful in gauging the degree to which CNS structures are mature in patients with West Syndrome and, quite possibly, in patients with other neurological conditions. We do believe this issue is worthy of further study and have incorporated circadian heart rate analysis as well as the measurement of other biological rhythms in our ongoing clinical studies to further elucidate their significance.

References

1.   Ardura J, Andres J, Aldana J, Revilla MA, Aragon MP. Heart rate biorhythm changes during the first three months of life. *Biol Neonate*, 1997;72:94–101.

2.   Bloom FE. Breakthroughs 1998. *Science* 1998;282:2193.

3.   Nelson W, Tong YL, Lee JK, Halberg F. Methods for cosinor-rhythmometry. *Chronobiologia* 1997;6:305–25.

80

Case 21

HYPERACTIVE BEHAVIOUR AND ATTENTIONAL DEFICIT IN A 7-YEAR-OLD BOY WITH MYOCLONIC JERKS

Johan Arends, Albert P Aldenkamp and Biene Weber

History

A 7-year-old boy was referred to our child neurological programme for learning disabilities with complaints about hyperactive behaviour, attention deficit, lack of concentration and unexplained fluctuations in school performance. Moreover, short periods (lasting some seconds) of sudden change of alertness were reported; the change in alertness was accompanied by loss of function. These short episodes occurred both at school and at home, mostly when the boy was watching television or playing computer games. There was no amnesia for these events or change of facial colour, but sometimes there were stereotyped movements. Most of these events were interpreted as symptoms of the attention-deficit–hyperactivity disorder (ADHD) and the movements were interpreted as 'tics'.

Hyperactive behaviour had started at a very young age and did not respond to treatment (e.g. with methylphenidate). After starting in regular education, the boy had been referred to special education because of the hyperactive behaviour, combined with conduct disorders. Psychomotor development was normal, although language development was delayed.

Examination and investigations

Neurological examination was normal. The patient was right-handed.

EEG showed normal background activity with frequent multifocal (poly)spike–waves (occurring six times in each 10 seconds). These waves were sometimes localized frontally and at other times they were generalized. During the recording, eight short seizures combined with epileptiform discharges were observed; these occurred only when the patient was watching television and they were accompanied by jerks. There was no specific photosensitivity to light

81

stimuli, but there may have been sensitivity to specific patterns (such as the red colours on the television screen).

Neuropsychological investigation showed subnormal intelligence (Wechsler full-scale IQ was 56), with corresponding verbal and performance scores (verbal IQ was 62 and performance IQ was 54). Beery tests for psychomotor development showed a psychomotor delay of about 3 years, a delay in language development, and symptoms of ADHD (especially attentional deficits and hyperactive behaviour) and conduct disorders. There was evidence that the ADHD is a secondary symptom. During several periods, the sudden drops in alertness were observed. After such episodes, the symptoms of ADHD increased.

EEG combined with neuropsychological assessment showed frequent multifocal epileptiform discharges of sharp waves, spike–waves and polyspike–waves. During this period, frequent myoclonic jerks were observed (74 jerks in a recording that lasted 30 minutes). These jerks especially involved the shoulders (the left and right shoulders independently) with hypertonia. In addition there were infrequent absence seizures (four were recorded in $\frac{1}{2}$ hour). The myoclonic jerks were most pronounced when the patient was watching television, but they were also present during absences seizures when he was not watching television. The myoclonic absences interfered significantly with cognitive function such that the patient did not react to questions during the myoclonic seizure and did not remember being questioned after the seizure. Simultaneously with these seizures the EEG showed generalized discharges with spike–waves and polyspike–waves over a period of 5–13 seconds; there was also sometimes localized activity of frontal origin. In addition, photosensitivity for patterns and bright colours was established. This was accompanied by self-induction. The patient reported feeling a pleasant sensation in his head during the seizures. Figure 21.1 shows a sample of the EEG discharges during the myoclonic absence seizures.

Magnetic resonance imaging scanning showed no abnormalities.

Diagnosis

Myoclonic absence epilepsy[1] with developmental delay and secondary ADHD symptoms with conduct disorders.

Treatment and outcome

Some antiepileptic drugs (e.g. carbamazepine, phenytoin, vigabatrin, gabapentin) may increase the frequency or severity of seizures. About 50 % of patients respond favourably to valproate, ethosuximide or lamotrigine, either in monotherapy or in combination.[2] However, treatment should be initiated

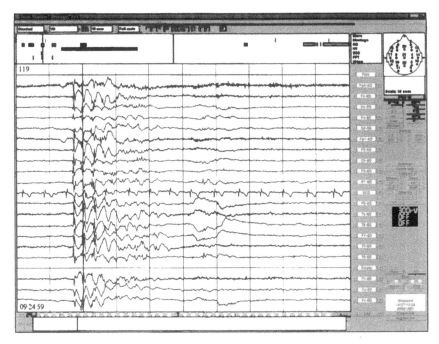

Figure 21.1: Ictal EEG during a myoclonic absence seizure.

carefully, since high doses of these drugs can also lead to an increase in seizure frequency, probably through the alteration of vigilance.

In this patient, treatment was initiated with ethosuximide 250 mg twice daily using 62.5 mg/ml syrup; however, the syrup was changed to tablets after poor drug compliance and the dose was increased to 750 mg/day. At this dose the patient was reported to be slow and tired, and seizure frequency increased. After the dose was lowered to 500 mg/day, his seizure frequency decreased. Because we considered the ADHD symptoms to be secondary, no pharmacological treatment for ADHD was started. To assist the patient's parents, practical counselling was provided in the home, especially focused on improving the family's strategies for coping with the epilepsy and the bad behaviour and on implementing strategies to improve drug compliance. A behaviour modification programme was also started to reduce self-induction. About 1½ years after starting this combined treatment strategy, the patient was considered almost seizure free.

Commentary

Why did we choose this case?

Although it is documented that the syndrome of myoclonic absence epilepsy is associated with mental retardation (in 45 % of patients at onset of the epilepsy, with a further 25 % developing mental retardation during the course of the disease),[3] our case illustrates that the myoclonic jerks can also interfere with cognitive function and thus cause state-dependent cognitive impairment in addition to the trait-dependent impairments caused by the syndrome. Although photosensitivity is described as a rare comorbid symptom, seizures may be precipitated by light stimulation. In this case, self-induction was also present. This may contribute to the intractability in some cases and therefore compliance should be carefully monitored. Family counselling may be needed as in this case.

The differential diagnosis of myoclonic absence epilepsy may be difficult. For example, when there is a myoclonic component, the differential diagnosis may involve childhood or juvenile absence epilepsies; these, however, rarely affect the upper limbs (unlike myoclonic absence epilepsy). Moreover, in myoclonic absence seizures almost no eyelid twitching is present, unlike classical absences. EEG recordings may also be misinterpreted as classical 3-Hz spike–waves of classical absence epilepsy. In myoclonic absences the discharges are more irregular, there are more polyspikes and often there is an asymmetry. When myoclonic absences are suspected, an electromyogram of the shoulder muscles can be helpful in the differential diagnosis since the myoclonias may be very subtle, especially when patients are already being treated with anti-epileptic drugs. Every patient with absences that prove to be therapy resistant has to be regarded as suffering from myoclonic absences. The syndrome of myoclonic–astatic epilepsy has a similar age of onset and also combines absences with myoclonic seizures. There are, however, tonic–clonic seizures in the period before the onset of the absences and drop-attacks, and massive myoclonus that develops soon after the appearance of the absences. The myoclonic jerks in juvenile myoclonus epilepsy are briefer, and not associated with loss of consciousness, but are associated with tonic–clonic seizures without absences, and they start at a later age.

What did we learn from this case?

Apart from the above comments, we were particularly surprised by the significant impact of the syndrome on intelligence. This may be partially caused by the interference of the myoclonic jerks with normal information processing and the development of ADHD as a secondary symptom. In particular, the cognitive effects of the myoclonic jerks may be substantial because of the high frequency of seizures.

84

Moreover, in this specific case the seizures may be confused with behavioural symptoms during longer periods – at the time of referral, all this boy's symptoms had been erroneously interpreted as being due to ADHD or as being repetitive tics.

Although the syndrome of myoclonic absence epilepsy is often associated with development delay, this is too often seen as an untreatable trait-factor. State-dependent factors such as high seizure frequency and conduct disorders should be vigorously treated. This may result in a normal or only slightly delayed development.

In a recent study, seven out of 14 patients with myoclonic absence epilepsy showed evidence of a chromosome abnormality syndrome (trisomy 12 p and Angelman syndrome).[4] In this patient no chromosomal investigations were performed. This should be done in patients with more than one seizure type, early-onset seizures or severe development delay.

References

1.   Tassinari CA, Lyagoubi S, Santos V, *et al*. Etude des décharges de pointes ondes chez l'homme. II. Les aspects cliniques et electroencephalographiques des absences myocloniques. *Rev Neurol* 1969;**121**:379–83.

2.   Perucca E, Gram L, Avanzini G, Dulac O. Antiepileptic drugs as a cause of worsening of seizures. *Epilepsia* 1998;**39**:5–17.

3.   Dulac O, Kaminska A. Intractable myoclonic absences. In: Schmidt D, Schachter SC. *Epilepsy: problem solving in clinical practice*. London: Martin Dunitz; 2000: 361–4.

4.   Elia M, Guerrini R, Musumeci SA, *et al*. Myoclonic absence-like seizures and chromosome abnormality syndromes. *Epilepsia* 1998;**39**:660–3.

Further reading

Aldenkamp AP, Overweg-Plandsoen WCG, Arends J. An open nonrandomized clinical comparative study evaluating the effect of epilepsy on learning. *J Child Neurol* 1999;**14**:795–801.

Overweg-Plandsoen WCG, Van Bronswijk JC, Arends J, Aldenkamp AP. The effect of epileptiform discharges and difficult-to-detect seizures on cognitive function. *Epilepsia* 1999;**40**(**suppl 2**):100–1.

Seizures With A Musical Association

Tim Betts

History

At the age of 12 years, a young girl had her first complex partial seizure while playing the piano. She had an aura of intense fear followed by a brief loss of consciousness and a flaccid fall from which she recovered after a brief period of postictal confusion. Attacks continued to occur despite trials of several antiepileptic drugs.

When I saw her for the first time, she was aged 18 and was taking a mixture of phenytoin, carbamazepine and valproate. She was an intelligent young woman who hoped to go to university, but she found studying and concentration difficult owing to the sedative effects of her medications.

There was no family history of epilepsy and no history of head injury or of a febrile convulsion. She was having up to 12 seizures a month and had noticed a recent increase in frequency because, whenever she heard a certain popular tune being played, she had one of her characteristic seizures. This tune, sung by a rather raucous group, was adapted from a well-known classical tune. She began to fear ambient music and began to avoid going to concerts in case she heard the tune. In time, her anxiety about hearing this particular tune had begun to generalize to all music, and the frequency of non-music-triggered seizures had also increased.

At presentation she wondered if her attacks were actually epileptic and requested drug withdrawal rather than other drugs and wished to be considered for alternative therapies. She knew of no emotional association with the tune.

Examination and investigations

Physical and psychiatric examinations were normal, apart from evidence of mild generalized anxiety. Bloods levels of her medications were in the therapeutic range. Two EEGs showed spike–wave activity localized to the right temporal lobe. A brain magnetic resonance imaging scan was normal.

A seizure was observed when the particular tune was played to her. (I was unable to obtain the co-operation of the EEG department, but I felt it necessary to induce a seizure to be sure of the diagnosis). She was lying down. She was apprehensive before the music started but was not hyperventilating. After the tune had played for some 60 seconds she suddenly seemed to lose concentration, looked completely terrified and became flushed. She did not reply when spoken to, seemed to lose awareness of her surroundings and then began to swallow and smack her lips. Her limbs were flaccid, she stopped breathing for about 30 seconds and her lips became cyanosed. She then took a breath and regained awareness but was a little confused and still apprehensive.

Diagnosis

Simple partial seizure evolving to a complex partial seizure, originating in the right temporal lobe and sometimes induced by a particular tune (musicogenic epilepsy).

Treatment and outcome

I decided against desensitization to the tune itself because her seizures also occurred spontaneously, but I considered that aura interruption (by teaching her to relax and drop her arousal at the instant the seizure started) might be helpful. I had just started to use aromatherapy and had found that an aromatherapy massage reduced seizure frequency in some patients for some weeks afterwards, and I had toyed with the idea of using the powerful smell of an aromatherapy oil as a counter-measure in a manner related to Efron's technique.

The patient agreed to try this approach and chose a relaxing oil (ylang ylang). After several massages with the diluted oil I taught her an autohypnotic technique so that she could immediately associate the smell of the gently inhaled oil (vigorous sniffing might trigger a seizure) with the intense relaxation induced by massage with the oil. Once relaxation seemed to occur automatically when she smelt the oil (which she carried round with her in a small bottle), she was instructed to inhale the oil gently as soon as she either felt a seizure starting (she had about 1 minute of warning with retained awareness) or if she heard the tune. When in a situation where she could not reach her bottle of oil she used a tactile memory of the masseur's thumb pressing on a particular relaxing acupressure point on her back as a counter-measure but this was more difficult to concentrate on.

There was a rapid and dramatic reduction in seizure frequency and after 4 months she became seizure-free and remained so even when her medication was slowly withdrawn over the next year (at her request). She learnt that she needed to practice the technique even when not having seizures but after a while she did not need to carry the bottle of oil with her but merely had to recall the smell of the oil (so called 'smell memory' – smell is the easiest of the senses to condition).

Later still she would occasionally smell the aroma of ylang ylang for no obvious reason and opined herself that her brain had learnt to automatically switch epileptic activity off without her needing to think about it.

During the treatment she suddenly remembered that the triggering tune was the one she had been playing (in its classical form) at the time she had her first seizure. When last seen, 3 years after obtaining seizure control, she was still seizure-free and off medication.

Why did I choose this case?

I chose this case because it reminds me that epilepsy has an important psychological side and is often mediated by arousal. Sometimes teaching the patient to modify arousal rapidly is more effective than any amount of medication.

What did I learn from this case?

I learned that most reflex epilepsies are triggered by an emotional response to the stimulus (particularly musicogenic epilepsy). Psychological (behavioural or cognitive) therapy for epilepsy has a long tradition but is under-researched and deserves to be more thoroughly assessed. This case set me thinking about how this might be done. Above all, in using a psychological therapy for epilepsy, one learns as much from the patient as the patient learns from the therapist – treatment should be a partnership. The patient also gains the feeling that he or she can do something about the seizures, thus enhancing feelings of mastery and control.

Further reading

Brown S. Other treatments for epilepsy. In: Hopkins A, Shorvon S, Cascino G, eds. *Epilepsy*, 2nd ed. London: Chapman and Hall; 1995:309–17.

Efron R. The conditioned inhibition of uncinate fits. *Brain* 1957;**80**:251–62.

Kirk Smith M, van Toller C, Dodd G. Unconscious odour conditioning in human subjects. *Biol Psychiatry* 1992;**17**:221–31.

Wolf P. Aura interruption: how does it become curative? In: Wolf P, ed. *Epileptic seizures and syndromes*. London: John Libbey; 1994:667–73.

Zifkin B, Zatorre R. Musicogenic epilepsy. In: Zifkin B, Andermann F, Beaumanoir A, Rowan J, eds. Reflex epilepsies and reflex seizures. *Advances in neurology*, vol 75. Philadelphia: Lippincott–Raven; 1998:273–81.

Case 23

Temporal Lobe Epilepsy, Loss Of Episodic Memory And Depression In A 32-Year-Old Woman

Christian G Bien

History

This previously healthy woman, a smoker for more than 10 years (one pack per day), experienced her first seizure (tonic–clonic) at the age of 32 years. Subsequently, she developed complex partial seizures, with features suggesting an origin in the dominant temporal lobe, at a frequency of three a day. Several anticonvulsive drug regimens (valproate, valproate plus phenytoin, lamotrigine) did not control the seizures. In parallel to the epilepsy, the patient developed severe loss of episodic memory and mood lability with a predominance of depression and – later on – verbal aggression.

Examination and investigations

The patient was admitted to the Epilepsy Center of the University of Bonn, Germany, 9 months after her initial seizure. Physical examination revealed no focal neurological deficits. She had severe affective abnormalities, consisting of major depression with lability of mood. Neuropsychological testing revealed verbal and visual memory deficits.

A magnetic resonance imaging (MRI) scan showed left-sided hippocampal volume loss with increased T2 signal, indicating hippocampal sclerosis. Interictal EEG revealed bilateral anterior temporal epileptiform discharges (sharp waves, sharp-and-slow waves). Recordings of five habitual seizures showed a uniform left temporal onset of rhythmic theta activity with spread to the contralateral temporal lobe contacts within 6–20 seconds. Positron emission tomography scanning revealed left temporal hypermetabolism. Ictal single photon emission computed tomography scanning showed left temporal hyperperfusion. A search for neoplasia, including serum testing for autoantibodies associated with paraneoplastic neurological syndromes, was negative. There were no abnormal values in standard tests of the cerebrospinal fluid, including an extensive serological search for neurotropic infectious agents.

Diagnosis

Temporal lobe epilepsy with complex partial and secondarily generalized tonic–clonic seizures, memory loss and organic affective syndrome, presumed to be due to limbic encephalitis.

Treatment and outcome

Owing to the severe memory deficits, resective epilepsy surgery was initially withheld. Several drug regimens failed to control the seizures. The patient's affective disorder was treated with mirtazapine and later with mirtazapine plus citalopram.

On the basis of the suspected diagnosis of a chronic encephalitic origin of the left temporomedial damage (non-paraneoplastic limbic encephalitis), immunosuppressive therapy was started 10 months after the first seizure. The patient received prednisolone 100 mg/day for 1 month. After this, the daily dose was reduced by 10 mg/month.

The patient became seizure-free for 3 months, but her memory function did not change and the affective abnormalities increased – suicidal tendencies as well as aggressive behavior were noted. A change of the antidepressant drug therapy to venlafaxine led to an improvement. However, the psychic abnormalities were still unbearable for the patient and her family. Since these problems were in part attributed to the high-dose corticosteroid treatment, prednisolone was tapered down.

The seizures recurred. A Wada test indicated left hemispheric language dominance. A left sided amygdalohippocampectomy was offered to the patient, but she and her family were thoroughly informed about the risk of a further decline of her verbal memory performance. The patient wished to be operated on, and 17 months after her first seizure, the procedure was performed.

Histopathological investigation of the hippocampal specimen obtained during epilepsy surgery revealed segmental neuronal loss and astrogliosis (hippocampal sclerosis) and perivascular and parenchymatous inflammatory infiltrates consisting of T lymphocytes (Fig. 23.1).

Eleven months after surgery, the patient was seizure-free apart from three complex partial seizures, which had occurred when the patient had not regularly taken her antiepileptic medication (lamotrigine 400 mg/day postoperatively). A renewed search for neoplasia was initiated.

90

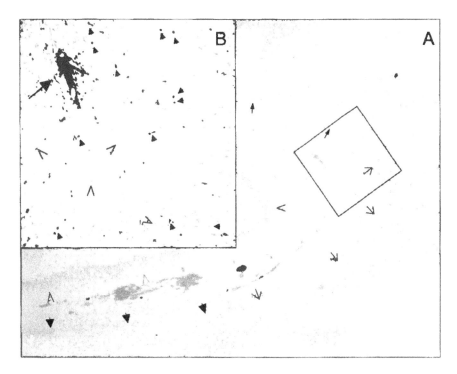

Figure 23.1: *(A) Hippocampus. Arrowheads: sector cornu ammonis (CA) 1, which is almost completely devoid of neurons. Arrows with wide angle: cornu ammonis 2, with neurons largely preserved. Arrows with filled head: cornu ammonis 3, with almost no neurons preserved. Open angles: dentate gyrus, preserved. Hematoxyline and eosin; original magnification ×25. (B) Detail of (A) (box). Large arrow: vessel and perivascular space containing numerous lymphocytes. Arrowheads: parenchymatous lymphocytes. Open angles: microglial cells. Immunohistochemical staining for leukocyte common antigen (CD45), slight counterstaining with hemalum; original magnification ×100.*

Commentary

The case illustrates that mediotemporal lobe epilepsy with hippocampal sclerosis may rarely present as an adult-onset disease on the basis of chronic limbic encephalitis. Limbic encephalitis is usually associated with a neoplasia and is then known as paraneoplastic limbic encephalitis. However, cases without neoplasia have been identified in a cohort of patients undergoing presurgical evaluation (non-paraneoplastic limbic encephalitis). Limbic encephalitis should be included in the differential diagnosis of temporal lobe epilepsy that is not typical for the 'classical' syndrome of temporal lobe epilepsy with medial sclerosis. Such cases are characterized by a subacute onset of pharmacoresistant temporal lobe seizures, affective abnormalities, severe memory loss, and limbic lesions on the MRI scan. A malignant condition, usually a small cell lung cancer in the presence of characteristic autoantibodies, needs to be excluded. Long-term follow-up in cases of suspected paraneoplastic limbic encephalitis is mandatory because the neurological syndrome may begin more than 2 years before the detection of the underlying tumor.

What did I learn from this case?

Even though the condition can be securely diagnosed only on the basis of a histological examination, clinical data and neuroradiological findings may suggest the diagnosis. Treatment of these pharmacoresistant syndromes is difficult, because not only the seizures but also the severe memory deficits and the affective disorder need to be accounted for when a regimen is planned. In cases of paraneoplastic limbic encephalitis, treatment of the underlying neoplasm is the most effective therapy. In patients with non-paraneoplastic limbic encephalitis, high-dose immunosuppression can be performed in addition to anticonvulsive and antidepressant pharmacotherapy. Patients with non-paraneoplastic limbic encephalitis (and paraneoplastic limbic encephalitis alike) usually present with bilateral mediotemporal lesions. However, unilateral cases may occur, as shown by the patient presented here. For patients with non-paraneoplastic limbic encephalitis who have unilateral lesions, resective temporal lobe surgery should be considered. The patient presented here became almost seizure-free after amygdalohippocampectomy.

Further reading

Bien CG, Schulze-Bonhage A, Deckert M, et al. Limbic encephalitis not associated with neoplasm as a cause of temporal lobe epilepsy. *Neurology* 2000;55:1823–8.

Gultekin SH, Rosenfeld MR, Voltz R, Eichen J, Posner JB, Dalmau J. Paraneoplastic limbic encephalitis: neurological symptoms, immunological findings and tumour association in 50 patients. *Brain* 2000;123:1481–94.

Case 24

Epileptic 'Dreamy States' In A Young Man

Warren T Blume

History

A 20-year-old left-handed, right-footed, right-eyed and previously neurologically healthy man began to have focal and generalized seizures without known cause at age 15 years.

The focal seizures began as a 'dreamy state', otherwise described as an unreal faint feeling or as a cephalic sensation followed by nausea and occasionally euphoria. The patient denied loss of awareness but stared straight ahead without oroalimentary or manual automatisms. He emerged gradually without postictal dysphasia or other Todd's phenomenon. These attacks had become more frequent over the years and were occurring about 35 times a month and clustering up to 17 a day.

Fear, olfactory or gustatory sensations, motor phenomena, intraictal language or speech impairment, and other experiential phenomena did not accompany these attacks.

About 20 generalized tonic–clonic (grand mal) seizures had occurred over the past 6 months, occasionally in sequences of up to 10–15 minutes in length.

The central nervous system functional enquiry was clear – his memory and judgement were subjectively intact although he found that the medications had slowed his ability to react.

The neurological history was also clear – febrile seizures, meningitis, encephalitis or major head injury had not occurred.

Examination and investigations

The neurological examination was normal. Visual fields, pupils and fundi were normal. There was no focal motor deficit, and his gait and co-ordination were normal. Neuropsychological testing revealed no abnormalities. Memory was normal.

His awake and sleep interictal EEGs were normal. A single clinical seizure was associated with 6-Hz rhythmic waves at Fz, Cz, C4, and F4 with spread to P4 and also involving F8 but with only slight involvement of M2, M1 and elsewhere. Therefore, the seizure appeared to have a parasagittal origin with greater

93

involvement of the right side. Nausea was the only clinical symptom of this attack.

A small, approximately circular mass lesion in the mesial aspect of the right parietal region was identified on magnetic resonance imaging without contrast enhancement (Fig. 24.1).

A habitual seizure was recorded by subdural EEG, revealing onset in the right posterior cingulate area (Fig. 24.2).

Histological examination of the completely resected focal right mesial parietal lesion disclosed a dysembryoplastic neuroepithelial tumor.

Diagnosis

Partial seizures secondary to a dysembryoplastic neuroepithelial tumor.

Treatment and outcome

No seizures have occurred since the right posterior cingulate lesion was resected.

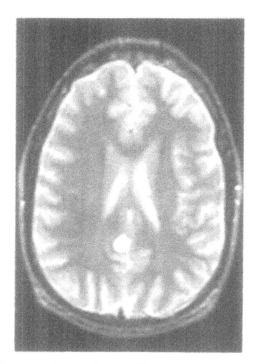

Figure 24.1 *Discrete right mesial parietal lesion on magnetic resonance imaging scan.*

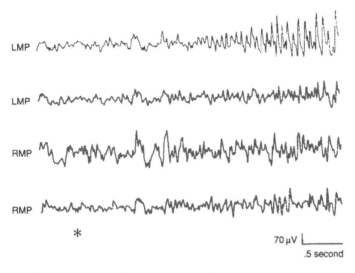

LMP

LMP

RMP

RMP

*

70 μV

.5 second

Figure 24.2 *Right subdurally recorded clinical seizure beginning in third channel (*) as irregularly sequential spikes spreading first ipsilaterally (fourth channel) and then contralaterally (first, then second channel) and becoming maximally expressed on left. LMP, left mesial parietal (cingulate gyrus); RMP, right mesial parietal (cingulate gyrus).*

Commentary

The limbic lobe comprises a ring of phylogenetically primitive cortex, including the cingulate gyrus, the parahippocampal gyrus (which is the anterior–inferior extension of the cingulate gyrus) and the hippocampal formation. The hippocampus connects with the anterior thalamic nuclei via the fornix and the mamillothalamic tract. The posterior cingulate receives afferents from the anterior thalamic nuclei, thus completing the Papez loop.[1] The posterior cingulate gyrus receives much more abundant afferents from the orbital frontal cortex, the parahippocampal gyrus, the dorsolateral frontal lobe and the parietal lobe than the anterior cingulate gyrus does. The posterior cingulate gyrus sends efferents to the hippocampus via the entorhinal cortex.

Reports describing semiology of seizures arising from the cingulate gyrus are few and often contain limited detail. Phenomena described include fear, aggressive verbalisations, staring, gestural automatisms, asymmetric tonic events, ocular and cephalic version, and autonomic phenomena involving the respiratory, cardiovascular and digestive systems. Some of these phenomena probably represent spread of the ictus to adjacent motor regions and even to other parts of the limbic system.[2-4]

95

What did I learn from this case?

Although the majority of seizures with experiential and epigastric phenomena arise from the temporal lobe, a minority of such attacks may involve other portions of the limbic system, which may have explained the symptomatology here. No clinical feature would specify the mesial parietal region as an origin for such attacks, but the very prominent tendency for generalized tonic–clonic seizures raises the possibility of a parasagittal focus. Limbic seizures that arise from one or both temporal lobes would probably be associated with interictal temporal spikes on at least one EEG, while neuropsychological testing would usually disclose a verbal or non-verbal memory impairment.[5]

Normal findings from these examinations would raise the possibility of an extratemporal origin for these seizures, including the cingulate gyrus or the orbital frontal area. Ictal propagation of posterior cingulate seizures to the supplementary sensory–motor areas could produce diffuse or unilateral sensory phenomena and progression to asymmetrical postural seizures.[6,7] However, such phenomena did not appear in this patient.

References

1. Papez JW. A proposed mechanism of emotion. *Arch Neurol Psychiatry* 1937;**38**:725–43.

2. Mazars G. Cingulate gyrus epileptogenic foci as an origin for generalized seizures. In: Gastaut H, Jasper H, Bancaud J, Waltregny A, eds. *The physiopathogenesis of the epilepsies.* Springfield, IL: Charles C Thomas; 1969:186–9.

3. Bancaud J, Talairach J. Clinical semiology of frontal lobe seizures. In: Chauvel AV, Delgado-Escueta AV, *et al.,* eds. *Advances in neurology* vol 57. New York: Raven; 1992:3–58.

4. Williamson PD. Frontal lobe seizures. Problems of diagnosis and classification. In: Chauvel P, Delgado-Escueta AV, Halgren E, Bancaud J, eds. *Advances in neurology* vol 57. New York: Raven; 1992:289–309.

5. Jones-Gotman M, Harnadek M, Kubu CS. Neuropsychological assessment for temporal lobe epilepsy surgery. *Can J Neurol Sci* 2000;**27(suppl 1)**:S39–S43.

6. Tukel K, Jasper H. The electroencephalogram in parasagittal lesions. *Electroencephalogr Clin Neurophysiol* 1952;**4**:481–94.

7. Penfield W, Jasper H. *Epilepsy and the functional anatomy of the human brain.* Boston: Little, Brown; 1954:94.

Case 25

Left Arm And Leg Shaking In A Patient With A History Of Treated Syphilis

Daniel J Brotman and Majid Fotuhi

History

A 65-year-old man presented to the emergency department in April 1999 for evaluation of possible seizures.[1] He had a history of treated hypertension and treated syphilis, and he was undergoing outpatient evaluation for an aortic arch aneurysm. His chief complaint was uncontrollable shaking of his left arm and leg. The first shaking episode had occurred 1 year earlier. At that time, he was walking when he suddenly developed uncontrollable shaking of the left arm and leg. This episode lasted for a few seconds and terminated spontaneously when the patient sat down. From that point onwards, the episodes occurred intermittently, about once or twice a week. The shaking would occur only when the patient was upright and always resolved when he sat or lay down.

He did not seek medical attention for these symptoms because he did not perceive them to represent a serious medical problem. However, during the month before admission the episodes had increased dramatically in frequency – they were occurring many times a day and had caused several falls. By the time of presentation, the patient was unable to walk and complained that every time he stood he would develop the shaking movements. The shaking would abate within seconds when he sat down, such that the duration of each episode was no more than 10 seconds. The character of the episodes was always the same: only the left arm and leg were affected, he always remained alert despite his inability to control the shaking, and he noted no weakness or paresthesias after episodes. He denied any history of seizures, stroke or syncope. He also denied headaches, fever, chest pain, arthralgias and skin rashes.

Examination and investigations

The patient appeared healthy and comfortable. Upper extremity blood pressures

97

were 162/54 mmHg on the left and 73/56 mmHg on the right. He was afebrile. Carotid and radial pulses were graded as 3+ on the left and 1+ on the right. Heart sounds were normal; there was an ejection murmur that radiated to the left carotid artery but not to the right. The lungs were clear, the neck veins were flat and there was no edema. There were no swollen joints or skin rashes. Neurological examination was normal while the patient was sitting or lying down. However, on each attempt to stand up, he developed large-amplitude 3–4 Hz shaking of his left arm and leg. He could not voluntarily control the shaking, yet he remained alert and conversant during each episode. He could not stand upright long enough for orthostatic measurements of blood pressure and pulse.

Brain magnetic resonance imaging (MRI) and magnetic resonance angiography were normal except for mild small vessel ischemic changes. An aortic angiogram (Fig. 25.1) revealed a proximal 5 cm aneurysm of the aorta involving the origin

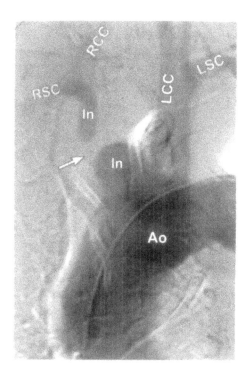

Figure 25.1: *Aortic angiogram showing a proximal 5 cm aneurysm of the aorta (Ao) involving the origin of the innominate artery (In) and obstructing its antegrade flow (arrow). However, there is flow in the right subclavian artery (RSC) via retrograde passage from the right common carotid artery (RCC). Circulation in the left common carotid (LCC) and left subclavian (LSC) is normal. The right vertebral artery is not visualized.*

98

of the innominate artery and obstructing its antegrade flow. However, there was flow in the right subclavian artery via retrograde passage from the right common carotid artery. Circulation in the left common carotid and left subclavian was normal. The right vertebral artery was not visualized.

Several hours after the aortic angiography, the patient developed weakness and numbness in his left arm and leg that were no longer postural but constant. A repeat diffusion-weighted brain MRI scan showed a new small infarct involving the right ventrolateral thalamus and posterior internal capsule (Fig. 25.2).

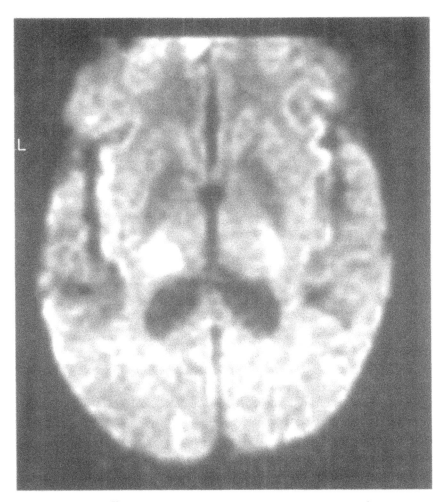

Figure 25.2: *Diffusion-weighted magnetic resonance imaging scan showing an acute infarct involving the right ventrolateral thalamus and posterior internal capsule.*

Diagnosis

Orthostatic limb-shaking transient ischemic attacks (TIAs).

Treatment and outcome

Because immediate cardiac surgery would risk hemorrhagic transformation of this patient's acute ischemic cerebrovascular accident (CVA), he was observed for a month before he underwent successful graft replacement of the aortic arch and great vessels. Examination of the pathological specimen revealed atherosclerotic changes and mild lymphocytic infiltration of the aortic wall, consistent with (but not specific for) treated syphilitic aortitis. Fortunately, his neurological deficits resolved almost completely with rehabilitation. The patient was last seen in April 2000, and at that time was ambulatory and without weakness or limb-shaking episodes.

Commentary

The patient's CVA led to symptoms in the same body distribution that had been involved in his preceding limb shaking episodes, indicating that the shaking probably represented recurrent TIAs.[1] Other authors have described limb shaking TIAs caused by internal carotid stenosis, sometimes postural and sometimes preceding ischemic CVAs.[2-4] This case demonstrates that such symptoms can also result from more proximal occlusions.

Although the pathogenesis of limb-shaking TIAs is not well understood, Baumgartner and Baumgartner studied cerebral vasomotor reactivity in a series of patients with this disorder.[2] They found that vasodilatation induced by carbon dioxide was absent in the cerebral vessels of the affected hemisphere, implying that the resistance vessels were already maximally dilated. This suggests that the presence of critical ischemia with limited collateralization may predispose to limb-shaking episodes in affected patients. These and other authors have found no evidence of seizure activity on EEG in patients affected by limb-shaking TIAs.[2,3,5,6]

Other explanations of this patient's symptoms could include focal seizures,[7] orthostatic tremor or pure neurosyphilis. Although no EEG was performed during a limb-shaking episode, focal motor seizures were unlikely because of the predictable onset and termination of limb-shaking with standing and sitting. Orthostatic tremor is unlikely because it typically involves both legs and has a higher frequency (13–18 Hz).[8] Neurosyphilis may have triggered inflammatory changes in the cerebral arteries, but is unlikely to have caused the CVA because it occurred shortly after angiography.

100

What did we learn from this case?

This case illustrates three important clinical points:

* TIAs may mimic seizures by presenting with shaking of the extremities;
* limb-shaking TIAs, like other TIAs, may signal an impending CVA and should be evaluated thoroughly; and
* postural limb-shaking is suggestive of severe impairment of the anterior cerebral circulation and should trigger evaluation of the carotid arteries as well as the proximal aorta if a patient has a history of syphilis or other risk factors for an aortic aneurysm.

How did this case alter our approach to the care and treatment of our epilepsy patients?

We now think of the possibility of limb-shaking TIAs in patients who are thought to have focal motor seizures when the movements are related to posture.

References

1. Brotman DJ, Fotuhi M. Syphilis and orthostatic shaking limbs. *Lancet* 2000;**356**:1734.

2. Baumgartner RW, Baumgartner I. Vasomotor reactivity is exhausted in transient ischaemic attacks with limb shaking. *J Neurol Neurosurg Psychiatry* 1997;**65**:561–4.

3. Baquis GD, Pessin MS, Scott RM. Limb shaking: a carotid TIA. *Stroke* 1985;**16**:444–8.

4. Firlik AD, Firlik KS, Yonas H. Physiological diagnosis and surgical treatment of recurrent limb shaking: case report. *Neurosurg* 1996;**39**:607–11.

5. Zaidat OO, Werz MA, Landis D, Selman W. Orthostatic limb shaking from carotid hypoperfusion. *Neurology* 1999;**53**:650–1.

6. Tatemichi TK, Young WL, Prohovnik I, Gitelman DR, Correll JW, Mohr JP. Perfusion insufficiency in limb-shaking transient ischemic attacks. *Stroke* 1990;**21**:341–7.

7. Kaplan PW. Focal seizures resembling transient ischemic attacks due to subclinical ischemia. *Cerebrovasc Dis* 1993;**3**:241–3.

8. McManis PG, Sharbrough FW. Orthostatic tremor: clinical and electrophysiologic characteristics. *Muscle Nerve* 1993;**16**:1254–60.

Case 26

NEW ONSET OF NOCTURNAL SEIZURES IN A 69-YEAR-OLD MAN

P Barton Duell

History

A 69-year-old man experienced three episodes of generalized tonic–clonic seizures that occurred at 3.00 or 4.00 AM, during sleep. The seizures were observed by his wife. His mental status after each seizure was consistent with a postictal state.

He had a history of stable asymptomatic coronary artery disease, combined hyperlipidemia, treated hypothyroidism and a mildly increased body mass index of 31 kg/m². He had undergone coronary artery bypass surgery at the age of 62 years but had no history of myocardial infarction. He subsequently had percutaneous coronary angioplasty three times between the ages of 67 and 68 years. He had been a non-smoker for 30 years. He rarely consumed alcoholic beverages.

His mother, father and paternal grandfather had died from cerebrovascular accidents at the ages of 94, 79 and 80, respectively. He had no personal or family history of seizures, but he had sustained mild head trauma without loss of consciousness 1½ years previously.

His medications were niacin (500 mg three times a day orally), aminosalicylic acid (81 mg/day orally) and thyroid (1.5 grain/day orally).

Examination and investigations

His neurological examination was unremarkable and non-focal. The results of brain computerized tomography and brain magnetic resonance imaging were normal. A cardiovascular evaluation did not reveal evidence of myocardial ischemia or cardiac arrhythmias.

He was subsequently found to have nocturnal hypoxemia caused by obstructive sleep apnea, which was ameliorated by treatment with continuous positive airway pressure (CPAP) during sleep.

102

Diagnosis

Generalized tonic–clonic seizures precipitated by nocturnal hypoxemia caused by obstructive sleep apnea.

Treatment and outcome

He was initially treated with phenytoin 400 mg/day in divided doses for control of seizures. CPAP used at night alleviated the episodic hypoxemia. He remained seizure-free for 1 year after discontinuation of phenytoin until he traveled to an altitude of about 2100 m and slept without using his CPAP machine. (The altitude at home was about 100 m). After that single seizure, he had no additional seizures during the subsequent 2.5 years.

Commentary

I chose this case for several reasons. First, the new onset of seizures in a 69-year-old man with coronary atherosclerosis is often attributable to causes such as cerebrovascular disease, cardiac arrhythmias, hypotension, embolic phenomena, metabolic abnormalities, and intracranial tumors or other intracranial pathology.[1] Despite the increased prevalence of obstructive sleep apnea among overweight patients, this diagnosis is often not considered in patients with seizure disorders. Moreover, patients are not always able to characterize the timing of their seizures well enough to delineate a purely nocturnal pattern of occurrence.

Secondly, although the patient's previous mild head trauma could have caused brain injury that resulted in the development of an epileptogenic focus, such pathology alone was insufficient to explain his seizures. It is plausible that an epileptogenic focus was unmasked by hypoxemia resulting from obstructive sleep apnea.

Thirdly, because the patient had only a limited number of seizures, it was not initially apparent that his seizures always occurred nocturnally during the middle of sleep. This observation narrowed the differential diagnosis and led to the diagnosis of obstructive sleep apnea.

What did I learn from this case?

Obstructive sleep apnea is an under-diagnosed condition that is associated with severe health consequences. Although this diagnosis is sometimes suggested by a characteristic constellation of symptoms, many of the symptoms are non-specific

103

and easily disregarded by health-care providers. In some cases, seizures are the presenting sign of sleep apnea,[2,3] as in this patient. Treatment of sleep apnea in children with epilepsy has been shown to improve seizure control,[4] as predicted. In addition, patients with a seizure disorder may experience an increase in the frequency of seizures if they develop obstructive sleep apnea, a situation that could occur as a consequence of marked weight gain.[5]

Patients who present with sleep apnea appear to have an increased risk of seizures. The results of a recent retrospective study from Prague suggest that 19 (4 %) out of 480 adult patients with sleep apnea had experienced at least two seizures in adulthood.[6] The mean age of the 19 patients at the time of the initial seizure was 48 ± 16 years; their mean body mass index was only 32 ± 10 kg/m^2. Despite the limitations of this study, the results suggested that patients with sleep apnea may have a higher prevalence of seizures than the general population, which has been estimated to be 0.5–1.0 % in Minnesota, USA.[7]

In summary, hypoxemia resulting from sleep apnea can precipitate seizures or exacerbate an underlying seizure disorder. Thus, it may be useful to consider the possibility of sleep apnea in patients who are being evaluated for seizures, particularly among those in whom seizures occur exclusively during sleep. In addition, patients who are being treated for sleep apnea and nocturnal hypoxemia but who are not known to have a seizure disorder may warrant careful assessment and monitoring for the possibility of hypoxemia-induced seizure activity.

References

1.   Stephen LJ, Brodie MJ. Epilepsy in elderly people. *Lancet* 2000;355:1441–6.

2.   McNamara ME. Detection of sleep apnea during standard ambulatory cassette EEG recording for seizures: two case reports. *Clin Electroencephalogr* 1990;21:168–9.

3.   Bradley TD, Shapiro CM. ABC of sleep disorders. Unexpected presentations of sleep apnoea: use of CPAP in treatment. *BMJ* 1993;306:1260–2.

4.   Koh S, Ward SL, Lin M, Chen LS. Sleep apnea treatment improves seizure control in children with neurodevelopmental disorders. *Pediatr Neurol* 2000;22:36–9.

5.   Lambert MV, Bird JM. Obstructive sleep apnoea following rapid weight gain secondary to treatment with vigabatrin (Sabril). *Seizure* 1997;6:233–5.

6.   Sonka K, Juklickova M, Pretl M, Dostalova S, Horinek D, Nevsimalova S. Seizures in sleep apnea patients: occurrence and time distribution. *Sb Lek* 2000;101:229–32.

7.   Hauser WA, Annegers JF, Kurland JF. Incidence of epilepsy and unprovoked seizures in Rochester, Minnesota. *Epilepsia* 1993;34:453–68.

Further reading

Duell PB. Role of sleep apnoea in epilepsy in elderly people. *Lancet* 2000;**356**:162. [A brief synopsis of this case was previously published in this paper.]

Case 27

NONCONVULSIVE STATUS EPILEPTICUS AND FRONTAL LOBE SEIZURES IN A PATIENT WITH A CHROMOSOME ABNORMALITY

Maurizio Elia

History

The patient is a 22-year-old man who developed normally until his first seizure at 3 years of age. Initially, his seizures were characterized by myoclonic jerks of the upper limbs. The seizures increased in frequency until they occurred many times a day during infancy. Over time the seizures changed and began to include impaired consciousness, pallor, abdominal pain, the expression of fear, mydriasis, motor automatisms and complex visual hallucinations. They often had a long duration and occurred in clusters. Other seizures were characterized by a staring gaze, diffuse hypertonia and clonic jerks of the upper limbs.

Polytherapy with phenobarbital, carbamazepine, valproate and phenytoin had little effect.

When the patient came to my attention, there were behavioral disturbances with frequent and sudden outbursts of rage. Daily episodes of non-convulsive status epilepticus occurred out of wakefulness, characterized by clouding of consciousness, unresponsiveness to stimuli, crying or expression of terror, gestures and verbal automatisms. He was also having several partial seizures a night that were characteristic of seizures of frontal lobe onset.

The patient was born at term and delivery was uneventful. His mother suffered from epilepsy and took antiepileptic drugs during pregnancy.

Examination and investigations

No gross dysmorphic features were evident. Neurological examination showed only a subtle postural tremor of the hands.

A magnetic resonance imaging (MRI) scan of the brain was normal. Evaluation with the Wechsler Adult Intelligence Scale revealed mild mental retardation (full-scale IQ 64, verbal IQ 60, performance IQ 73). Interictal EEG was

106

characterized by long sequences of slow spike-and-wake complexes that were more prominent over the frontal regions of both hemispheres. During non-convulsive status epilepticus, diffuse slow spike-and-wake complexes and slow waves were quasi-continuous and sometimes intermixed with brief runs of 4–5 Hz spike-and-wave complexes (Fig. 27.1). Ictal EEG showed an initially diffuse low-voltage fast activity, which was more evident over the frontal leads, followed by a short burst of rhythmic spike-and-wave complexes and then by pseudoperiodic runs of slow waves for many seconds. The recruiting rhythm was accompanied by a tonic contraction of deltoid muscles.

The patient's karyotype showed 46, XY/46, XY, r(20) (p13q13.3) 90 % mosaic.

Diagnosis

Non-convulsive status epilepticus and frontal lobe seizures due to ring chromosome 20 syndrome.

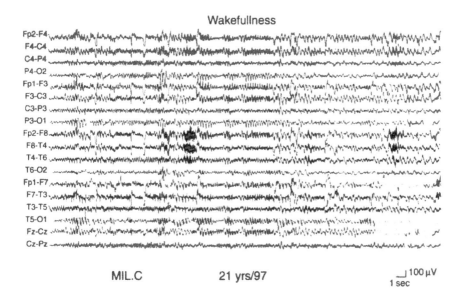

Figure 27.1: EEG recording during non-convulsive status epilepticus showing quasi-continuous diffuse slow spike-and-wave complexes and slow waves, which are sometimes intermixed with brief runs of 4–5 Hz spike-and-wave complexes.

Treatment and outcome

Treatment with phenytoin 300 mg/day, lamotrigine 200 mg/day, felbamate 2100 mg/day) and vigabatrin (3000 mg/day) in different combinations did not control the episodes of status epilepticus or the partial seizures.

Commentary

In recent years, several chromosomal syndromes have been identified that seem to show a peculiar clinical and EEG picture, such as Angelman syndrome, fragile X syndrome, Miller–Dieker syndrome and Wolf–Hirschhorn syndrome. However, on very few other occasions have seizures and EEG characteristics been described in detail, which would be necessary to define an electroclinical phenotype and eventually to classify the epilepsy syndrome. Furthermore, it is conceivable that other chromosomal abnormalities would manifest a specific electroclinical picture that could help the epileptologist to choose the genetic analysis to be carried out as well as helping to identify specific genes that influence the process of epileptogenesis.

This case fully confirms that ring 20 syndrome represents a new model of a symptomatic partial epilepsy, which certainly deserves to be included in a future classification of epileptic syndromes and diseases.

What did I learn from this case?

This case aroused my interest for several reasons. Ring 20 syndrome has been reported in more than 30 cases, mostly sporadic or mosaic. Patients with ring 20 syndrome present with mental retardation of varying degree and no gross dysmorphic features apart from rare heart or urogenital anomalies. Seizures are present in 90 % of cases and are invariably intractable. They begin at between 1 month and 21 years of age and are mostly complex partial seizures or partial seizures with secondary generalization.

Ring 20 syndrome represents a newly described and peculiar combination of clinical findings and seizure patterns, including episodes of non-convulsive status epilepticus that often herald the onset of seizures and that occur in many cases with a daily or weekly frequency, lasting 10–50 minutes. It should be emphasized that some ictal manifestations, such as those observed in this case, could be misdiagnosed as behavioural changes. Interictal EEG shows slow waves, spikes, sharp waves, or spike-and-wave complexes over the frontal regions. The ictal EEG is characterized by long runs of slow waves intermixed with high-voltage spikes, which are diffusely prominent over the frontal regions and changing in

108

frequency during the discharges. Moreover, bursts of 5-Hz theta-waves, sometimes without apparent clinical manifestations, have been reported in ring 20 syndrome. MRI evidence of frontal lobe dysplasias has been sporadically reported.

The pathophysiology of (frontal) epilepsy in ring 20 syndrome is not clearly understood, although it is known that the gene for autosomal-dominant nocturnal frontal epilepsy (CHRNA4) maps at the 20q13.2–q13.3 region.

I think that routine cytogenetic studies should be performed in all patients who present with this clinical picture, particularly in the absence of clear malformations on MRI.

Further reading

Inoue Y, Fujiwara T, Matsuda K, *et al*. Ring chromosome 20 and nonconvulsive status epilepticus. A new epileptic syndrome. *Brain* 1997;**120**:939–53.

Kobayashi K, Inagaki M, Sasaki M, Sugai K, Ohta S, Hashimoto T. Characteristic EEG findings in ring 20 syndrome as a diagnostic clue. *Electroencephalogr Clin Neurophysiol* 1998;**107**:258–62.

Canevini MP, Sgro V, Zuffardi O, *et al*. Chromosome 20 ring: a chromosomal disorder associated with a particular electroclinical pattern. *Epilepsia* 1998;**39**:942–51.

Petit J, Roubertie A, Inoue Y, Genton P. Non-convulsive status in the ring chromosome 20 syndrome: a video illustration of 3 cases. *Epil Dis* 1999;**1**:237–41.

Case 28

AN UNUSUAL CAUSE OF NOCTURNAL ATTACKS

Donald W Gross, Eva Andermann, David C Reutens,
François Dubeau and Frederick Andermann

History

A 32-year-old right-handed man developed nocturnal attacks at the age of 6
months. These attacks were brief and associated with stiffening of the limbs
without loss of consciousness. A diagnosis of nocturnal paroxysmal dystonia was
entertained. Despite multiple trials of antiepileptic drugs, the attacks continued
in clusters of 10–20 per night with several weeks between bouts.

Examination and investigations, treatment and outcome

Neurological examination, interictal EEG and magnetic resonance imaging (MRI)
were normal. Because of the uncertainty of the diagnosis, the patient had
prolonged video-EEG monitoring. A total of 46 seizures with stereotyped clinical
manifestations were recorded. The seizures started with facial movements and
were sometimes associated with a groan. The patient would then sit up from
sleep, stiffen and flex his upper limbs, and become apneic. Most attacks lasted
less than 30 seconds, and longer attacks were associated with perioral cyanosis.
During the seizures he retained awareness, and on some occasions he was able to
respond to questioning. The postictal period was brief and there was no postictal
slowing.

On reduced doses of antiepileptic drugs, the patient had two flurries of over
50 attacks a night, each bout being associated with a single generalized
tonic–clonic seizure. During both these episodes, he required intubation and
mechanical ventilation and developed a transient hypoxic encephalopathy.

After each flurry the seizures stopped spontaneously, but because of the
dramatic history, carbamazepine 1000 mg/day and phenytoin 200 mg/day were
continued.

Six years after the episode of status epilepticus, his nearly 4-year-old daughter
developed similar nocturnal attacks. They were also associated with respiratory

distress and tonic posturing, and they also occurred in clusters. Sleep EEG was normal. After the introduction of carbamazepine 200 mg/day she had a few attacks and then became seizure-free.

Diagnosis

Familial frontal lobe epilepsy with nocturnal attacks.

Commentary

Familial frontal lobe epilepsy with nocturnal attacks is being increasingly diagnosed. Patients have normal MRI scans and often do not show interictal or ictal EEG abnormalities. Some of these patients, but not all, respond to anticonvulsants.[1,2]

We report an apparently sporadic case that for many years had presented a problem in diagnosis. The familial nature of this patient's epilepsy became apparent only when his younger daughter developed identical nocturnal attacks. Both had clusters of stereotyped nocturnal seizures with tonic posturing and respiratory distress.

The clinical syndrome in this family was that initially described as sporadic paroxysmal nocturnal dystonia.[1,2] The identity of this syndrome is now in doubt and the attacks are currently considered to represent focal frontal epilepsy (Lugaresi E, personal communication). A clue to the epileptic nature of the disorder in the father was the occurrence of a generalized tonic–clonic seizure during a flurry of attacks.

Another interesting finding is the striking remission in the father, which has also been previously reported.[3] In this patient a spontaneous remission is suspected, but owing to the severity of the previous symptoms, it has not been possible to withdraw the anticonvulsants.

Previously reported families have shown autosomal-dominant inheritance of the disorder.[2,4] It is possible that the proband in this family had a spontaneous mutation of the responsible gene; however, previous families have been reported to have a penetrance of 69%. The mutation could have occurred in a recent ancestor with lack of expression, or there may have been a failure of recognition of the syndrome in previous generations.[4]

A mis-sense mutation of the nicotinic acetylcholine receptor on chromosome 20q13.2–13.3 has been found in two families with familial frontal lobe epilepsy.[5] This mutation was not found in this family. More recently there has been a suggestion of genetic heterogeneity in familial frontal lobe epilepsy.[6]

111

What did we learn from this case?

As the proband of this family presented as a sporadic case, it is possible that other sporadic cases may also prove to be familial, highlighting the importance of considering the diagnosis in apparently sporadic patients with frontal lobe epilepsy who do not have a demonstrable structural lesion.

References

1.   Lugaresi E, Cirignotta F, Montagna P. Nocturnal paroxysmal dystonia. *J Neurol Neurosurg Psychiatry* 1986;**49**:375–80.

2.   Lee BI, Lesser RP, Pippenger CE, *et al*. Familial paroxysmal hypnogenic dystonia. *Neurology* 1985;**35**:1357–60.

3.   Reutens DC, Andermann F, Olivier A, Andermann E, Dubeau F. Unusual features of supplementary sensorimotor area epilepsy: cyclic pattern, unusual sensory aura, startle sensitivity, anoxic encephalopathy, and spontaneous remission. In: Lüders HO, ed. *Advances in neurology*, vol 70. Philadelphia: Lippincott–Raven: 1996;293–300.

4.   Scheffer IE, Bhatia KP, Lopes-Cendes I, *et al*. Autosomal dominant nocturnal frontal lobe epilepsy. A distinctive clinical disorder. *Brain* 1995;**118**:61–73.

5.   Steinlein OK, Mulley JC, Propping P, *et al*. A missense mutation in the neuronal nicotinic acetylcholine receptor alpha 4 subunit is associated with autosomal dominant nocturnal frontal lobe epilepsy. *Nature Genet* 1995;**11**:201–3.

6.   Berkovic SF, Scheffer JE. Genetics of human partial epilepsy. *Curr Opin Neurol* 1997;**10**:110–4.

Case 29

ANGER AND FRUSTRATION FOLLOWED BY A SEIZURE

Sunao Kaneko

History

The patient is an 18-year-old woman who began having tonic–clonic seizures at the age of 2 years in the setting of measles. Her seizures initially responded well to treatment with phenytoin 100 mg/day and phenobarbital 100 mg/day, but when she was aged 14, her seizures began to occur the instant she became angry, usually out of frustration.

For a number of years, family members, as well as medical and nursing personnel, considered these seizures to be hysterical. They consisted of brief tonic extensions of both legs and tremulous movements of her extremities while she was lying down, or sudden falling down if she was walking. Often, she could talk during these seizures. The attacks lasted about 10 seconds. The family history was negative for epilepsy and mental retardation.

Examination and investigation

The general examination showed bowlegs. Cranial nerves were intact as were reflexes and the remainder of the neurological examination. The patient's IQ could not be examined – her mental age was 4½ years. Computed tomography scans of the brain and a chromosomal analysis were normal. Intraictal EEG recordings revealed diffuse and bilateral spikes, sharps and multiple spike–wave complexes that were predominant in the right frontotemporal areas.

When the patient was calm and cheerful, emotional stimulation was conducted with simultaneous EEG recording (anger was induced by verbal stimulation) (Fig. 29.1). Seizures occurred the moment that the patient felt anger.[1]

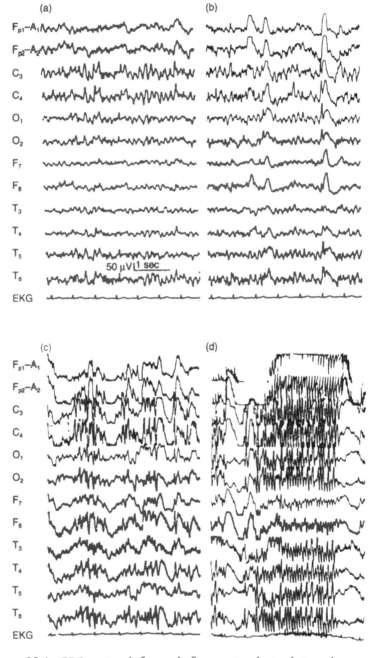

Figure 29.1: *EEG tracings before and after emotional stimulation, showing the appearance of clinical seizures and epileptic discharges. (a) EEG at resting state. (b) EEG 5 minutes after hyperventilation. (c) EEG during emotional stimulation. (d) Occurrence of epileptic seizures after emotional stimulation.*

114

Diagnosis

Complex partial seizures with secondary generalization. Moderate mental retardation.

Treatment and outcome

The seizures responded well to phenytoin 200 mg/day, primidone 200 mg/day, carbamazepine 1000 mg/day and diazepam 10 mg/day, together with teaching the patient how to deal with family problems and interpersonal relationships. Seizures have been completely controlled as long as she takes her medication regularly.

Commentary

Stress is one of the most important causes of seizures in people with epilepsy, particularly patients with complex partial seizures. A patient's emotional state can profoundly influence the frequency of their epileptic seizures; indeed, emotional management was important and effective in this case.

Emotionally induced seizures usually do not occur the moment the patient senses the anger or other emotion. However, there are exceptions, as illustrated by this patient. The treatment strategy varies – patients with mental retardation usually need a supportive approach, family and social intervention, and the support of medical, nursing and family members. Patients with normal intelligence may respond to neurobehavioural management interventions.[2] There is abundant evidence that a significant degree of seizure control for many patients with focal epilepsy can be established by altering their thinking and behaviour.[3]

What did I learn from this case?

Some patients with epilepsy are misdiagnosed as suffering from other conditions such as hysteria, as was the case here, and consequently are not correctly treated.

When I first met this patient I was in my second year as a postgraduate neuropsychiatry student. By examining and treating her, I realized that epilepsy lay in the borderland between what was conventionally understood as the provinces of neurology and psychiatry. I discovered that psychological care was indeed important in the management of epilepsy. As a result of my experiences in treating this patient, I made up my mind to specialize in epileptology.

References

1. Ishihara O, Kaneko S, Wazima A, Fukushima Y. Emotional activation of EEG in an epileptic patient. *Clin Electroencephalogr* 1976:6;378–88.

2. Joy Andrews D, Reiter JM, Schonfeld W, Kastel A, Denning P. A neurobehavioural treatment for unilateral complex partial seizure disorders: a comparison of right and left hemisphere patients. *Seizure* 2000:9;189–97.

3. Fenwick PB. Behavioural treatment of epilepsy. *Postgrad Med J* 1990:66;336–8.

116

Case 30

MYOCLONIC JERKS IN A COMPUTER SPECIALIST

Dorotheé GA Kasteleijn-Nolst Trenité

History

A 32-year-old man was referred for evaluation of myoclonic jerks and dizziness while working in front of a computer. He owned his own computer firm.

He had experienced myoclonic jerks of the arms from the age of 8 years. These jerks generally occurred 1 minute after he got out of bed and lasted from a few minutes to several hours. As a boy, he was noted to 'spill his milk' and sometimes his legs 'gave way'. The myoclonic jerks occurred with or without loss of consciousness. Sleep deprivation, and more especially, stressful situations such as examinations, provoked seizures.

On his 16th birthday he had his first tonic–clonic seizure while driving his new motorcycle to school; according to his parents the road was 'shiny.' Within a period of 3 weeks, another two tonic–clonic seizures occurred without an aura. Treatment with valproate changed the seizure pattern. For the past 7 years he has had no more tonic–clonic seizures. However, myoclonic jerks and dizziness have continued to occur once in a while, such as shortly after wakening, but mainly when he works in front of a computer screen, particularly a bad quality black and white screen or a screen with a frequency of less than 70 Hz, regardless of colour. He prefers to work with a grey background, without bright colours or pictures with colours and high contrast, such as a combination of yellow and blue. Furthermore, fast movements on the screen have caused dizziness.

Seizures have never occurred in front of a television set; in general, he avoids watching television but if he does, he keeps a distance between him and the set.

In addition, he has had myoclonic jerks triggered by malfunctioning fluorescent lighting. Other visual stimuli, such as sunlight through trees or on water, or black and white striped patterns (closing blinds, escalators) have never caused myoclonic jerks. Sailing is his hobby and he has never had seizures while doing this. Neither has driving been a problem – however, he nearly always wears dark brown sunglasses.

His current medication is valproate 2300 mg/day (the serum valproate concentration is 114 mg/l).

His family history is positive for epilepsy in his grandfather and uncle on his father's side. No further description is available.

Examination and investigations

On investigation, no neurological abnormalities were found and intelligence was normal. A computed tomography scan was normal. An EEG showed alpha activity, which was intermingled with sharp components; the alpha activity increased after hyperventilation. There were no spontaneous epileptiform discharges. Photic stimulation with flash frequencies between 2 and 60 Hz in the conditions eye closure, eyes closed and eyes open was performed; pattern stimulation with black and white striped patterns was tested; and the patient was asked to watch a 50-Hz television showing various programmes. Finally, a 70-Hz computer screen with scrolling text and graphic elements was used.

Generalized epileptiform discharges, which were maximal over the occipitotemporal areas, were recorded with photic stimulation at 30 and 40 Hz during eye closure; these discharges were associated with consistent dizziness. Epileptiform discharges, which were confined to the occipital area, occurred during photic stimulation at 23, 25, 30 and 50 Hz during eye closure, during photic stimulation at 25–40 Hz with eyes closed, and at a distance of 50 cm from the 50-Hz television set, which displayed a computer game, a flashing black and white video clip and an advertisement. Dizziness was again noted. The pattern on the 70-Hz computer monitor did not evoke abnormalities.

Diagnosis

Juvenile myoclonic epilepsy with photosensitivity, and sensitivity for specific visual stimuli.

Treatment and outcome

At work, the patient started to use only a 135-Hz monitor and his complaints of dizziness and jerks disappeared. His morning jerks continued.

Commentary

This case shows that a history of dizziness and jerks, eyelid myoclonia or loss of consciousness should be taken seriously. As in this case, most patients note

118

myoclonia or dizziness during diffuse or generalized epileptiform discharges evoked by photic stimulation or other visual stimuli such as television (only classical absence seizures are not noticed by the patients themselves). This is very useful knowledge for patients. They can find out what visual stimuli in daily life cause risks. By closing one eye or switching off the television or computer screen as soon as signs and symptoms occur, they can reduce the risk of having a tonic–clonic seizure, unless they are extremely photosensitive and not taking anti-epileptic medication.

Another reason I chose this case is that this patient had a combination of spontaneous seizures, typical for juvenile myoclonic epilepsy, and a clear history of photosensitive epilepsy. Although it is known that 30 % of patients with juvenile myoclonic epilepsy show a photoparoxysmal response in their EEG, a history of visually induced seizures is often lacking. This could result from difficulty in discriminating between seizures that occur spontaneously and seizures that are visually induced, or from lack of knowledge about the possibility of provocation of seizures by television, sunlight or visual patterns.

Finally, this case shows how patients can learn to avoid certain situations; this patient restricted his proximity to a television screen and wore dark sunglasses while driving or sailing.

What did I learn from this case?

I learnt that patients can be sensitive to very specific visual stimuli. This patient had a history of computer-induced seizures but not television-induced seizures, which to my knowledge was very unlikely. He had myoclonic jerks caused by malfunctioning fluorescent lighting but never had seizures elicited by sunlight on water or sunlight through trees. This apparent inconsistency in clinical history proved to be in line with the EEG investigations in which all kinds of visual stimuli were used to provoke photosensitivity.

This case also taught me that even with a very high dosage of valproate (2300 mg/day), a reaction to visual stimuli was still present. The tonic–clonic seizures disappeared but the myoclonic jerks (both the spontaneous jerks and the visually induced jerks) did not change with valproate therapy.

Further reading

Harding GFA, Jeavons PM. *Photosensitive epilepsy*. London: Heinemann; 1994.

Kasteleijn-Nolst Trenité DGA, Binnie CD, Meinardi H. Photosensitive patients. Symptoms and signs during intermittent photic stimulation and their relation to seizures in daily life. *J Neurol Neurosurg Psychiatry* 1987;**50**:1546–9.

Kasteleijn-Nolst Trenité DGA. Reflex seizures induced by intermittent light stimulation. In: Zifkin BG, Andermann F, Beaumonoir A, Rowan AJ, eds. *Reflex epilepsies and reflex seizures. Advances in neurology*, vol. 75. Philadelphia: Lippincott–Raven; 1998:99–121.

Ricci S, Vigevano F, Manfredi M, Kasteleijn-Nolst Trenité DGA. Epilepsy provoked by television and video games: safety of 100 Hz screens. *Neurology* 1998;**50**:790–3.

Ricci S, Vigevano F. The effect of video-game software in video-game epilepsy. *Epilepsia* 1999;**40(suppl 4)**:31–7.

Wilkins AJ, Darby CE, Binnie CD, Stefensson SB, Jeavons PM, Harding GFA. Television epilepsy: the role of pattern. *Electroencephalogr Clin Neurophysiol* 1979;**47**:163–71.

Wilkins AJ. *Visual stress*. Oxford: Oxford University Press, 1995.

Zifkin BG, Kasteleijn-Nolst Trenite DGA. Reflex epilepsy and reflex seizures of the visual system: a clinical review. *Epileptic disorders* 2000;**2**:129–36.

Acknowledgement

I would like to thank P Voskuil, neurologist from the Hans Berger Clinic in Breda, Holland for referring this patient to me. I am also grateful to the EEG technician, E Dekker (SEIN).

Cases 31 and 32

Issues In Epilepsy And Pregnancy

Ronald E Kramer and Kirsten A Bracht

History

The first case (case 31) involves a 39-year-old right-handed woman who presented for evaluation of uncontrolled seizures. Seizure onset had been at age of 10 years, when she had presented with a generalized tonic–clonic convulsion. She was placed on medication at that time but her seizures continued.

Her seizures were described as generalized tonic–clonic convulsions. They occur approximately once a year. In addition, the patient has seizures that are thought to be possible complex partial seizures. These are characterized as a change in mental status with a behavioral arrest, followed by eye fluttering and some subtle picking motions of the upper extremities. These seizures last less than 30 seconds. They tend to occur in clusters that last for 1–2 hours, and they occur on a monthly basis.

The seizures were thought to be related to menstrual periods but she was unable to document any such correlation on seizure logs. Sleep deprivation did exacerbate the patient's tonic–clonic seizures.

The patient had a history of a vascular headache disorder, which was quiescent. She was gravida 0, para 0. She was a high school graduate who was attending a business school to become a court reporter. She denied tobacco or alcohol use. A maternal first cousin suffered from recurrent generalized tonic–clonic seizures. Her brother had suffered one generalized tonic–clonic seizure but was not being treated. Her mother had a history of migraine headaches.

Her previous physicians had told her that she should not become pregnant because she has epilepsy.

The second case (case 32) also involves a 39-year-old right-handed woman, who presented with two unprovoked generalized tonic–clonic seizures at the age of 37. She had been placed on valproate after her second seizure and remained seizure-free on valproate monotherapy.

Her past medical history was notable for two episodes of deep vein thromboses in the left lower extremity, at the ages of 23 and 37, which had been treated with aspirin. Coagulopathy work-up had been negative. The patient had a 2-year history of a vascular headache disorder. While on valproate she remained free of headaches.

The patient was a gravida 2, para 1 female at presentation. She had a 7-year-

121

old daughter who was alive and well. She was a college graduate working as an accountant. Her family history revealed a migraine headache disorder in her mother. Coronary artery disease had occurred in a brother at the age of 46 and in her father at the age of 51.

The patient had recently been told by her referring physicians that because she now had a seizure disorder and was on seizure medications she could not get pregnant.

Examinations and investigations

In the first patient, the neurological examination was unremarkable. A previous computed tomography scan and EEG were reported as normal. The patient had a magnetic resonance imaging (MRI) scan, which was also normal. Video-EEG monitoring demonstrated generalized spike–wave discharges interictally as well as in association with her clinical events.

In the second patient, the neurological examination was also unremarkable. MRI showed non-specific white matter changes consistent with small vessel disease that was felt to be mildly excessive for her age. Routine sleep-deprived EEG showed a bilateral, intermittent frontotemporal dysrhythmia, maximal over the left frontotemporal region.

Diagnoses

The first patient was diagnosed with primary generalized epilepsy characterized by primary generalized tonic–clonic seizures and atypical absence seizures.

The second patient was diagnosed with seizure disorder secondary to small vessel disease of the brain. It was unclear whether chronic epilepsy existed in the patient and needed treatment.

Treatments and outcomes

The first patient had been previously maintained on a four-drug regimen: carbamazepine 800 mg/day, acetazolamide 200 mg/day, ethosuximide 500 mg/day and phenobarbital 60 mg/day.

After our diagnosis had been established, medication simplification and switches were attempted. Side effects occurred with valproate monotherapy and then with felbamate monotherapy. Monotherapy with lamotrigine and with topiramate were each unsuccessful because of lack of seizure control. The patient was maintained on a regimen of lamotrigine 500 mg/day and topiramate

122

200 mg/day. She did not suffer any further generalized tonic–clonic seizures and her atypical absence clusters were reduced to occasional isolated seizures every few weeks.

After her first evaluation and visit, issues of epilepsy and pregnancy were discussed. The patient was told about her options and placed on supplemental folic acid. Once the patient had been stabilized on a combination of lamotrigine and topiramate, she became pregnant. Amniocentesis and ultrasound performed at 18 weeks' gestation were normal and no complications or malformations are expected according to the obstetrician in the high-risk obstetrical clinic.

The second patient was told that she was a candidate for medication withdrawal since she had remained seizure free for over 2 years and her diagnosis was somewhat in doubt. She had been maintained on valproate monotherapy 1250 mg/day with levels running approximately 40 µg/ml. Because of her concerns regarding recurrent seizures, this was continued and she was placed on supplemental folic acid.

On follow-up, she is pregnant with twins and is 2 months away from her estimated date of confinement. During the end of her first trimester she suffered another deep venous thrombosis in her left lower extremity and was placed on heparin for the remainder of her pregnancy. Repetitive ultrasounds have all been normal and no complications are expected by the obstetrical staff.

Commentary

The first patient had seizures that were uncontrolled with polypharmacy whereas the second patient had significant systemic disease and seizures that were controlled with monotherapy. Both women had been explicitly instructed by previous physicians not to have children because they had epilepsy and were following these instructions when they arrived at our center, although they both wished to become pregnant. After several counseling sessions, they chose to become pregnant in full understanding and acceptance of the risks involved.

The majority of pregnancies in women with epilepsy proceed without complications. There are, of course, increased risks to both mother and child. Historically, there were prejudices against any person with epilepsy becoming pregnant and there were laws in the USA to regulate fertility and marriage as late as the 1980s.[1]

An increase in seizure frequency during pregnancy occurs in only 20–30 % of patients.[2,3] This increase may reflect altered metabolism or altered pharmacokinetics of antiepileptic drugs during pregnancy. Non-compliance is an important issue to address. Women with seizures have an increased risk of obstetrical complications, including anemia, hyperemesis gravidarum, pre-eclampsia, premature labor and abruptio placentae from trauma.[1]

123

Congenital malformations are more frequent in the offspring of women with epilepsy and risks are further enhanced by antiepileptic drugs. Minor and major anomalies can occur up to three times more often in women with epilepsy, with risks increasing almost exponentially as the number of drugs increases.[4] Although fetal exposure is usually an unavoidable risk, drug withdrawals before conception should always be considered in women whose seizures have been controlled or in whom the diagnosis is suspect.

Prenatal counseling is the most critical aspect in managing women of child-bearing potential. Physicians should follow published guidelines.[3,4] The goals of these guidelines are:

- to obtain patient compliance with a proactive treatment plan;
- to minimize drug burden;
- to maximize seizure control;
- to monitor fetal development with the patient's goals in mind; and
- to communicate frequently and often with the obstetrical team prior to delivery.

What did we learn from these cases?

Even as we begin the new century, older approaches and historic biases in regard to epilepsy and pregnancy still exist in the medical community. Some physicians may feel the need to provide guidance that absolutely guarantees a good outcome – a goal that is, of course, impossible to achieve. Physicians may also feel pressured to make decisions that are really best left to the patient in regard to the issues that surround epilepsy and pregnancy.

How did these cases alter our approach to the care and treatment of our epilepsy patients?

Similar cases and issues come up frequently in our clinic. As a result, we now discuss family planning issues at the very first visit with all women of child-bearing potential. A separate visit is set aside solely to discuss the issues of pregnancy and epilepsy. Such an approach is especially needed in today's medical environment in which time pressures for clinicians keep increasing.

We now understand that there are never any absolute right or wrong answers about epilepsy and pregnancy. The physician's roles are to provide education, statistics and a risk–benefit analysis that helps the patient make decisions, and to implement the safest and most medically sound treatment plan with the patient's goals in mind. It is up to the patient to make an informed decision. Some patients may require a more active level of leadership from the physician, but we believe that most patients can integrate the information in the context of their own life choices.

References

1. Yerby MS. Treatment of epilepsy during pregnancy. In: Wyllie E, ed. *The treatment of epilepsy: principles and practice*, 2nd ed. Baltimore: Williams and Wilkins; 1996:785–98.

2. Cantrell DC, Riela SJ, Ramus R, Riela AR. Epilepsy and pregnancy: a study of seizure frequency and patient demographics. *Epilepsia* 1997;**38(suppl 8)**:231.

3. Morrell MJ. Guidelines for the care of women with epilepsy. *Neurology* 1998;**51(suppl 4)**:517–21.

4. Delgado-Escueta AV, Janz D. Consensus guidelines: preconception counseling, management, and care of the pregnant woman with epilepsy. *Neurology* 1992;**42(suppl 5)**:149–60.

Addendum

Since going to press, both of these women completed their pregnancies. Both underwent C-sections without complication. The babies have normal examinations and are obtaining normal milestones on time.

125

Case 33

STATUS EPILEPTICUS AFTER A LONG DAY OF WHITE-WATER RAFTING IN THE GRAND CANYON

David M Labiner

History

The patient was a 31-year-old woman who was vacationing in Arizona. After a long day of white-water rafting on the Colorado River in the Grand Canyon, she developed her first-ever seizures. They were described by a paramedic that witnessed them as being generalized tonic–clonic events that were associated with aspiration. She was taken to the closest hospital and treated with phenytoin and phenobarbital. After an initial improvement, she developed status epilepticus and was transferred to my facility. She was treated with pentobarbital for her status epilepticus and her seizures were controlled, but attempts to decrease the barbiturates caused further partial seizures with secondary generalization characterized by focal motor activity as well as generalized convulsive activity. Attempts to use both carbamazepine and valproate were not successful, owing to a marked increase in hepatic enzymes.

Family history was notable for psychiatric disease in two brothers.

Examination and investigations

The patient was intubated and on a ventilator. There were no focal neurological findings. Neuroimaging studies were negative. When the barbiturates were reduced, the EEG was compatible with status epilepticus, with multifocal epileptiform features.

Extensive evaluation of serum, spinal fluid and urine were initially unrevealing. After approximately 90 days, a diagnosis of aminolevulinic acid dehydratase deficiency porphyria was made by red blood cell enzyme analysis.

Diagnosis

Status epilepticus associated with aminolevulinic acid dehydratase deficiency porphyria.

Treatment and outcome

Once the diagnosis of porphyria was made, the patient was tapered off barbiturates and switched to intravenous lorazepam and then to oral clonazepam. She awoke from the prolonged drug-induced coma and was discharged from the hospital on clonazepam. However, she complained of memory problems and intermittent confusion as well as seizures. The seizures were characterized as periods of behavioral arrest and staring associated with automatisms, followed by up to 30 minutes of confusion. These events were felt to be consistent with complex partial seizures occurring up to 15 times a day.

Because of its cognitive side effects, the dose of clonazepam was slowly reduced. The patient was readmitted to hospital with convulsive status epilepticus that was treated with lorazepam and paraldehyde. She was started on gabapentin 300 mg/day and her dose was rapidly increased to 900 mg/day. The patient had no further convulsive activity once the gabapentin was initiated. Her dose was further increased in increments of no greater than 300 mg twice a week. Seizure control was significantly improved at 1800 mg/day with no significant side effects. At higher doses, the patient had significant side effects, particularly somnolence and confusion.

The patient remained under adequate control for the next 9 months, when she developed pneumonia in the setting of an exacerbation of her porphyria and subsequently died. Her death was unrelated to seizures or the use of gabapentin.

Commentary

This case represented an unusual case of partial epilepsy caused by a metabolic disorder. Seizures are not a major manifestation of the porphyrias, and the diagnosis was not made for 3 months despite appropriate screening 2 weeks after the onset of her symptoms. Porphyria syndromes are inherited in an autosomal-dominant fashion except for congenital erythropoietic porphyria, which is autosomal-recessive. Although the abnormalities are present from birth, the symptoms typically do not appear until after puberty. The syndromes are characterized by acute attacks separated by latent periods. The primary neurological and psychological manifestations of the disorder are peripheral

127

neuropathy, weakness, paresis, sensory abnormalities, respiratory paralysis, seizures, hyporeflexia, cranial nerve palsies, behavioral changes, irritability or anxiety, hallucinations and depression.

Seizures associated with porphyria can be especially difficult to treat because many of the commonly used antiepileptic drugs can cause exacerbations of the syndrome. This phenomenon has been well documented for the barbiturates, phenytoin and carbamazepine. Benzodiazepines, valproate and even bromides have been advocated for treating seizures associated with porphyria.

What did I learn from this case? How did this case alter my approach to the care and treatment of my epilepsy patients?

Often we do not consider metabolic etiologies as a major cause of partial seizures and therefore miss the diagnosis of the underlying etiology. Apart from reacquainting myself with the diagnosis and features of porphyria, I realized that some of the treatments that were given to this patient (barbiturates and phenytoin) probably caused an exacerbation of her underlying disorder. Moreover, the nature of the disease often requires persistence and repeated testing to establish the diagnosis.

Additionally, gabapentin was not yet available in the USA nor was it known to be safe in treating seizures related to porphyria. Because of the desperate situation of this patient, we sought and obtained compassionate use of this drug based on what was known at the time about its lack of hepatic metabolism. We correctly reasoned that it would be safe to try gabapentin in this patient, and it turned out to be effective. Not only did we learn that gabapentin was a good anticonvulsant, we were able to use it as monotherapy to control this patient's seizures.

Further reading

1. Desnick RJ. The porphyrias. In: Isselbacher KJ, Braunwald E, Wilson JD, Martin JB, Fauci AS, Kasper DL, eds. *Harrison's principles of internal medicine*. New York: McGraw Hill; 1994:2073–9.

2. Krauss GL, Simmons-O'Brien E, Campbell M. Successful treatment of seizures and porphyria with gabapentin. *Neurology* 1995;**45**:594–5.

3. Labiner DM, Ahern GL, Kolb MA, Johnson DS, Vengrow MI. Gabapentin is both safe and effective in treating seizures associated with porphyria. *Epilepsia* 1994;**35(suppl 8)**:53.

4. Reynolds NC Jr, Miska RM. Safety of anticonvulsants in hepatic porphyrias. *Neurology* 1981;**31**:480–4.

128

Case 34

A FARMER WHO WATCHED HIS OWN SEIZURES

Gerhard Luef

History

The patient was a 37-year-old man with a history of epilepsy since the age of 3. Two different seizure types were described – episodes of altered consciousness and abnormal behaviour, and transient loss of consciousness associated with tonic posturing and clonic limb movements and sometimes with loss of bladder control and lacerations of the tongue.

There was no family history of seizures. Pregnancy and delivery were normal; however, he had low birth weight and needed to be observed in an incubator. Developmental milestones in the first 3 years were unremarkable.

The patient had been treated with a number of different antiepileptic drugs including phenytoin, carbamazepine, valproate, primidone, vigabatrin and topiramate, either alone or in combination, but he still had uncontrolled seizures. On a combination of topiramate 600 mg/day and phenytoin 350 mg/day (giving serum levels for phenytoin of 18.5 μg/ml and for topiramate of 6.9 μg/ml), his seizure severity was markedly reduced, but he still suffered from between about seven and 10 complex partial seizures a month. The combination did, however, render him free of generalized tonic–clonic seizures.

The major problem for this patient, a farmer with poor educational background, was that he could not find a wife because of his seizures. After 8 months on stable dosages and plasma concentrations, he underwent a presurgical evaluation.

Examination and investigations

Clinical examination revealed no pathological findings. Neuropsychological examination found verbal and visual memory deficits and cognitive deficits. Several EEGs demonstrated diffuse slowing and intermittent theta-wave activity in the left frontotemporal region. Magnetic resonance imaging scanning demonstrated gliosis in the left posterior cruz.

129

After withdrawal of his antiepileptic drugs, two seizures were recorded with video-EEG monitoring. The first event occurred while the patient was lying in bed. There were chewing automatisms followed by complex fine motor automatisms and dystonic posturing of the right arm and left leg, vocalization and arrhythmic head movements. There was no response to an examining nurse and consciousness was impaired. The second event started from a sitting position and was similar to the first with automatisms, but this one was followed by a tonic–clonic seizure. Both seizures started with left frontal theta rhythm, followed by slowing in the left temporal region and ending with diffuse slowing.

Diagnosis

Frontal lobe epilepsy with complex partial and secondary generalized seizures.

Treatment and outcome

Since medical treatment did not achieve complete seizure control, I recommended a presurgical evaluation. During 1 week of video-EEG monitoring, we recorded only two seizures and so monitoring was continued for another week. The patient was discharged on the same antiepileptic drug combination – topiramate and phenytoin – and a new date for epilepsy monitoring was set in 6 months.

During a lecture to students, he was asked if he would like to see the two seizures that had been recorded by video-EEG monitoring. He agreed. He was deeply impressed by seeing his own seizures and did not stop talking about his seizures over the next few days.

During a follow-up appointment 3 months after being sent home from the hospital, he reported having had six observed seizures in the first 3 weeks after discharge, with freedom from seizures since then. He went another 3 months without a seizure, and so the scheduled admission for repeat video-EEG monitoring was cancelled.

He was last seen in November 2000 (3 years later) on the original combination of 600 mg topiramate and 350 mg phenytoin, and he was satisfied because his seizures had been completely eliminated.

Commentary

Intractability is not an absolute phenomenon. Some patients are inadequately treated. Other patients who are labeled with chronic epilepsy do not in fact have

130

epilepsy (e.g. some have pseudoseizures). As in this case, a small fraction of patients with intractable epilepsy will be rendered seizure-free by adjunctive therapy such as vagus nerve stimulation, EEG biofeedback, transcranial magnetic stimulation or self-control techniques.

More than 50 % of patients with seizures preceded by auras reported they were able to avoid complex partial seizures or secondary generalization by engaging in special behaviours.[1] These are very individual methods such as complex motoric manœuvres, relaxation techniques and sensory stimulation (e.g. smell). Self-assertion might be another such method, as I believe occurred in this case.

What did I learn from this case?

Epilepsies are a heterogeneous group of disorders. The prognosis depends more on the aetiology of the seizures and the clinical background of the patient than on the seizures or the treatment prescribed. Psychosocial aspects of the disorder frequently have the most far-reaching implications for the patient and family, and this should be borne in mind when planning comprehensive management.

Present-day pharmacological and neurosurgical options offer more solutions for our patients than ever before. However, it is the information about the various aspects of epilepsy that we provide patients that helps them the most in achieving optimal seizure control. In this case, the information that made the greatest difference was having the patient watch the video-EEG recording.

This case taught me that patients undergoing a presurgical evaluation should always be offered the opportunity of watching their own seizures. In my experience, patients respond in one of two ways. Some deny that they have seizures, but most others are impressed by the experience, and some of them might have a therapeutic benefit, as in this case.

Reference

1.   Wolf P. Aura interruption: How does it become curative? In: Wolf P, ed. *Epileptic seizures and syndromes. With some of their theoritical implications.* London: J Libbey, 1994;667 73.

131

Case 35

THE BORDERLAND OF NEUROLOGY AND CARDIOLOGY

Martha J Morrell

History

FH is a 35-year-old right-handed woman entrepreneur who presented because of recent episodes of altered awareness. She had an unremarkable past medical history until 5 months before presentation, when the first episode occurred. She and her husband were dining out when she suddenly developed nausea and a headache. Although she had consumed one or two glasses of wine, she did not feel intoxicated. She requested that they leave and, while walking through the parking lot, became dizzy and diaphoretic. Her husband helped her to the car. While they were driving home, she became limp and pale and did not respond to her husband's voice or touch for at least 4 minutes. He called for emergency help and was met by an ambulance on the way home.

She was transported to a nearby hospital where she appeared groggy but oriented. Blood pressure and heart rate were normal, as was an electrocardiogram (ECG). She quickly returned to normal and was released home. She recalls nothing from the time she left the restaurant until she was in the emergency room.

The second episode occurred 2 weeks before her presentation. Her husband returned from an early Saturday morning errand and found her lying on the bathroom floor. She was confused and slow to respond, and said repeatedly, 'I really feel sick' and 'my head really, really hurts'. There were no signs of trauma. The patient recalled being in the bedroom and did not know how she had got to the bathroom, which was on the other side of the house. As her husband helped her up, she vomited and was incontinent of urine.

She was taken by ambulance to her community hospital. For approximately 6 hours she appeared confused. In the hospital, they noted that her tongue was bitten. Blood pressure and heart rate were unremarkable and an ECG was normal. A head computed tomography scan was negative. She returned home and fell deeply asleep for several hours. When she awoke, she remembered nothing of the event or the hospital evaluation.

Past medical history was remarkable for a 1-year history of bifrontal headaches with nausea. She had a syncopal episode in 1990 on a train, when she had become diaphoretic, complained, 'I am not feeling well' and lost awareness. Her husband put her head down and she returned to normal within 1 minute. She had no risk factors for epilepsy. She took no medications or recreational drugs.

Review of systems revealed episodes of mild light-headedness associated with menses. She recalled several nights of intense dreams, diaphoresis and disrupted sleep over the past year.

Family history was negative for epilepsy, although her 55-year-old mother had a history of syncope and hypoglycemia as well as headaches. Her father, two brothers, one sister and 18-month-old son were all in good health.

Examination and investigations

General and neurological examinations were unremarkable. A brain magnetic resonance imaging scan was normal, as was an ECG and awake and sleeping EEG. A tilt table test was normal.

In the midst of this evaluation, the patient had a third and fourth event. Both were preceded by nausea, an intense feeling of illness, diaphoresis and pallor. The third occurred while at the hairdresser. She appeared groggy but conscious for 20 minutes and then returned to baseline. The fourth episode occurred at dinner. She was groggy and confused for 20 minutes, even though her husband lay her down on the floor and elevated her legs. While in this position, she stiffened and had a generalized tonic–clonic seizure with tongue biting and incontinence. She was taken by ambulance to her local emergency room, received phenytoin intravenously and was admitted for 3 days. No further episodes occurred. Both ECG and EEG were normal, as were thyroid function tests and a glucose tolerance test. The patient declined her cardiologist's recommendation to have a cardiac pacemaker installed.

Three days later, she was taken off phenytoin and admitted for 5 days of continuous video-EEG monitoring with simultaneous ECG monitoring. No events occurred and no ECG or EEG abnormalities were detected. A second tilt table test was positive because of a typical event and significant bradycardia induced with isoproterenol.

Initial diagnosis, treatment and outcome

The patient was diagnosed with cardiogenic syncope. After obtaining a second and third cardiology consultation, she had a cardiac pacemaker implanted.

Eight months after the initial presentation, the patient's husband called and reported that she had perimenstrual episodes of confusion and memory loss.

Blood pressure (taken several times by him) was 110–120/50–60 mmHg each time and heart rate was 65–80 beats per minute. He was very concerned because of 2 days of repeated episodes of confusion and poor responsiveness with continuous profound memory impairment.

She was admitted to hospital, where examination was remarkable for psychomotor retardation and amnesia. An EEG showed rhythmic right temporal delta. The patient and the EEG cleared with intravenous lorazepam, although she remained amnestic for events over 4 days. The pacemaker was interrogated and was functioning normally but was being repeatedly activated for heart rates less than 65 beats per minute.

Second diagnosis, treatment and outcome

The patient was diagnosed with right temporal lobe onset seizures and treated with carbamazepine. She continues to have one or two brief episodes at menses every two to four menstrual cycles. She has declined to change her medication regimen. The pacemaker is in place and working.

Commentary

This patient has localization-related epilepsy of right anterior temporal lobe origin that causes cardiac rhythm disturbance. Her presentation was most consistent with decreased cerebral perfusion pressure leading to an alteration in consciousness and, on several instances, generalized tonic–clonic seizures. The diagnosis was difficult to make because of the unusual presentation and because sophisticated EEG and cardiac diagnostic testing were initially negative. Persistence paid off and a final diagnosis was ultimately achieved.

Cardiac rhythm changes are common with seizures. Nearly 40 % of patients with medically intractable localization related epilepsy display cardiac rhythm or repolarization abnormalities during or immediately after seizures recorded with continuous monitoring with ECG and EEG.[1] These cardiac rhythm and conduction abnormalities are seen more often in generalized tonic–clonic seizures than in complex partial seizures.

Ictal tachycardia is the most typical ictal cardiac rhythm disturbance. In one study of 92 seizures in 41 patients,[2] 82.5 % developed ictal tachycardia. Changes in heart rate occurred before the onset of EEG seizure in 76.1 % of seizures. Early tachycardia was more common in seizures of temporal lobe onset.

Ictal bradycardia is less common but not unusual; 3.3 % of persons monitored during seizures with continuous video-EEG monitoring showed bradycardia just before or during the seizure.[2]

134

This patient had an ictal bradycardia syndrome that led to vasovagal syncope and a syncopal convulsion. This syndrome is seen most often in people with temporal lobe epilepsy.[3] Whether these cardiac rhythm disturbances increase the risk of sudden unexplained death is not known. However, given the potentially catastrophic consequences of this abnormality of cardiac rhythm, it seems prudent to implant a cardiac pacemaker, in addition to providing antiepileptic drugs.

Epileptic discharges may alter cardioregulatory regions of the brain, including the limbic cortex and hypothalamus. These autonomic changes may present as simple partial seizures or may occur without obvious ictal manifestations. Therefore, autonomic simple partial seizures can be difficult to diagnose.

Another interesting feature of this case is the catamenial pattern to her seizures. Between one-third and one-half of women with epilepsy have catamenial seizure patterns.[4] Cardiac events that display cyclical patterns associated with menstruation may represent autonomic seizures, and epilepsy should be considered in the differential diagnosis.

What did I learn from this case?

This case reinforced my appreciation of the importance of entertaining a broad differential diagnosis whenever a patient presents with paroxysmal episodes of altered consciousness. It may be very difficult to establish a definitive diagnosis in these cases. For this woman, the diagnosis could not be made definitely until the cardiac rhythm abnormality was controlled. The EEG changes induced by the cerebral hypoperfusion would most likely have obscured an ictal pattern. Therefore, re-evaluation with video-EEG monitoring after the pacemaker was implanted was appropriate.

How did this case alter my approach to the care and treatment of my epilepsy patients?

I believe that dual therapy – treatment of the seizures and the cardiac rhythm disturbance – is appropriate for seizures with autonomic features. For this patient, the after-effects of seizures included days of amnesia. This frightened her and affected her work performance, which required excellent recall of intricate financial dealings. My impression was that the prolonged amnesia was a consequence of the cerebral hypoperfusion rather than the ictal discharge itself. Since at least 30 % of patients with localization-related epilepsy are not completely controlled with antiepileptic drugs, I think it is wise to provide prophylactic treatment for bradycardia in order to lessen the postictal symptoms. Although this approach is speculative, I believe that a patient like this is also at higher risk of sudden unexplained death and that the pacemaker provides a degree of protection.

135

References

1. Nei M, Ho RT, Sperling MR. EKG abnormalities during partial seizures in refractory epilepsy. *Epilepsia* 2000;**41**:542 8.

2. Schernthaner C, Lindinger G, Potselberger K, *et al.* Autonomic epilepsy: the influence of epileptic discharges on heart rate and rhythm. *Wien Klin Wochenschr* 1999;**111**:392–401.

3. Reeves AL, Nollet KE, Klass DW, Sharbrough FW, So EL. The ictal bradycardia syndrome. *Epilepsia* 1996;**37**:983–7.

4. Morrell MJ. Epilepsy in women: the science of why it is special. *Neurology* 1999;**53(suppl 1)**:S42–S48.

Case 36

A MAN WITH SHOULDER TWITCHING

Erasmo A Passaro and Ahmad Beydoun

History

A 52-year-old left-handed man presented to the emergency room because of near-continuous twitching of his left shoulder. This shoulder twitching was irregular in frequency, lasted several minutes at a time, and waxed and waned in intensity. The twitching ceased when he was asleep and decreased in intensity when he was distracted.

With detailed questioning, the neurology house officer learned that the patient had intermittent twitching of his left calf muscle while gardening 5 days earlier. The following day, this twitching spread to his left quadriceps muscle and his abdominal muscles. He and his wife visited a local emergency room, at which time the twitching involved the entire left side of his body. He was placed on clonazepam and was scheduled for an outpatient neurology appointment. The report of the non-contrast brain computed tomography (CT) scan from the local emergency room was unremarkable except for a questionable right parietal hypodensity on a single slice. He denied loss of awareness, motor weakness or sensory changes with these events.

The past medical history was unremarkable. There was no recent history of head trauma, fever or headache. There were no risk factors for stroke except for a history of heavy cigarette smoking, and no past history of transient ischemic attack or cerebral infarction. There was no history of alcohol or drug abuse. He had never experienced a similar type of event in the past.

His social history revealed that he had been happily married for several years and had a multiple pack–year smoking history. He had recently retired from the local fire department after several years of service.

Examination and investigations

The patient was afebrile with normal vital signs. Both his general physical examination and his neurological examination, which included normal strength and symmetric deep tendon reflexes, were unremarkable. The observed left shoulder twitching caused his proximal arm to move in an irregular manner. There was no clonic twitching in the proximal or distal arm or hand. The left shoulder twitching ceased when he was asleep or distracted. The twitching increased if he was asked to move his left arm voluntarily. The intensity of the twitching was variable. Suspecting that the events might be non-epileptic, the neurology house officer applied a saline patch to the patient's shoulder and the twitching appeared to subside. Interestingly, he was not significantly distressed about the twitching, although his wife was visibly upset.

A 21-channel digital EEG was performed. The left shoulder twitching was recorded. The EEG showed electromyographical artifact that correlated with the shoulder twitching; however, no significant change in the EEG activity from baseline was noted. Although this EEG was normal, he was admitted for video-EEG long-term monitoring because of the history earlier in the week of twitching in his calf with subsequent involvement of his left hemibody. Futhermore, the CT scan report of an equivocal hypodensity in the right parietal region raised further suspicion that these events might be epileptic in origin.

While he was monitored with video-EEG, his head was kept stationary to reduce movement artifact and to increase the possibility of identifying an EEG correlate. Furthermore, to facilitate the identification of an EEG correlate in the central region, the EEG was reformatted with a montage consisting of a longitudinal bipolar chain over the parasagittal region and transverse bipolar chains across the frontal, central and parietal regions. The EEG sensitivity was increased to 5 μV/mm and the high frequency filter was reduced to 15 Hz. With these maneuvers, a sharp wave was observed with maximal negativity at the right central electrode and the vertex electrode. This discharge occurred a few milliseconds before each left shoulder twitch.

Diagnosis

Epilepsia partialis continua (EPC) involving the left deltoid muscle.

Treatment and outcome

The EPC persisted despite a phenytoin level of 18 μg/ml. A magnetic resonance imaging (MRI) scan with gadolinium enhancement revealed a large ring-enhancing lesion involving the high convexity of the right parietal lobe with significant surrounding edema. Twenty-four hours later, the patient developed progressive left hemiparesis over several hours. A repeat brain MRI showed that the lesion had doubled in size.

138

On the basis of this rapid increase in the size of the lesion, a brain abscess was suspected, and the patient was brought to the operating room for right parietal craniotomy and needle aspiration of the lesion. Neuropathology confirmed the presence of a brain abscess. He was placed on intravenous antibiotics for several weeks. Several months later, in follow-up, he had a mild decrease in the fine motor skills of his left hand that made it difficult for him to play the guitar. He has had no further seizures since his surgery.

Commentary

The unusual features of this patient's left shoulder twitching raised the possibility that this event was non-epileptic in origin. In particular, the twitching was irregular and frequent but intermittent; it disappeared in sleep and decreased with distraction or when a sensory stimulus was applied to the shoulder.

EPC is a rare type of localization-related motor epilepsy; it is defined as spontaneous regular or irregular clonic twitching of cerebral cortical origin, sometimes aggravated by action or sensory stimuli, that is confined to one part of the body and that continues for a period of hours, days or weeks.[1] EPC was initially described by the Russian neurologist Kojewnikow in children with the Russian spring–summer tick-borne viral encephalitis.

EPC may present with unusual features. For example, EPC may be reduced or disappear in sleep[2] and increase with movement. The muscle twitches are sometimes irregular and can vary in intensity. Approximately one patient in three has the entire side of the body involved. However, a single part of the body may be involved, such as the hand or fingers (or both) or, less commonly, proximal muscles, such as the deltoid, pectoralis or triceps muscle.[2] In some patients, when multiple muscles are involved, asynchrony of muscle twitching may be present. These unusual features often confound the diagnosis and sometimes suggest a movement disorder or a psychogenic etiology.

Furthermore, the routine EEG during these events does not show an epileptiform correlate in over half of cases.[3] An EEG correlate is not observed because a large area of cortical neurons need to be firing synchronously for the amplitude of the EEG activity to be large enough for a scalp EEG correlate to be observed.[4] Often an EEG correlate is obtained only with EEG back-averaging techniques. In some cases, the jerks can be induced with transcranial magnetic stimulation.[3]

In children, the most common cause of EPC is Rasmussen's encephalitis.[3] In adults, the most common etiologies include a cerebral infarct or a neoplasm. It is less commonly seen in focal cortical dysplasia,[5] infectious mass lesion (especially tuberculosis[6]) and non-ketotic hyperglycemia.[7] Rarely, EPC is caused by neurotoxicity arising from penicillin, azlocillin or cephotaxime in high doses or diagnostic use of metrizamide.[4] EPC due to anti-Hu associated paraneoplastic encephalomyelitis has also been reported.[8]

EPC is usually refractory to antiepileptic drugs. When EPC is refractory to medications and a structural etiology is present, neurosurgical removal is most effective but may result in a fixed motor deficit.[4]

What did I learn from this case?

EPC may present with irregular clonic twitching of a single muscle group, which may be irregular in frequency and vary in intensity. In addition, the twitching may be reduced in sleep, aggravated by movement or, occasionally, improved by a sensory stimulus. Furthermore, sometimes a patient's unique emotional reaction to an illness, which in this case was indifference, may incorrectly suggest a psychogenic etiology.

Since many cases do not show an EEG correlate, an alternate diagnosis might be incorrectly considered. Maneuvers to eliminate movement artifact that obscure the recording and digital EEG reformatting are necessary to increase the yield of routine EEG. In cases where the routine EEG shows no epileptiform correlate and an epileptic process is being considered, EEG back-averaging may be helpful. Neuroimaging to exclude a structural cause should be performed.

How did this case alter my approach to the care and treatment of my epilepsy patients?

Seizures may have unusual manifestations that can mimic non-epileptic conditions such as movement disorders and psychogenic seizures. A clinician must always keep an open mind and take a meticulous history from the patient and family about the description, onset and evolution of the event. For example, in this case the earlier history of jacksonian spread raised the suspicion of epileptic seizures. In addition, careful correlation of clinical behavior with the EEG, montage reformatting and maneuvers to reduce movement artifact were necessary to increase the yield of non-invasive ictal EEG.

References

1.   Obeso JA, Rothwell JC, Marsden CD. The spectrum of cortical myoclonus from focal reflex jerks to spontaneous motor epilepsy. *Brain* 1985;**108**:193–224.

2.   Thomas JE, Reagan TJ, Klass DW. Epilepsia partialis continua. A review of 32 cases. *Arch Neurol* 1977;**34**:266–75.

3.   Cockerell C, Rothwell J, Thompson PD, Marsden CD, Shorvon SD. Clinical and

140

physiologic features of epilepsia partialis continua. Cases ascertained in the UK. *Brain* 1996;**119**:393–407.

4. Biraben A, Chauvel P. Epilepsia partialis continua. In: Engel J Jr, Pedley TA, eds. *Epilepsy: a comprehensive textbook.* Philadelphia: Lippincott–Raven; 1997:2447–53.

5. Kuzniecky R, Berkovic S, Andermann F, Melanson D, Olivier A, Robitaille Y. Focal cortical myoclonus and rolandic cortical dysplasia: clarification by magnetic resonance imaging. *Ann Neurol* 1988;**23**:317–25.

6. Juul-Jensen P, Denny-Brown D. Epilepsia partialis continua. *Arch Neurol* 1966;**15**:563 78.

7. Singh BM, Strobos RJ. Epilepsia partialis continua associated with non-ketotic hyperglycemia: clinical and biochemical profile of 21 patients. *Ann Neurol* 1980;**8**:155–60.

8. Shavit YB, Graus F, Probst A, Rene R, Steck AJ. Epilepsia partialis continua: a new manifestation of anti-Hu associated paraneoplastic encephalomyelitis. *Ann Neurol* 1999;**45**:255–8.

141

Case 37

EPILEPTIC FALLS DUE TO THE HEART

Steven C Schachter

History

The patient is a 43-year-old white woman who had a convulsion at the age of
9 months in association with a high fever. Because of recurrent febrile
convulsions, she was begun on mephobarbital at the age of 4 years.

On the first day of her first menstrual period, at the age of 11, she had her first
afebrile seizure. Over the ensuing years, she experienced two different types of
seizures at an average frequency of four times a month each. The first type
consisted of the feeling that she is being forced or pushed down. This would last
five seconds without postictal symptoms. The second type began without a
warning: she lost consciousness and then was observed to stare for up to
30 seconds and then to fall abruptly to the ground, usually with no apparent
rhythmic or tonic motor movements. She regained consciousness approximately
10–20 seconds later. Postictally, she was tired, hungry and frustrated.

Previous trials of medication included various combinations of maximally
tolerated dosages of mephobarbital, carbamazepine, phenytoin, phenobarbital,
ethotoin, clonazepam, acetazolamide, valproate, lamotrigine, felbamate and
gabapentin.

Her past medical history was significant for an occipital hemorrhage secondary to
a seizure-related head injury at the age of 26, ovarian cysts and a transiently positive
antinuclear antibody that was thought to be secondary to phenytoin. Family history
was negative for epilepsy. Her father died from a myocardial infarction.

Previous evaluation consisted of an EEG (which showed left temporal
interictal epileptiform discharges) and a normal routine brain magnetic resonance
imaging scan.

Examination and investigations

The patient's general, cardiological and neurological examinations were
unremarkable.

142

Because her seizures were medically intractable, she was admitted to the hospital for video-EEG monitoring to determine whether epilepsy surgery was possible. Her antiepileptic medications were tapered and several seizures of the second type described above were recorded while she was in bed. The ictal EEG recordings demonstrated electrographic seizure activity confined to the left anterior to mid-temporal region. In addition, electrocardiographic (ECG) monitoring showed progressive bradycardia leading to complete asystole for up to 14 seconds before a normal heart rate was resumed. The change in cardiac rhythm began after the initial clinical manifestations of the seizures (staring and unresponsiveness). The ECG findings prompted a cardiology consultation.

Diagnosis

Cardiological diagnosis was asystole secondary to enhanced vagal tone from the left temporal lobe-onset seizures.

Treatment and outcome

The patient underwent implantation of a dual-chamber pacemaker. Since then, she has continued to have both types of seizures but has not fallen to the ground in association with the second type. She has elected to defer epilepsy surgery at this time.

Commentary

This patient had medically refractory simple partial and complex partial seizures. The latter type was often associated with abrupt falling to the ground if she was standing during the seizure. Over the years, it was assumed that the patient's falls to the ground were a direct effect of the seizures on the strength and tone in her lower extremities. Only when she underwent ictal EEG monitoring did it become apparent that there was an alternative explanation – cardiac asystole. This conclusion is supported by the fact that she has not fallen since implantation of a cardiac pacemaker even though she continues to have the other typical manifestations of her seizures. Independent of her seizures, the patient had no other clinical evidence of cardiac arrhythmias.

Ictal-induced changes in heart rate and rhythm are among the many possible autonomic manifestations of seizures.[1] Sinus tachycardia is the most frequent disturbance of cardiac rate that accompanies seizures.[2] In one series of 12 consecutive patients with temporal lobe seizures, ictal tachycardia was associated with left-sided seizure onset in four patients and right temporal lobe onset in eight patients.[3]

Bradyarrhythmias, including bradycardia, sinus arrest, atrioventricular block and asystole, occur much less frequently than tachyarrhythmias.[2-6] In some patients with ictal-induced bradyarrhythmia, loss of consciousness may be due to syncope and not to the seizure. In this patient, a change in consciousness (manifested by staring and unresponsiveness) preceded the change in heart rate, although it is likely that her falls were associated with cardiac asystole.

Recognition of the cardiovascular manifestations of seizures requires a high index of suspicion. This case illustrates that patients with abrupt falls following the onset of typical complex partial seizures should be evaluated for possible ictal-related cardiac conduction disturbances with simultaneous ECG and EEG monitoring.

What did I learn from this case?

I learned that a fall in conjunction with a seizure may result from cardiogenic syncope. In this case, the falls to the ground posed the risk of injury to the patient (as had happened, for example, with the traumatic occipital hemorrhage at the age of 26); moreover, the falls were preventable even if the seizures were not fully controlled. I also realized that I would have missed this diagnosis if the patient had not undergone simultaneous ECG and EEG monitoring.

How did this case alter my approach to the care and treatment of my epilepsy patients?

I now take a more thorough history from patients who fall as a result of their seizures about the circumstances immediately preceding the fall. Was there stiffening or muscle twitching? Was there facial pallor? Did someone take a pulse as the patient was falling or immediately before or after? If the answers are suggestive of cardiac arrhythmia as a cause for the falls, then I recommend simultaneous ECG and EEG monitoring and a cardiological consultation when appropriate.

References

1. Freeman R, Schachter SC. Autonomic epilepsy. *Semin Neurol* 1995;15:158–66.

2. Devinsky O, Price BH, Cohen SI. Cardiac manifestations of complex partial seizures. *Am J Med* 1986;80:195–202.

144

3.   Marshall DW, Westmoreland BF, Sharbrough FW. Ictal tachycardia during temporal lobe seizures. *Mayo Clin Proc* 1983;**58**:443–6.

4.   Constantin I, Martins JB, Fincham RW, Dagli RD. Bradycardia and syncope as manifestations of partial epilepsy. *J Am Coll Cardiol* 1990;**15**:900–5.

5.   Smaje JC, Davidson C, Teasdale GM. Sino-atrial arrest due to temporal lobe epilepsy. *J Neurol Neurosurg Psychiatry* 1987;**50**:112–13.

6.   Howell SJ, Blumhardt LD. Cardiac asystole associated with epileptic seizures: a case report with simultaneous EEG and ECG. *J Neurol Neurosurg Psychiatry* 1989;**52**:795–8.

Case 38

A YOUNG MAN WITH NOISE-INDUCED PARTIAL SEIZURES

Bettina Schmitz

History

A 34-year-old Turkish man started having seizures at the age of 16 years. Most of his seizures were induced by unexpected noises, like the opening of a door or the ringing of a bell. These acoustic triggers could be relatively subtle, such as the sound induced by the clumsy handling of cutlery by the patient himself. Seizures occurred exclusively when the patient was awake and increased in frequency over the years.

When he was first seen in my clinic in 1988 he was 22 years old and was having up to 10 seizures every day. He had been treated by a number of neurologists, all of whom had diagnosed psychogenic seizures. Drug treatments had included tranquilizers, neuroleptic drugs and antidepressants, but none of these therapies had a significant effect on the frequency of his seizures.

The patient was born in Turkey. Pregnancy and delivery were described as normal, but he had delayed development of motor and verbal skills. He had been a moderate scholar and finished school at the age of 16, the same year his seizures first started.

He was married and had a 2-year-old healthy child but had been out of work since the age of 18 on account of his seizures. He lived with his family. Owing to the frequency of his seizures, which often caused the patient to fall and had produced multiple injuries in the past, he was looked after in a highly protective manner.

Examination and investigations

Neurological examination revealed a hypotrophy of the right arm and leg and a mild right-sided central hemiparesis.

Cranial computed tomography (CT) scanning showed a left frontoparietal hypodense region suggestive of infarction and ipsilateral hemispheric atrophy (Fig. 38.1). These findings were confirmed on magnetic resonance imaging. HMPAO

146

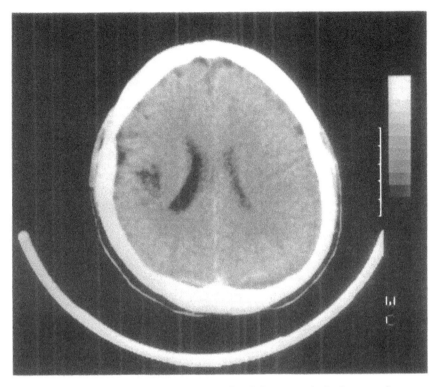

Figure 38.1: *CT scan demonstrating a left-sided porencephalic lesion and ipsilateral hemispheric hypotrophy.*

(= 99mTc-hexamethyl propyleneamine oxime) single photon emission CT scanning showed the extensive area of hypoperfusion in the left hemisphere, most marked in the frontoparietal region, and hypoperfusion in the contralateral right cerebellum.

Interictal EEGs were normal except for a mild slowing in the left frontocentral region. Five seizures were recorded during video-telemetry. Seizures were all induced by an unexpected acoustic stimulus (Fig. 38.2). The seizures started with a startle reaction, followed by tonic posturing with symmetrical extension of arms and legs, accompanied by a loud, undulating, high pitched vocalization. This was followed by rhythmic pelvic movements, a rolling of the body, and frenetic, thrashing movements of all limbs. There was also enuresis associated with long seizures. There was no postictal confusion – the patient was immediately able to act and speak, and he claimed to be aware of everything that happened during the seizure. Seizure duration was always less than 1 minute. The duration and severity of seizures were inconstant; however, the sequence of motor elements was highly stereotypic. Ictal surface EEGs were unrevealing beyond movement artifacts.

147

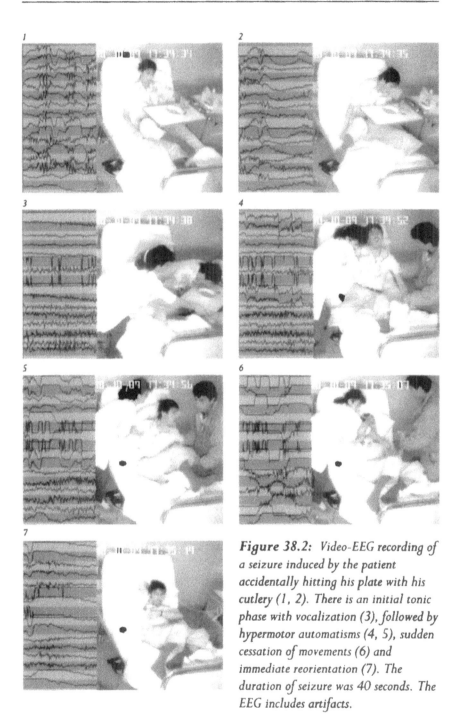

Figure 38.2: *Video-EEG recording of a seizure induced by the patient accidentally hitting his plate with his cutlery (1, 2). There is an initial tonic phase with vocalization (3), followed by hypermotor automatisms (4, 5), sudden cessation of movements (6) and immediate reorientation (7). The duration of seizure was 40 seconds. The EEG includes artifacts.*

Diagnosis

Symptomatic frontal lobe epilepsy with startle-induced tonic and hypermotor seizures secondary to perinatal brain damage with left frontoparietal infarction.

Treatment and outcome

After I had first seen this patient in 1988 and made the diagnosis of epilepsy, he was put on carbamazepine monotherapy, which reduced the frequency and severity of his seizures for only a short period. He then was put on add-on propranolol 40 mg/day with mild benefit. Following the introduction of clobazam, seizure frequency was markedly reduced, and after a gradual increase to 80 mg/day he became seizure-free. Since then, seizures have recurred only twice, the first time during a period of fever, the second time in relation to non-compliance. He has slowly stopped his comedication and is now on monotherapy with clobazam 40 mg/day, which has slowly been decreased over the past 12 years. He is back at work, is seizure-free and has no side effects from his medication.

Commentary

This patient is a typical case of startle-induced frontal lobe epilepsy. Startle-induced seizures were classified among the reflex epilepsies by Alajouanine and Gastaut in 1955.[1] The most common trigger is a sudden auditory stimulus. Onset is in the first 20 years of life. Startle epilepsy occurs almost exclusively in patients with brain lesions, which usually date back to the prenatal or perinatal period. In most cases lesions are unilateral and consist of porencephalic cysts or local atrophy. Many patients have hemiparesis and some degree of mental retardation. Seizures start with an abrupt startle reaction followed by a tonic phase. Both cortical and subcortical structures may be involved in the pathophysiology of startle-induced seizures. It has been postulated that the startle response triggers an epileptogenic region, which in turn activates an epileptogenic region that may be located near the supplementary motor cortex.[2]

Response to conventional drug treatment is poor. The best results have been reported with a combination of carbamazepine and benzodiazepines.[3]

The first modern report of a series of patients with frontal lobe seizures that had been carefully studied with intracranial electrodes appeared in 1985.[4] Subsequent reports confirmed the existence of this peculiar type of seizure disorder with prominent motor automatisms, and three major subtypes have now been well defined.[5] Many neurologists were unfamiliar with frontal lobe

149

epilepsies and, because of the often bizarre and expressive seizure phenomena, frontal lobe seizures (also called pseudopseudoseizures) were often misdiagnosed as pseudoseizures until the late 1980s.

What did I learn from this case?

In one's first year of training one learns from every patient. This case taught me a number of lessons.

First, this patient had a disorder that I had never heard of in medical school. It was exciting to learn that, although his syndrome is rare, there had been a number of then recent studies that showed that he was not at all unique but a rather typical case. Thus, I learned that in medicine we may still discover distinct syndromes provided we look for typical patterns.

Second, it is a good example of the challenge in making the diagnosis of epileptic seizures versus psychogenic seizures. My immediate impression had been that his seizures were not organic because they looked very dramatic and they were always triggered by an external stimulus. Startle epilepsy is an example of a seizure disorder in which psychological and organic mechanisms are closely intertwined, because seizures are triggered by a psychophysiological reflex mechanism. I was also misled by the fact that the patient's consciousness was preserved throughout the seizure. The fact that these frontal hypermotor automatisms can occur with intact consciousness shows that the brain still has lessons to teach us about clinical–anatomical relationships.

Third, although for pragmatic reasons it might be preferable to have a limited number of antiepileptic drugs, there are always patients who may profit from one of the old or second-line drugs and who respond differently from the majority of patients. This patient did not develop cognitive problems and did not become tolerant when treated with clobazam. These side effects have caused many epileptologists to exclude clobazam completely from their drug repertoire.

Fourth, even patients with difficult-to-treat seizures that seem desperate do not justify therapeutic nihilism. Severe epilepsy leads to behavioural problems and social difficulties, as in this case. His marriage was threatened by his disabling seizure disorder and a regular job seemed impossible, owing to cultural reasons as well as to the realistic risks of frequent motor seizures. However, social development may normalize after seizure control. It happened in this case because the patient's role was not fixed and adjusted to his seizure disorder when he was successfully treated.

How much did this case alter my approach to the care and treatment of my epilepsy patients?

This patient was one of my first telemetry cases in my first year of work in a specialized epilepsy unit. Back then I witnessed discussions about the then-novel concept of frontal lobe epilepsies and can remember senior epileptologists admitting that they had falsely diagnosed cases in the past as psychogenic seizures. (Dieter Janz referred to a patient of his with nocturnal hypermotor seizures as the 'werewolf-man' who, in retrospect, had had typical nocturnal frontal lobe seizures.)

I hope that this case contributed to my self-criticism with respect to the firmness of my clinical diagnoses. More generally, this case is a good example of the fact that it is always justified to keep an open mind about what is claimed to be medical fact and about the opinions of authorities, because these 'facts' and opinions obviously can be wrong. I hope that cases like this one have made me a more tolerant teacher – especially when young doctors in my courses do not simply accept my 'epileptological wisdom' but request evidence, which I am often not able to provide.

Certainly, each time this patient visits my clinic, which he does once a year with one of his children, he nourishes and renews my endurance and optimism when planning and modulating treatment strategies for patients with complicated epilepsies.

References

1. Alajouanine A, Gastaut H. La syncinésie-sursaut et l'épilepsie-sursaut à déclanchement sensoriel ou sensitif inopiné. *Rev Neurol* 1955;**93**:29–41.

2. Tassinari CA, Rubboli G, Michelucci R. Reflex epilepsies. In: Dam M, Gram L, eds. *Comprehensive epileptology*. New York: Raven Press; 1990:233–46.

3. Sáenz-Lope E, Herranz-Tanarro FJ, Masdeu JC, Chacon Pena JR. Hyperekplexia: a syndrome of pathological startle responses. *Ann Neurol* 1984;**15**:36–41.

4. Williamson PD, Spencer DD, Spencer SS, Novelly RA, Mattson RH. Complex partial seizures of frontal lobe origin. *Ann Neurol* 1985;**18**:497–504.

5. Williamson PD, Engel J, Munari C. Anatomic classification of localization-related epilepsies. In: Engel J, Pedley TA, eds. *Epilepsy: a comprehensive textbook*. Philadelphia: Lippincott–Raven; 1997:2405–16.

151

Case 39

THE GIRL WITH VISUAL SEIZURES WHO WASN'T SEEING THINGS – TRANSIENT BLINDNESS IN A YOUNG GIRL

Carl E Stafstrom

History

Lauren, a 10-year-old girl, presented with a several month history of episodes that she described as follows: 'I see floating colored dots. Then my eyes cross and I suddenly can't see – I just see black in both eyes' (Fig. 39.1). 'I get real scared when things go blank. I feel like I'm in La-La Land.'

The first spell occurred a few days after her dog was killed by a car. She had about 30 or 35 spells over the 3 months before presentation at the clinic; each spell was identical. The spells lasted from 30–60 seconds and she recovered quickly, but they were often followed by an occipital or retro-orbital throbbing headache, nausea and vomiting. Witnesses confirmed that Lauren was lucid during a spell – she can reply to questions and follow instructions. She recalls each spell clearly afterwards ('My mind was playing tic-tac-toe'). Witnesses also describe that her eyes 'dart back and forth rapidly' during a spell and Lauren describes 'shaky vision.' Spells seem to be more frequent when she is outside in the sun, looking out a window or watching television.

Lauren is a healthy, normally developing girl. Pregnancy, labor and delivery were uneventful. She reached all developmental milestones on time and is a good student. She is active in dance. Her mother recently divorced and remarried. There is no family history of epilepsy or migraine.

Past evaluations included a normal brain magnetic resonance imaging (MRI) scan and a routine EEG. Previous physicians concluded that Lauren suffered from a combination of migraine and depression, with psychosomatic spells related to post-traumatic stress (resulting from her parents' divorce and the death of a pet).

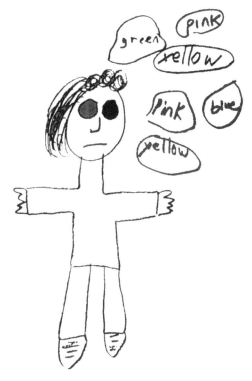

Figure 39.1 *The patient's diagram of her spells of visual obscurations. The child was asked, 'Please draw a picture of what it is like to have one of your spells'. Her first subjective symptom was of colored spots floating in her left visual field. A few seconds later, vision in both eyes became obscured (note the blackened eyes).*

Examination and investigations

Lauren was a delightful, articulate girl with age-appropriate cognitive skills. Her general physical examination and detailed neurological examinations were normal. She became tearful when discussing the recent death of her dog. When asked to draw a picture describing her symptoms during a spell, she produced the drawing shown in Figure 39.1.

The routine EEG (see Fig. 39.2) showed frequent right occipital spike wave and polyspike discharges, single or in trains up to 1.5 seconds, with amplitudes up to 200 µV. The posterior dominant rhythm was slower on the right. During the EEG, Lauren fortuitously had one of her typical spells. She suddenly announced, 'I'm having one,' whereupon right-beating nystagmus was seen for

153

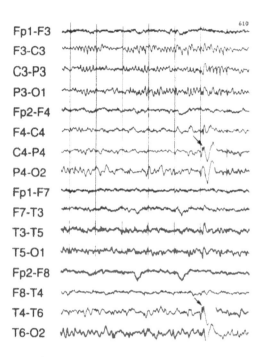

Figure 39.2 *Interictal EEG recording (awake, eyes closed) showing right occipital high-voltage spike–wave complexes (arrows), superimposed on right posterior slowing.*

the next 15 seconds. During the spell she counted to 15 but could not count fingers; she followed an instruction to stick out her tongue and was able to state her name and age correctly. She recalled a spoken phrase afterwards. Fifty seconds after the onset, she announced, 'It's over'. The EEG correlate began with a burst of polyspike–wave activity in the right posterior quadrant. This evolved into diffuse low-voltage fast activity that increased in amplitude, becoming 8–10 Hz spike–waves, maximal in the right posterior region. After 30 seconds, the spikes dissipated, and were replaced by diffuse slowing that was maximal in the right occipital area.

Diagnosis

Benign occipital epilepsy of childhood, also known as benign childhood epilepsy with occipital paroxysms[1] and late-onset benign occipital seizures.[2,3]

Treatment and outcome

Lauren was initially treated with valproate. Her spells subsided promptly, but returned several months later and did not respond to increasing doses. She was switched to carbamazepine with excellent results until a few breakthrough seizures prompted the addition of gabapentin. On this regimen she has remained seizure-free for the past 4 years. She is now 14 years old and is doing well academically and socially.

Commentary

This patient presented with brief, stereotypic episodes of visual obscuration with mild confusion but preserved awareness. Her seizures are therefore complex partial in type. The clinical symptomatology and interictal and ictal electrographic localization suggest an occipital origin. Her normal development and neurologic status and the lack of any lesion on MRI suggest an idiopathic etiology.

Lauren's initial complaints were considered by several physicians to be psychological in origin on the basis of their onset after psychosocial stressors and her dramatic self-reports (e.g. 'I'm going blind again!'). Indeed, many patients with seizures, particularly complex partial seizures, present with vague complaints or behaviors that are considered psychogenic until further detailed history and investigations establish the correct diagnosis.

Other practitioners suggested that Lauren had migraines, a plausible diagnosis given her transient visual loss followed by throbbing headache and nausea. However, several features in this case suggested that epilepsy should have been included in the differential diagnosis. Lauren's spells were stereotyped and frequent. The entire episode was brief, with visual symptoms lasting less than 1 minute and the headache persisting for only a few minutes.

Benign occipital epilepsy of childhood is an idiopathic, localization-related age-specific epilepsy syndrome.[1,4] Several subtypes may exist, based on age of onset, daytime versus night-time occurrence and subtleties of symptoms.[2,3,5,6] Given Lauren's age and clinical features, she best fits the late-onset form of benign occipital epilepsy of childhood.[3] Clinical symptoms vary widely.[7,8] Typical features may include elementary visual hallucinations, blindness, head or eye deviation, alteration of consciousness, generalized or hemiclonic seizures, and postictal headache, nausea or vomiting. Interictal electrophysiological investigations reveal high-amplitude sharps or spike–waves in the occipital or posterotemporal regions, usually suppressed by eye opening. However, the proportion of cases of benign occipital epilepsy of childhood among children who

155

present with occipital spikes is small.[9] Treatment with carbamazepine or clobazam is often successful. At least 60 % of children remit spontaneously by their late teenage years.[3]

What did I learn from this case?

I learned that one must not be biased by earlier medical evaluations and that one should bear in mind that epilepsies present with a wide variety of clinical manifestations, including subtle alterations of mental status and what may seem like 'hysterical' symptoms. We should pay particular attention to a child's own description of the symptoms. Although several authors have commented that a child's lack of verbal sophistication, especially at young ages, may make an accurate diagnostic assessment difficult,[2,6] with concerted effort one can often obtain a wealth of information from the child. In this case, previous physicians either considered Lauren's symptoms to be psychogenically based, given the proximate psychosocial stressors, or else lumped her symptoms into migraine. Although it is important to consider the psychosocial factors that may contribute to a child's symptoms, we must carefully sort out the ictal details before assuming causality. The aura of migraine typically consists of scotomata, scintillations or visual obscurations. Occipital seizures more commonly present as transient colored circular patterns, as seen in this child's drawing (see Fig. 39.1); zig-zag and achromatic patterns are distinctly unusual.[2,10]

How did this case alter my approach to the care and treatment of my epilepsy patients?

I try to keep an open mind and pay particular attention to the child's description of his or her event. Having the child illustrate his or her symptoms by drawing a picture may be useful diagnostically. This technique is simple, involves no expense and may be particularly useful in younger children who cannot verbalize their symptoms well. Lauren's depiction of her initial visual symptoms (colored spots) is very similar to those drawn by much older patients with this syndrome.[2,3]

This case also emphasizes the importance of EEG evaluation of spells of uncertain etiology. Although we were fortunate to obtain an ictal recording of Lauren's spell, which clinched the diagnosis, such serendipity rarely occurs. Newer methods, including home ambulatory EEG monitoring (now available with video), should enhance our yield of diagnosing the wide variety of spells that occur in children.

References

1. Commission on Classification and Terminology of the International League Against Epilepsy. Proposal for revised classification of epilepsies and epilepsy syndromes. *Epilepsia* 1989;**30**:389–99.

2. Panayiotopoulos C. Elementary visual hallucinations, blindness, and headache in idiopathic occipital epilepsy: differentiation from migraine. *J Neurol Neurosurg Psychiatry* 1999;**66**:536–40.

3. Panayiotopoulos C. *Benign childhood partial seizures and related epileptic syndromes. Current problems in epilepsy*, vol 15. London: John Libbey; 1999.

4. Gastaut H. A new type of epilepsy: benign partial epilepsy of childhood with occipital spike-waves. *Clin Electroencephalogr* 1982;**13**:13–22.

5. Ferrie C, Beaumanoir A, Guerrini R, *et al*. Early-onset benign occipital seizure susceptibility syndrome. *Epilepsia* 1997;**38**:285 93.

6. Andermann F, Zifkin B. The benign occipital epilepsies of childhood: an overview of the idiopathic syndromes and of the relationship to migraine. *Epilepsia* 1998;**39(suppl 4)**:S9–S23.

7. Maher J, Ronen G, Ogunyemi A, Goulden K. Occipital paroxysmal discharges suppressed by eye opening: variability in clinical and seizure manifestations in childhood. *Epilepsia* 1995;**36**:52 7.

8. van den Hout B, van der Meij W, Wienke G, *et al*. Seizure semiology of occipital lobe epilepsy of children. *Epilepsia* 1997;**38**:1188–91.

9. Libenson M, Caravale B, Prasad A. Clinical correlations of occipital epileptiform discharges in children. *Neurology* 1999;**53**:265–9.

10. Panayiotopoulos C. Visual phenomena and headache in occipital epilepsy: a review, a systematic study and differentiation from migraine. *Epileptic Disord* 1999;**1**:205–16.

Case 40

SYNCOPE IN A PATIENT WITH TEMPORAL LOBE EPILEPSY

Paolo Tinuper

History

A 42-year-old right-handed woman began having attacks at 38 years of age. Seizures were characterized by a feeling of something warm flushing from her chest to the face. Then she lost consciousness and fell if she was standing up. No automatisms or other ictal signs were reported. Seizures occurred monthly, clustering around the time of her menses. Because her attacks were believed to be of cardiac origin, cardiological tests, including 24-hour electrocardiographic monitoring and autonomic investigations, were performed. These tests were normal. The patient was therefore referred to a neurologist.

Examination and investigations

Neurological examination was normal. Interictal EEG showed focal spikes in the left temporal region. Brain magnetic resonance imaging showed a left mesiotemporal lesion, probably a low grade astrocytoma.

A seizure was recorded during video-polygraphic monitoring with the patient lying down. At the beginning of the seizure, the EEG showed low amplitude fast activity over the left temporal area, which was then replaced by a prolonged run of sharp discharges in the same region. The beginning of the discharges coincided with a progressive slowing of heart rate, at which time the patient reported the usual sensation of flushing in her face and faintness. Normal heart rate was regained at the end of the seizure (Fig. 40.1).

Diagnosis

Lesional left temporal lobe epilepsy with arrhythmogenic seizures.

158

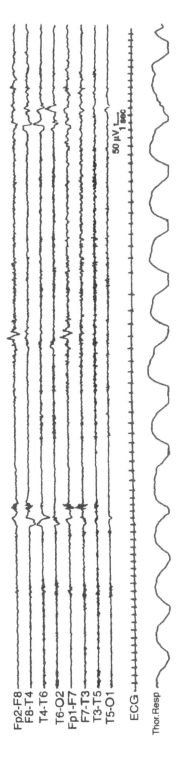

Figure 40.1: *Video-polygraphic monitoring of a seizure with the patient lying down. Ictal EEG at the beginning of the seizure showed a low amplitude fast activity over the left temporal areas, replaced by a prolonged sharp wave discharge on the same region. The beginning of the discharge coincided with a progressive slowing of heart rate. At this point the patient reported the usual sensation of flushing in her face and fainting. Normal heart rate was regained at the end of the seizure.*

159

Treatment

Phenytoin was started without any improvement in seizure frequency.

Commentary

In clinical practice, the differential diagnosis between syncopal attacks and epileptic seizures is a frequent problem and the semiological and anamnestic data are not always sufficient to clarify the picture. In this case, the simultaneous EEG and electrocardiography documented the change in heart rate during the seizure. Had the patient been standing up instead of lying on the laboratory bed, she would have fallen to the ground with a syncopal attack.

An increase in heart rate is commonly reported during epileptic seizures; this is probably related to adrenergic activation. Arrhythmogenic seizures, in particular bradycardic, are rarely described in the literature, probably owing to the lack of polygraphic (extracephalic) parameters during prolonged video-monitoring sessions.

For many reasons, it is important to be aware of the possibility of ictal modifications of heart rate during seizures. First, ictal arrhythmias are potentially dangerous and affected patients must be considered at risk of life-threatening episodes. Secondly, commonly used antiepileptic drugs (such as carbamazepine or phenytoin) have some effect on heart conduction and may worsen the picture. Finally, in those patients with frequent and drug-resistant arrhythmogenic attacks, the need for a cardiac pacemaker must be evaluated.

What did I learn from this case?

This case enhanced my interest in vegetative changes during partial epileptic seizures. The mesial structures of the temporal lobes are densely interconnected with the central autonomic structures, and consequently mesial temporal epileptic foci may influence autonomic parameters such as heart rate and blood pressure, either interictally or, more dramatically, during seizures. Because most partial seizures are recorded during long-term video-monitoring as patients with drug-resistant seizures undergo presurgical evaluation, I recommend adding an electrocardiographic tracing to the recording montage. Otherwise, arrhythmogenic seizures may be missed. Patients with this unusual type of seizure must be investigated accurately and treated appropriately.

Further reading

Benarroch EE. The central autonomic network: functional organisation, dysfunction, and perspective. *Mayo Clin Proc* 1993;**68**:988–1001.

Blumhardt LD, Smith PEM, Owen L. Electrocardiographic accompaniments of temporal lobe epileptic seizures. *Lancet* 1986;1(8489):1051–5.

Devinsky O, Pacia S, Tatambhotla G. Bradycardia and asystole induced by partial seizures: a case report and literature review. *Neurology* 1997;**48**:1712–4.

Jallon P. Arrhythmogenic seizures. *Epilepsia* 1997;**38**:43 7.

Reeves AL, Nollet KE, Klass DW, Sharbrough FW, So EL. The ictal bradycardia syndrome. *Epilepsia* 1996;**37**:983–7.

Van Buren JM, Ajmone-Marsan C. A correlation of autonomic and EEG components in temporal lobe epilepsy. *Arch Neurol* 1960;**3**:683–703.

Wannamaker BB. Autonomic nervous system and epilepsy. *Epilepsia* 1985;**26(suppl 1)**:S31–S39.

Case 41

ATTACKS OF RISING SENSATIONS, PALLOR AND LOSS OF CONSCIOUSNESS

Torbjörn Tomson

History

A 32-year-old previously healthy female nurse sought medical advice because of repeated episodes of clouded consciousness during the previous 2 months.

She had a total of four attacks and described them as beginning with a strange rising sensation that started from the neck or even the feet and spread to the head within a few seconds. The sensation was difficult to describe but rather pleasant. Once the sensation reached her head, there was blurring of vision and loss of consciousness.

Friends who witnessed the attacks reported that her face turned pale and she sweated profusely and fell to her right side while sitting. No jerks were noted and she recovered promptly after some 30 seconds of unconsciousness. Two of the attacks were associated with urinary incontinence. Two episodes occurred when she was standing upright, and two attacks came on while she was seated. All four occurred during menstruation but apart from that no particular precipitating factors could be identified. One distant relative had epilepsy but otherwise the family history was negative for epilepsy.

Examination and investigations

Physical and neurological examination was completely normal, although the blood pressure was somewhat low at 100/70 mm Hg. Computed tomography and magnetic resonance imaging scans of the brain were normal. An interictal scalp EEG revealed epileptiform activity over the right frontal temporal region. During long-term monitoring with EEG and electrocardiography, the patient had the initial symptoms of her habitual attacks. After having experienced the pleasant rising sensation, she felt that she was going to faint and lay down on a sofa, whereby the symptoms gradually disappeared without the patient losing consciousness. At the time of the symptoms, EEG revealed seizure activity mainly over the right temporal region, which after some seconds was followed by pronounced bradycardia (26–30 beats per minute) for 15 seconds (Fig. 41.1).

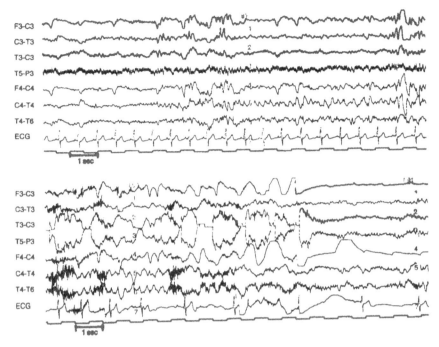

Figure 41.1: Scalp EEG recording with seven channels and a simultaneous electrocardiograph. The upper panel shows onset of seizure activity in the form of an initial bilateral frontotemporal rhythm of 6–7 Hz followed by continued seizure activity over the right temporal region. A pronounced bradycardia with a heart rate below 30 beats per minute is recorded on the electrocardiograph several seconds after seizure onset (lower panel). (Courtesy of Associate Professor Bengt Y Nilsson, Department of Clinical Neurophysiology, Huddinge University Hospital, Sweden.)

Diagnosis

Complex partial seizures with ictal bradycardia.

Treatment and outcome

Implantation of a cardiac pacemaker was seriously considered, but it was decided to evaluate the effect of treatment with antiepileptic drugs first. Valproate was chosen because of the risk of cardiodepressive effects of carbamazepine. The patient was put on valproate 1200 mg/day, which has rendered her completely seizure-free.

163

Commentary

One of the most frequent tasks for anyone involved in the evaluation of patients with unclear attacks of altered consciousness is to distinguish between syncope and epileptic seizures. This case illustrates that sometimes it is not 'either–or' but 'both', not only in the same patient but even during the same single attack. The patient suffered from partial seizures with ictal bradycardia that led to syncope. Indeed, the two components of the attack can be distinguished in the history. The first part, the aura with the rising sensation, suggests a partial seizure originating from medial temporal structures, whereas the symptoms that follow are more compatible with syncope. As usual, the clues to a correct diagnosis were available in the history.

It is well known that partial seizures may be accompanied by changes in heart rate. In one study, ictal arrhythmias were found in 42 % of temporal lobe seizures recorded with simultaneous EEG and electrocardiography.[1] An increase in heart rate is by far the most frequent finding, but many other types of arrhythmia have been reported, although ictal bradycardia is comparatively rare.[1][3] This syndrome, which indicates seizure onset in the temporal lobe, should be considered in patients with a history that is suggestive of both epilepsy and syncope.[2]

What did I learn from this case?

This case reminded me of the importance of taking a careful history and of paying close attention to details in the patient's report. Furthermore, it demonstrated the value of including an ECG channel in the recording montage when using video-EEG monitoring to investigate a patient with unclear attacks of impaired consciousness. Finally, the case highlights that it is sometimes necessary to consider potential cardiac effects of antiepileptic drugs when treating epilepsy.

References

1. Blumhardt LD, Smith PEM, Owen L. Electrocardiographic accompaniments of temporal lobe epileptic seizures. *Lancet* 1986;1:1051–6.

2. Reeves AL, Nollet KE, Klass DW, Sharbrough FW, So EL. The ictal bradycardia syndrome. *Epilepsia* 1996;**37**:983–7.

3. Jallon P. Arrhythmogenic seizures. *Epilepsia* 1997;**38 (suppl 11)**:S43–S47.

Case 42

NON-CONVULSIVE STATUS EPILEPTICUS IN A PATIENT WITH IDIOPATHIC GENERALIZED EPILEPSY

Eugen Trinka

History

A 50-year-old otherwise healthy woman had a history of generalized tonic–clonic seizures (GTCS) since she was 19 years old. At that time, a computed tomography scan of the brain, her neurological examination and her family history were all unremarkable. The EEG showed generalized spike–wave discharges, and a diagnosis of idiopathic generalized epilepsy with GTCS was made. Valproate was introduced and her seizures were well controlled with a daily dose of 1800 mg.

After the onset of intolerable tremor, valproate was discontinued slowly and lamotrigine was gradually introduced, with an increase in dose of 25 mg every second week up to 400 mg/day (serum concentration 7.26 mg/l).

She tolerated the medication well without any side effects but the characteristics of her seizures changed. In addition to her usual GTCS, she developed frequent episodes of impaired cognition, disturbed behavior and myoclonic jerks that affected her arms and face, lasted for 2–6 hours and sometimes evolved into a GTCS. These episodes occurred approximately every 2 weeks. Clobazam was added, up to 30 mg/day, without success. The patient was admitted to our hospital in a confusional state with psychomotor slowing, slight myoclonias and disturbed behavior.

Examination and investigations

On neurological examination the patient was confused and only partly responsive. There were slight myoclonias in her face and arms. The EEG showed continuous generalized spike–wave activity and generalized fast polyspike activity. A magnetic resonance imaging scan of the brain was normal.

Diagnosis

Non-convulsive status epilepticus caused by iatrogenic exacerbation of idiopathic generalized epilepsy.

Treatment and outcome

Intravenously administrated lorazepam (4 mg) stopped these episodes and normalized the EEG. Lamotrigine was stopped and topiramate was slowly introduced (with a 25 mg increase in dose per week). Repeated EEGs were normal and the patient was seizure-free. Unfortunately, she developed intolerable psychomotor slowing and speech problems that led to discontinuation of topiramate.

Primidone was started and titrated to 750 mg/day without any side effects. Her seizures remained well controlled for the next 6 months and the EEG was normal.

Commentary

I chose this case, first, because it shows that even after a long course of good seizure control, severe worsening may occur if there are any precipitating factors – in this case a change of medication from valproate to lamotrigine.

Lamotrigine is often used in the treatment of idiopathic generalized epilepsy. Its efficacy is well documented in open-label studies and in one double-blind placebo-controlled study. However, it is not clear which patients will respond promptly and which patients will not be controlled with this new drug. There are some reports of seizure aggravation with lamotrigine, although the mechanisms and the incidence are not well known. Whether the seizure aggravation was due to the introduction of lamotrigine or to discontinuation of valproate remains unclear in this case.

Secondly, this case demonstrates that careful monitoring of clinical symptoms, seizure frequency and the EEG is helpful in determining the cause of aggravation or worsening of seizures when an effective antiepileptic drug is being discontinued and another drug is being introduced.

What did I learn from this case?

Apart from the seizure aggravation during the discontinuation of valproate and the introduction of lamotrigine, I was impressed by the change in seizure type. The patient had previously suffered from GTCS. After the introduction of lamotrigine the patient experienced frequent episodes of confusion and

166

myoclonic jerks in her face and arms, resembling non-convulsive status epilepticus. The EEG showed runs of polyspikes followed by slow spike–waves. The seizure semiology was previously not experienced by the patient and closely corresponds to Oller-Daurella's 'tonic–automatic crises'. The seizure type was completely suppressed by topiramate, although at the price of side effects. Primidone was introduced with success. It seems curious to me that although there are many new antiepileptic drugs, there are at least some patients who end up with older drugs after failure or side effects with the newer ones.

Further reading

Buchanan N. The use of lamotrigine in juvenile myoclonic epilepsy. *Seizure* 1996;**5**:149–51.

Buoni S, Grosso S, Fois A. Lamotrigine in typical absence epilepsy. *Brain Dev* 1999;**21**:303–6.

Catania S, Cross H, deSousa C, Boyd S. Paradoxical reaction to lamotrigine in a child with benign focal epilepsy of childhood with centrotemporal spikes. *Epilepsia* 1999;**40**:1657–60.

Frank M, Enlow T, Holmes G, *et al*. Lamictal (lamotrigine) monotherapy for typical absence seizures in children. *Epilepsia* 1999;**40**:973 9.

Gericke CA, Pickard F, deSaint-Martin A, *et al*. Efficacy of lamotrigine in idiopathic generalized epilepsy syndromes: a video–EEG-controlled, open study. *Epileptic Dis* 1999;**1**:159–65.

Guerrini R, Dravet C, Genton P, *et al*. Lamotrigine and seizure aggravation in severe myoclonic epilepsy. *Epilepsia* 1998;**39**:508–12.

Guerrini R, Belmonte A, Parmeggiani L, Perucca E. Myoclonic status epilepticus following high-dosage lamotrigine therapy. *Brain Dev* 1999;**21**:420–4.

Oller-Daurella L. [Tonic-automatic crises: clinical and EEG description. Discussion of their place in the epileptic crises classification and their representation in different potentials]. *Arch Neurobiol [Madrid]* 1970;**33**:303–16.

Case 43

IF AT FIRST YOU DON'T SUCCEED ...

Andrew N Wilner

History

F came to the office for his first visit when he was 40 years old. His mother's pregnancy was unremarkable, but he was premature by 6 weeks and blue at birth. He did not walk until 16 months of age or speak until 3 years of age.

F's first convulsion occurred at 15 months of age. He also had brief spells where he appeared afraid and ran to his mother. Despite phenobarbital and phenytoin, he continued to have seizures. After his physician switched him to primidone at the age of 12 years, F became violent and attacked a neighbor with a hatchet. He required institutionalization until he was aged 18.

While taking valproate 2 years ago he again became aggressive and was said to have a 'psychotic reaction'. His behavior improved when he began phenytoin. However, he continues to have seizures three times a month, although they can occur as often as nine times a day. According to his parents, he has right hand jerks, which sometimes proceed to a generalized convulsion. He also has other spells where he smacks his lips and stares. His seizures have failed to improve with acetazolamide, carbamazepine, chlordiazepoxide, clorazepate, diazepam and ethosuximide. He had an episode of status epilepticus when an intercurrent illness resulted in protracted nausea and vomiting.

His past medical history includes hyperthyroidism and hypertension, which he treats with medications. As a result of his seizures, he has fractured both wrists and his right foot and has suffered numerous lacerations on his face and scalp. He has no allergies and does not abuse drugs; nor does he drink alcohol or smoke. F is the only one in his family with epilepsy. His social life is very limited because of his seizures and limited cognitive and social skills. His mother is overprotective. His stepfather mostly ignores him. A prior evaluation included a normal EEG and a normal magnetic resonance imaging (MRI) study. He takes phenytoin (100 mg four times daily) and primidone (250 mg four times daily).

Examination and investigations

F answers questions slowly, but appropriately. His Mini Mental State Examination score is 25/30. His physical examination is normal and his neurological examination is non-focal. Video–EEG monitoring of eight seizures failed to reveal lateralization or localization (because of muscle artifact produced by grimacing and chewing at the onset of each seizure). Depth electrode monitoring revealed that 12 of 13 seizures originated from his right temporal lobe. The origin of the remaining seizure was unclear.

F's repeat MRI scan demonstrated right hippocampal atrophy with increased T2-weighted signal consistent with mesial temporal sclerosis. Positron emission tomography was normal. Neuropsychological testing did not lateralize or localize. The IQ was 83. A Wada test determined that he was left hemisphere dominant for language. Using his left hemisphere, he was able to remember 11 of 12 items. Using his right hemisphere, F couldn't answer any questions correctly.

Diagnosis

Intractable epilepsy caused by partial complex seizures and partial seizures with secondary generalization from the right temporal lobe.

Treatment and outcome

F had a right anterior temporal lobectomy without complication. Postoperatively, primidone was discontinued and he had two breakthrough seizures. I restarted the medication and he remains seizure free on two antiepileptic drugs. He attended adult education classes and passed his high school equivalency exam. He has been to vocational rehabilitation and found some part-time work. He also volunteers at the local hospital. He has learned to drive and can do errands, but he continues to live at home. He has made some friends at the epilepsy support group and has a girlfriend. He has been fishing with his stepfather for the first time.

Commentary

F presented with seizures that failed to respond to treatment. His stepfather considered him little more than a nuisance, and his mother worried about him daily. At the age of 40, there seemed little hope that he would ever live independently or become seizure-free. However, after a new and extensive evaluation, I was able to define an epileptic syndrome that was amenable to surgical treatment.

Many patients who appear 'hopeless' can be helped, whether by new

169

antiepileptic drugs, vagus nerve stimulation or epilepsy surgery. In F's case, a right temporal lobectomy resulted in a 99 % reduction of his seizures and a significant improvement in his quality of life.

What did I learn from this case?

First, I learned that although witnessed reports of seizures can be valuable, they pale in comparison to ictal videotapes. F's convulsions beginning with 'right hand jerks' reported by his family suggested Jacksonian seizures from a left frontal lobe lesion, unlikely to be amenable to seizure surgery. But video—EEG monitoring revealed that F's seizures consisted primarily of chewing and bouncing movements, with additional automatisms of right hand trembling, swinging and kicking of the right leg.

Second, I learned that antiepileptic drugs can subtly – or not so subtly – affect a patient's personality. In F's case, two drugs, primidone (which is notorious for its negative affect on behavior) and valproate (which is not usually associated with behavior abnormalities) altered his personality for the worse. When he was not on either of these drugs, F usually had a very placid disposition.

Third, I learned that if an imaging study is more than a few years old and there is reason to believe the patient has a lesion, a MRI scan with state-of-the-art equipment should be performed. F's first MRI was 'normal'. A follow-up scan revealed clear-cut mesial temporal sclerosis. Many older MRI scans did not have the resolution of today's scans, and significant pathology can be missed.

How did this case alter my approach to the care and treatment of my epilepsy patients?

F's case reinforced the concept that one must always ask: 'why does this patient have epilepsy?' I think that physicians tend to neglect this question because the answer in the past usually was 'I don't know,' as in F's case, even after a thorough evaluation. Now, with modern imaging, we can often answer that question and arrive at a more accurate diagnosis and prognosis. Learning why F had epilepsy permitted me to offer him the appropriate treatment.

Further reading

Benbadis SR. Is the underlying cause of epilepsy a major prognostic factor for recurrence? *Neurology* 1999;**53**:440.

Engel J. Etiology as a risk factor for medically refractory epilepsy. *Neurology* 1998;**51**:1243–4.

170

Semah F, Picot MC, Adam C, *et al.* Is the underlying cause of epilepsy a major prognostic factor for recurrence? *Neurology* 1998;**51**:1256–62.

Mattson RH, Cramer JA, Collins JF. Prognosis for total control of complex partial and secondarily generalized tonic clonic seizures. *Neurology* 1996;**47**:68–76.

Case 44

GYRATORY SEIZURES, ATAXIA AND DYSARTHRIA IN A YOUNG ADULT

Kazuichi Yagi

History

A 35-year-old woman had suffered her first generalized tonic convulsion at the age of 9 years when she was in bed soon after falling asleep. One month later, she had another generalized tonic convulsion, and treatment with antiepileptic drugs was started. She developed gyratory seizures several times a day.

She was admitted to the epilepsy center at the age of 12 because of status epilepticus. She was ataxic and dysarthric. Five seizures were recorded during routine video–EEG monitoring. Her seizure manifestations were conscious versive seizures and gyratory seizures to the left. With treatment the seizure frequency was reduced to one or two nocturnal seizures a week. She was a good student before the onset of epileptic seizures and finished middle school and got a job in a car factory. She was kept on her antiepileptic drug therapy but the versive seizures were not completely controlled until the age of 30.

Examination and investigations

Her EEGs showed constant continuous slow and sharp waves over the right frontal region. Computed tomography (CT) scans were uninformative, but magnetic resonance imaging (MRI) revealed abnormal irregular cortical formation in the right frontal lobe. MEG showed clusters of MEG spike equivalent-current dipoles (ECDs) in the right lateral frontal lobe where the abnormal cortical lesion was localized (Fig. 44.1). Single photon emission computed tomography (SPECT) with PAO showed regional hyperperfusion in the right frontal region during seizures; no abnormality was noted in the interictal period.

172

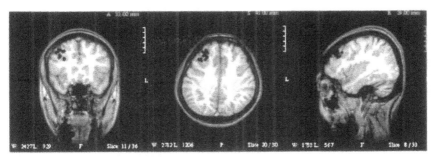

Figure 44.1: *Superimposed ECDs of MEG spikes on coronal, axial and sagittal MRI scans. A dark dot on the MRI scan represents one ECD of an MEG spike. These dots cluster in the right frontal lesion of the scan.*

Diagnosis

Frontal lobe epilepsy due to cortical dysplasia.

Treatment and outcome

Surgical treatment was recommended to her when she was 28. She hesitated to undergo surgical treatment and postponed it until the age of 30. A right frontal resection was undertaken after the epileptogenic zone was studied with intracranial EEG recordings, and functional mapping was performed with electrical stimulation in order to minimize postsurgical neurological deficits.

Since her operation she has been completely free from seizures and the antiepileptic drugs have been gradually reduced. She now has a better job at the car factory.

Commentary

There are several reasons why I chose this case. First, her seizures occurred only during sleep and didn't disturb her daily life. However, her parents were concerned about what would happen to her after their deaths, and I also thought that she withdrew from social life.

When I initially recommended surgical treatment to her, she told me that she would go through with it only if her seizures disappeared completely without any neurological deficits. I could not promise that she would become seizure-free

173

after surgery. I told her, however, that I couldn't control her seizures by drug therapy.

I suggested that we further examine her epileptogenic lesion. She agreed and after the evaluation she decided to undergo surgical treatment. The resected tissue showed cortical dysplasia. She has been free from seizures for 5 years now without any neurological deficit. She was lucky, considering that only 45 % of patients with extratemporal epileptogenic lesions become seizure-free after surgery.[1]

Second, MRI was more helpful than CT in identifying the lesion. In addition, the clustering region of MEG spike equivalent-current dipoles on MRI and the regional hyperperfusion on SPECT in the ictal period coincided well with the presumed epileptogenic zone from ictal and interictal EEG findings in this patient.

What did I learn from this case?

I learnt that detailed examinations should be carried out when seizures are resistant to antiepileptic drugs. Further, I learned that neuroimaging studies with CT, MRI, SPECT, and MEG, in addition to precise analysis of seizure manifestations by long-term video–EEG monitoring, are useful for detecting epileptogenic lesions. Finally, I realized that the best time to recommend surgical treatment is when all members of the family agree to it.

How did this case alter my approach to the care and treatment of my epilepsy patients?

Because of the successful surgical outcome in this patient, I now regularly suggest MRI in drug-resistant patients. In some patients, MRI detects abnormal lesions; however, only a few patients with extratemporal lesions undergo surgery.

This patient's case illustrates the importance of timing for surgical intervention. If the surgery had been done when she was aged 12, perhaps her life during adolescence would have been more pleasant. Recently, I have started to consider surgery earlier in a patient's course if the patient is a candidate for surgical treatment.

Reference

1. Engel J, Van Ness PC, Rasmussen TB, Ojemann LJ. Outcome with respect to epileptic seizures. In: Engel J, ed. *Surgical treatment of the epilepsies*. New York: Raven; 1993:609–21.

III

Surprising Turns and Twists

Case 45

RECURRENT AMNESTIC EPISODES IN A 62-YEAR-OLD DIABETIC PATIENT

Christine Adam, Claude Adam and Michel Baulac

History

In December 1996, after a recent diagnosis of type 2 diabetes, a 62-year-old right-handed man began to experience episodes resembling 'transient global amnesia', lasting 15 minutes to 1 hour. The episodes started on waking, with the loss of ability to plan his activities, followed by his asking a series of questions about what he had done the previous day, accompanied by a feeling of perplexity. Otherwise his behaviour seemed normal. There were no automatisms or other motor signs. He was not able to recall any details of the amnesic episode.

Examination and investigations

Two EEGs showed ictal discharges from the right frontotemporal region, but a subsequent 24-hour ambulatory EEG was normal. Magnetic resonance imaging (MRI) scanning of the brain showed right hippocampal atrophy with a high T2 signal.

The patient received valproate for 2 months, and he seemed to improve during that time. Meanwhile, his diabetes worsened, blood glucose levels fluctuating between 0.5 g/l and 3.5 g/l were noted, and insulin was started. He continued to have both hypoglycaemic episodes as well as marked hyperglycaemic episodes. The amnestic episode was thought to be caused by transient hypoglycaemia at the time, which could not be confirmed later with concomitant measurements.

The patient was seen in our hospital in May 1997 for evaluation of a few further similar episodes. A first EEG captured some slow spikes as well as a 'subclinical' right temporal lobe seizure on a later, standard EEG whose interpretation was uncertain. Nonetheless, vigabatrin was added to valproate. The amnestic episodes were infrequent during the following 6 months (occurring about once every 2 months), and they happened during periods of normal or high blood glucose levels.

In October 1997, the events shortened to a few minutes but increased dramatically in frequency, leading to a quasi-permanent amnestic state in which both anterograde and retrograde memory was affected. The patient was able to retain only very small

176

amounts of information. He complained of gait trouble, behavioural changes and a mild temporal–spatial disorientation. EEGs established a definite diagnosis of simple partial status epilepticus, showing temporal lobe seizures on both sides independently (but predominantly on the left). Up to three events in 30 minutes were recorded. Each seizure remained largely confined to one temporal lobe, although they would propagate mildly to neighbouring regions without any further clinical symptomatology. There was no evidence of impairment of consciousness. On admission the cerebrospinal fluid (CSF) was found to contain 0.4 g/l of protein per cell and normal glucose levels (the patient was hyperglycaemic at the time). Interferon-α was undetectable. The CSF remained normal 3 days and 1 week later. Herpes simplex virus-1 antibodies and the polymerase chain reaction were negative in the CSF. Other laboratory tests (including virology, bacteriology, autoimmunity, and inflammatory and paraneoplastic markers) were negative.

The seizures remained very active for 2 weeks despite clonazepam followed by intravenous phenytoin, together with high doses of oral antiepileptic drugs in combination (valproate, phenytoin, vigabatrin and clonazepam). Over the next 2 weeks the seizures disappeared, as shown by EEG monitoring. Despite the resolution of the status epilepticus, the amnestic and behavioural symptoms regressed slightly during the 2 months of hospitalization. A MRI scan of the brain 5 months later confirmed the presence of a small right hippocampus, which was hyperintense on FLAIR imaging; there was also notable volume loss in the left hippocampus (Fig. 45.1). The latest MRI (November 1998) confirmed bilateral hippocampal atrophy.

The clinical evolution was poor, with persistent anterograde amnesia, spatial–temporal disorientation and behavioural disorders with disinhibition and joviality.

Diagnosis

Temporal lobe epilepsy with simple partial status epilepticus and subsequent hippocampal atrophy.

Commentary

Why did we choose this case?

There are three reasons why we chose this case. First, it is well known that the epileptic origin of amnestic episodes may be difficult to recognize, especially in older patients.[1] In our observation, these episodes were initially misdiagnosed for hypoglycaemias, owing to the existence of difficult-to-treat diabetes. These manifestations were quite different from those of typical medial temporal lobe epilepsy (MTLE)[2,3] despite the presence of unequivocal hippocampal sclerosis on the first MRI scan. MTLE with hippocampal sclerosis is known to begin at about

177

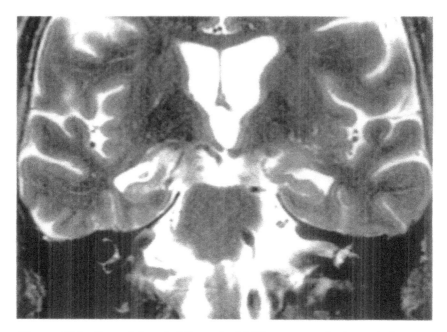

Figure 45.1: *Coronal slice of a T2-weighted MRI scan perpendicular to the long axis of hippocampus, 5 months after the occurrence of an amnestic simple partial status epilepticus in this 62-year-old patient. The left hippocampus is dramatically atrophic and the right hippocampus (originally affected) also showed a notable loss of volume.*

9 years of age with a large range of age of onset, but it is not known to have its onset at the age of 62, nor to cause seizures with aura that are of short duration and not purely amnestic.

Moreover status epilepticus is exceptional in classical MTLE. Our patient is much closer to the clinical entity reported under the term 'transient epileptic amnesia', which is defined by specific characteristics – onset in middle or old age, amnestic seizures lasting for 10 minutes or so that occur during wakefulness, and sometimes simple partial status epilepticus of very long duration (lasting days).[1] In this context, Lee *et al.*[4] have reported a transient MRI abnormality, but no evidence of hippocampal damage has been described until now.

What did we learn from this case?

We learnt that epileptic events can create acute hippocampal damage. Three types of events have been incriminated: early (most often febrile) convulsions;[5,6,7] rarely tonic–clonic status epilepticus;[8] and even a single, brief tonic–clonic seizure.[9] This case of hippocampal damage seems to be the first reported such case associated with simple partial status epilepticus. In this case, there is no

178

argument in favour of other underlying mechanisms such as a meningoencephalitis or anoxic–ischaemic factors of systemic origin. This indicates that very focal epileptic activity may be deleterious *per se*.

Hippocampal damage as a consequence of epileptic activity has generally been reported early in life, in young children[5,6,7] or in children, adolescents or young adults[8,9] and after single epileptic events. Our case is remarkable in that it occurred in an older adult and after repeated seizures over several weeks. This long duration was probably important in the development of this seizure-induced hippocampal damage. By contrast, the adult case reported by Jackson *et al.*[9] experienced only a short tonic–clonic seizure, but this was combined with severe respiratory disorders.

References

1. Zeman AZJ, Boniface SJ, Hodges JR. Transient epileptic amnesia: a description of the clinical and neuropsychological features in 10 cases and a review of the literature. *J Neurol Neurosurg Psychiatry* 1998;**64**:435–43.

2. French JA, Williamson PD, Thadani VM, *et al*. Characteristics of medial temporal lobe epilepsy: I. Results of history and physical examination. *Ann Neurol* 1993;**34**:774–80.

3. Williamson PD, French JA, Thadani VM, *et al*. Characteristics of medial temporal lobe epilepsy: II. Interictal and ictal scalp electroencephalography, neuropsychological testing, neuroimaging, surgical results, and pathology. *Ann Neurol* 1993;**34**:781–7.

4. Lee BI, Lee BC, Hwang YM, *et al*. Prolonged ictal amnesia with transient focal abnormalities on magnetic resonance imaging. *Epilepsia* 1992;**33**;1042–6.

5. Nohria V, Lee N, Tien RD, *et al*. Magnetic resonance imaging evidence of hippocampal sclerosis in progression: a case report. *Epilepsia* 1994;**35**:1332–6.

6. Perez ER, Maeder P, Villemure KM, *et al*. Acquired hippocampal damage after temporal lobe seizures in 2 infants. *Ann Neurol* 2000;**48**:384–7.

7. Van Landingham KE, Heinz ER, Cavazos JE, Lewis DV. Magnetic resonance imaging evidence of hippocampal injury after prolonged focal febrile convulsions. *Ann Neurol* 1998;**43**:413–26.

8. Tien RD, Felsberg GJ. The hippocampus in status epilepticus: demonstration of a signal intensity and morphological changes with sequential fast spin-echo MR imaging. *Radiology* 1995;**194**:249–56.

9. Jackson GD, Chambers BR, Berkovic SF. Hippocampal sclerosis: development in adult life. *Development Neurosci* 1999;**21**:207–14.

Case 46

ATTACKS OF NAUSEA AND PALPITATIONS IN A WOMAN WITH EPILEPSY

Jørgen Alving

History

The patient was a 28-year-old woman referred for evaluation of seizures. Her seizures had begun when she was 12 years of age with generalized tonic–clonic seizures and, allegedly, psychomotor seizures that were not further described. Seizures usually occurred just after awakening.

She was initially treated with carbamazepine and then with phenytoin, but she was changed to valproate because of side effects and insufficient seizure control. Valproate was reasonably effective, but because of unacceptable weight gain she was changed to a combination of lamotrigine and vigabatrin.

At the time of the referral, she was having approximately one seizure a month. She gave the following descriptions of her seizures: 'nausea, palpitations and an urge to urinate or defecate, sometimes ending in a generalized convulsion', and 'difficulty concentrating and understanding others, talking "gibberish", and a strong urge to urinate, lasting 15–20 minutes'.

Her family history was positive for unspecified epilepsy in an aunt and a cousin. Her birth, developmental milestones and school performance were unremarkable and there was no previous neurological illness.

Examination and investigations

Her neurological examination, including mental status examination, was normal. The initial EEG showed generalized paroxysmal abnormalities, and the brain magnetic resonance imaging scan was normal.

She was admitted to the hospital for EEG monitoring. A routine EEG, including a sleep EEG, was normal. A 96-hour ambulatory eight-channel cassette-EEG (while she was still on 2000 mg vigabatrin and 300 mg lamotrigine) showed no abnormality despite two episodes with nausea.

During a second admission, she had a cluster of the seizures described above. Video-EEG recording showed innumerable generalized bursts of 4–6 Hz spike–polyspike and waves (Fig. 46.1), each burst lasting 1–2 seconds and

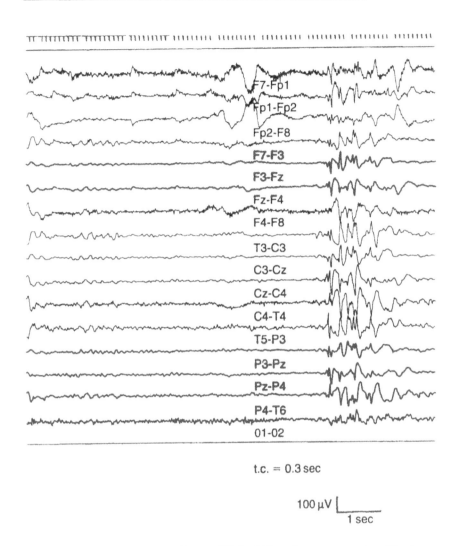

t.c. = 0.3 sec

100 µV ⌊_____
                1 sec

Figure 46.1: *(a) Generalized burst of 3.5–6 Hz spike–wave occuring 20 minutes before a tonic–clonic seizure, with very minor clinical accompaniments.*

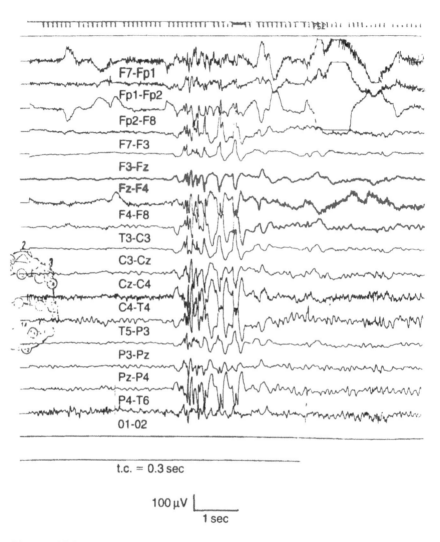

Figure 46.1: (b) *Generalized burst of polyspike–wave occurring 1 minute before a tonic–clonic seizure, with more marked clinical features (upward eye deviation).*

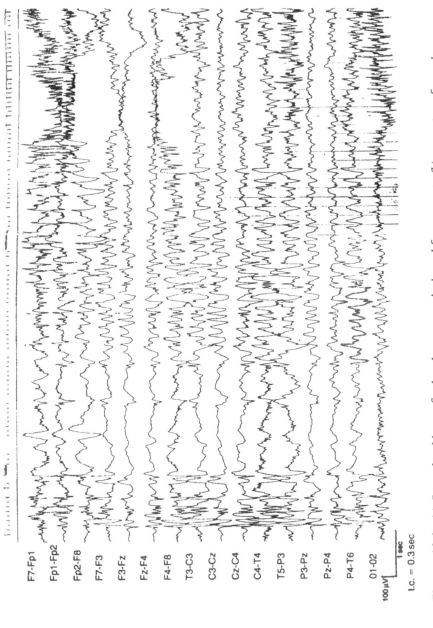

Figure 46.1: (c) Generalized burst of polyspike–wave with clinical features as in (b), occurring after a short generalized flattening and followed by tonic–clonic seizure.

183

accompanied by a slight lapse of consciousness and upward deviation of the eyes with blinking, but no clonic movements in the extremities. Over a 2-hour period, the paroxysmal bursts became more intense and frequent, finally terminating in a generalized tonic–clonic seizure, initiated by massive clonic movements in her face.

Diagnosis

Idiopathic generalized epilepsy (juvenile absence epilepsy, cycloleptic type), with some features of juvenile myoclonic epilepsy.

Treatment and outcome

After the video-EEG, valproate was re-instituted, and ethosuximide was subsequently added, with much improved seizure control. Because of recurrent problems with weight gain, valproate was replaced by lamotrigine. For the past 2 years, on a combination of lamotrigine 600 mg/day and ethosuximide 1000 mg/day, she has had only one generalized tonic–clonic seizure and two episodes with clustered absences.

Commentary

This patient's aura-like phenomena with strong autonomic components had obviously been misinterpreted as evidence of focal seizures. Furthermore, several normal EEGs despite prolonged monitoring made a diagnosis of idiopathic generalized epilepsy less likely, until a rather short but intensive session of video-EEG monitoring together with the history (including the age at onset) led to the correct classification of her seizure types and epilepsy syndrome.

The paradoxical exacerbation of generalized seizures with vigabatrin and carbamazepine is well known, but there is no evidence in this case to suggest that vigabatrin was responsible for the massive EEG abnormalities (and seizures) seen during intensive monitoring. The 96-hour cassette-EEG was performed on the same medication, and she had paroxysmal EEG abnormalities before vigabatrin treatment.

What did I learn from this case?

I learned that an incessant search for an exact seizure and syndrome diagnosis is essential, especially if the clinical semiology is equivocal. This case reinforced the concept that aura-like phenomena may be seen in idiopathic generalized epilepsies.

I also learned that a prolonged EEG recording performed at the 'wrong' time may not be informative in patients with idiopathic generalized epilepsies.

Finally, I learned that a prolonged EEG is not identical with intensive monitoring! I am now more careful to plan EEG monitoring when the chance of capturing clinical events is at its maximum.

Further reading

Janz D. *Die Epilepsien. Spezielle Pathologie und Therapie.* Stuttgart: Thieme; 1969.

Lee AG, Delgado-Escueta AV, Maldonato HM, Swartz B, Walsh GO. Closed-circuit television videotaping and electroencephalographic biotelemetry (video/EEG) in primary generalized epilepsies. In: Gumnit RJ, ed. Intensive neurodiagnostic monitoring. *Advances in neurology* vol 46. New York: Raven; 1987:27 68.

Pacia SV, Gueyikian V, Devinsky O. Auras in primary generalized epilepsy. *Epilepsia* 1996;**37(suppl 5)**:30.

Parker APJ, Agathonikou A, Robinson RO, Panaiyotopoulos CP. Inappropriate use of carbamazepine and vigabatrin in typical absence seizures. *Dev Med Child Neurol* 1998;**40**:517 9.

Case 47

ABSENCE STATUS EPILEPTICUS IN A 60-YEAR-OLD WOMAN

Gerhard Bauer

History

In 1974, a 60-year-old woman was admitted to hospital in a peculiar state. She was partially responsive and able to follow simple commands but unable to follow a conversation. She frequently smiled inappropriately and complained about dizziness. Eyelid fluttering was observed.

No neurologist had seen her before and her medical practitioner did not know of any history of paroxysmal events in the past. She was taking antihypertensive and cardiac medications.

Examination and investigations

The EEG showed continuously repeated runs of generalized 3-Hz spike-and-waves lasting up to 10–20 seconds. The short periods of interspersed activity revealed no gross abnormalities. Absence status was diagnosed and intravenous diazepam was administered, with prompt resolution of the status epilepticus.

The neurological examination after the episode resolved showed some mental slowing, exaggerated tendon reflexes and a Babinski sign on the right side.

Pneumoencephalograpy revealed mild brain atrophy (ascribed to vascular encephalopathy) but was otherwise normal. Cerebrospinal fluid was also normal.

Diagnosis

Absence status epilepticus occurring *de novo* in later life.

Treatment and outcome

The patient was put on a combination of ethosuximide and phenobarbital, which at the time was the recommended therapy for epilepsies with absence seizures.

Two years later, I saw her in the outpatient clinic and she reported having had her first generalized tonic–clonic seizure at the age of 36 years, which was 24 years before her presentation with absence status epilepticus. Since that time, sporadic tonic–clonic seizures had occurred every year, but she never reported them to her family or to her doctors. Seizures occurred without exception in the morning hours, when she was alone at home.

She reported that no further seizures had occurred since the start of antiepileptic medications. The EEG at this time showed generalized spikes and slight diffuse slowing.

During the visit the patient was in an elated mood. She was accompanied by a schoolfriend and the two women joked in the waiting room. I tried to find out why she had never reported her seizures and found myself dragged into a pleasant chat. To gain more information, I invited her schoolfriend to take part. During the conversation, the patient's friend stated that the patient had always been a *Blinzelgeiß* (blinking goat). With this term the conversation turned serious, and it became clear that during her school years the patient had suffered daily absence seizures until they resolved spontaneously at the age of 14 years. No prolonged absence status epilepticus had occurred until the episode that had led to hospital admission in 1974. I also learned that a sister of the patient had experienced absences and generalized tonic–clonic seizures.

In light of this new information, I diagnosed generalized idiopathic epilepsy, childhood absence epilepsy followed by generalized tonic–clonic seizures on awakening and absence status epilepticus. In addition, a diagnosis of vascular encephalopathy, hypertonia and coronary heart disease was made.

On a subsequent visit, the patient noted mood changes and reported that she had been diagnosed with depressive mood disorder associated with menopause ('involutional depression') by a psychiatrist. Antidepressant medication was prescribed, but she was non-compliant with both the psychotropic and antiepileptic medications. She continued to have generalized tonic–clonic seizures, scattered absence seizures and prolonged periods of 'dizziness'. Because these episodes of 'dizziness' had been treated successfully by her medical practitioner with intravenous diazepam, the diagnosis of repeated absence status epilepticus seemed to be justified.

In 1982, she was admitted to the hospital with cervical radiculopathy. Brain computed tomography showed slight brain atrophy. A trial of valproate led to an increase in absence seizures, and the former combination of ethosuximide and phenobarbital was re-established. After this admission the patient became

187

compliant and free of seizures. The mood changes stabilized without antidepressant medication, and the patient lived a decent life until she died from a cerebrovascular accident at the age of 75 years.

Commentary

Since the reappraisal of absence status by Andermann and Robb,[1] many forms of prolonged states of altered mental functions accompanied by ongoing spike activities in the EEG have been differentiated. Non-convulsive status epilepticus is now understood to include generalized absence status epilepticus and focal complex partial status epilepticus. Furthermore, it has become clear that generalized non-convulsive status epilepticus (absence status epilepticus) includes status epilepticus that occurs in association with known absence epilepsies, in Lennox–Gastaut syndrome, and de novo in later life.[2,3] Complex partial status epilepticus may be difficult to differentiate from absence status epilepticus during the episode, but the distinction usually becomes clear after clinical investigations have been performed.

When this patient first presented, absence status epilepticus occurring de novo in later life was diagnosed – this was a diagnosis that had been established in the literature three years earlier.[3] The EEG exhibited generalized 3-Hz spike-and-waves without any focal elements and against normal background activity. Although a focal component could not be excluded, the EEG and the prompt recovery led to the diagnosis of absence status epilepticus. Signs of a vascular encephalopathy were considered a comorbidity.

After learning of the patient's history of childhood absence epilepsy and generalized tonic–clonic seizures, the correct diagnosis was changed. The generalized character of the non-convulsive episode was confirmed, but it became clear that absence status epilepticus was not the presenting symptom but rather a manifestation of an idiopathic generalized seizure disorder.

Why absence status occurs as the late complication of an otherwise mild seizure disorder, which in this case was kept a secret by the patient (even from her family), remains an enigma. Some authors[4,5] consider that the condition is usually situational. Psychotropic drugs and withdrawal from benzodiazepines seem to be the most frequently observed precipitating factors.[2,6,7] Another entity – non-convulsive status epilepticus in a critically ill elderly patient – is unrelated to this discussion.[8]

This patient also suffered from cerebrovascular disease and a mood disorder. In the search of factors that may have triggered absence status, psychotropic agents could be ruled out, but the role of cerebrovascular insufficiency remains a speculation. Although the pathogenesis of absence status as a late complication of generalized idiopathic epilepsy is unknown, it is nonetheless a well-documented fact and might be syndrome-related.[9] In rare cases, absence status epilepticus represents the very first symptom of a generalized idiopathic epilepsy with late onset.[10]

What did I learn from this case?

I learned a number of lessons from this case. First, I learned that the diagnostically relevant information was gained during an informal chat with the patient and her schoolfriend. Besides a strictly medical interview, a personal conversation in a relaxed atmosphere represents an important part of taking a thorough history.

Second, her childhood absence seizures stopped spontaneously, without any medication. Her first generalized tonic–clonic seizure occurred many years later, at the age of 36. Thus, offering a good prognosis in cases of absence epilepsy, as is frequently done by pediatricians, may neglect the late complications, as in this case.

Third, if some patients with daily absence seizures do not come to medical diagnosis, as in this case, then the 'true' incidence, prevalence and natural history of the epilepsy is open to question. Since this case is not a single observation, the figures given in the published literature might be too low.

Fourthly, these uncertainties may also concern genetic studies. My patient's positive family history for seizures was only reported after repeated examinations. The degree to which a patient is affected may also be disguised in patients with a self-limited course that does not come to medical attention.

Fifthly, elderly people often suffer from multiple diseases. A seizure disorder occurring in an elderly patient cannot be uncritically assumed to be symptomatic of an acute or remote brain insult. Likewise, labeling a mild brain condition as a triggering factor remains speculative. With late seizures, the possibility of an idiopathic seizure disorder in earlier life cannot be ruled out categorically. The second age peak can be due to an exaggeration of a pre-existing idiopathic generalized epilepsy (as in this case), or it can really be *de novo*.[10]

How did this case alter my approach to the care and treatment of my patients with epilepsy?

I do not draw final conclusions after the first visit even if my conclusion fits nicely with recently published papers. If a patient wants to have a personal conversation besides the formal interview, I indulge the patient and take my time. Decisive information is sometimes reported only in a relaxed atmosphere.

I realize now that patients with generalized idiopathic epilepsies are prone to seizures throughout their lives. Therefore, before I consider withdrawing antiepileptic drugs, I take a careful history, with special attention to 'minor seizures'. If appropriate, I also obtain long-term EEG monitoring to look for generalized paroxysmal EEG abnormalities. I recognize that an EEG is crucial in evaluating patients with altered states of consciousness during the episode. Finally, even though multiple comorbidities are common in elderly patients, the causal relationship of these conditions to seizures should be judged critically.

References

1. Andermann F, Robb JP. Absence status. A reappraisal following review of thirty-eight patients. *Epilepsia* 1972;**13**:177–87.

2. Bourrat Ch, Garde P, Boucher M, Fournet A. États d'absence prolongée chez des patients agés sans passé épileptique. *Rev Neurol* 1986;**142**:696–702.

3. Schwartz MS, Scott DF. Isolated petit-mal status presenting de novo in middle age. *Lancet* 1971;**ii**:1399–401.

4. Thomas P, Beaumanoir A, Genton P, *et al.* 'De novo' absence status of late onset: report of 11 cases. *Neurology* 1992;**42**:104–10.

5. Thomas P, Andermann F. Late-onset absence status epilepticus is most often situation-related. In: Malafosse A, Genton P, Hirsch E, *et al.*, eds. *Idiopathic generalized epilepsies: clinical, experimental and genetic aspects*. London: John Libbey and Company; 1994:95–109.

6. Brodtkorb E, Sand T, Kristiansen A, Torbergsen T. Non-convulsive status epilepticus in the adult mentally retarded. *Seizure* 1993;**2**:115–23.

7. Rumpl E, Hinterhuber H. Unusual 'spike–wave stupor' in a patient with manic–depressive psychosis treated with amitryptiline. *J Neurol* 1981;**226**:131–5.

8. Litt B, Wityk RJ, Hertz S, *et al.* Nonconvulsive status epilepticus in the critically ill elderly. *Epilepsia* 1998;**39**:1194–202.

9. Agathonikou A, Panayiotopoulos CP, Giannakodimos S, Koutroumanidis M. Typical absence status in adults: diagnostic and syndromic considerations. *Epilepsia* 1998;**39**:1265–76.

10. Luef G, Bauer G. Idiopathic generalized epilepsy in adult-onset. *Epilepsia*, in press.

Case 48

HEMIPLEGIA IN A 76-YEAR-OLD WOMAN WITH STATUS EPILEPTICUS

Christoph Baumgartner

History

A 76-year-old woman was admitted to the emergency department because of focal motor status epilepticus consisting of clonic activity of the left face, arm and leg. On admission the patient was stuporous. The patient was treated intravenously with clonazepam and phenytoin, which stopped the focal motor activity. However, the patient developed a left-sided hemiplegia and remained stuporous.

The patient experienced her first seizure half a year before this admission. This first seizure consisted of focal motor seizures that evolved into a generalized tonic–clonic status epilepticus necessitating intubation and artificial ventilation. At that time a computed tomography (CT) scan showed a right posterior borderzone infarction and multiple lacunar vascular lesions that had not previously caused any transient or permanent neurological deficits. The patient recovered completely from status epilepticus and remained seizure-free on phenytoin. A follow-up CT scan performed 2 months before this admission showed a right parietal subdural hygroma (maximum width 15 mm). Because the hygroma did not exhibit a significant mass effect and the patient was completely asymptomatic and had no focal neurological signs, a conservative approach was undertaken.

Examinations and investigations

On transfer to my ward (on day 2 after admission to the emergency department), the patient was stuporous (Glasgow coma scale 8) and showed a left sided hemiplegia. A CT scan on admission was unchanged compared with the previous scan performed 2 months ago. Control CT scans performed on the following days also showed no significant changes. A magnetic resonance imaging scan essentially confirmed the CT scan findings. Cerebrospinal fluid showed a mild pleocytosis (14 cells/mm^3) consisting of granulocytes and lymphocytes as well as

191

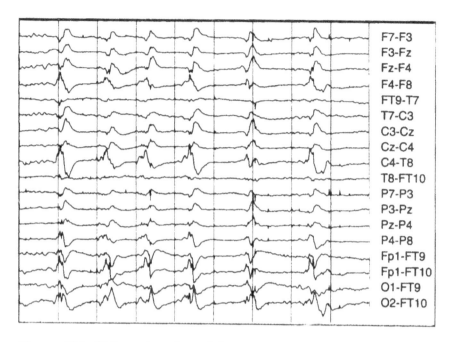

Figure 48.1: *EEG recording obtained during ictal hemiplegia showing periodic lateralized epileptiform discharges over the right hemisphere with maximum activity in the right central region.*

a total protein of 82 mg/dl, which was considered to be consistent with a non-specific meningeal irritation. An EEG showed periodic lateralized epileptiform discharges (PLEDs) over the right hemisphere (Fig. 48.1). A SPECT study showed marked hyperperfusion of the entire right hemisphere.

Diagnosis

Non-convulsive focal status epilepticus with ictal hemiplegia.

Treatment and outcome

After the diagnosis of focal status epilepticus the patient was treated with high dose benzodiazepines and intravenous phenytoin. However, while the state of vigilance slightly improved after this treatment, the hemiplegia remained unchanged. On day 5, therefore, it was decided to evacuate the hygroma via a

192

burr-hole using a Jackson–Pratt drainage. The hygroma completely resolved after this intervention. On EEG, the PLEDs disappeared and the patient gradually woke and she completely recovered from her hemiplegia over the next 2 weeks. A repeat single-photon emission CT (SPECT) study performed after her recovery showed – besides hypoperfusion in the right posterior borderzone a normal perfusion pattern and, specifically, no evidence of a hyperperfusion within the right hemisphere.

Commentary

Why did I choose this case?

I chose this case for several reasons. First, this case shows that convulsive status epilepticus can evolve into non-convulsive status epilepticus after what seems like successful treatment. Thus, in a recent study,[1] 48 % of 164 patients showed persistent EEG seizure activity after clinical control of convulsive status epilepticus and 14 % of patients developed non-convulsive status epilepticus. Persistent EEG seizure activity was associated with a significantly higher mortality and a poorer outcome in this study, which underlines the importance of EEG monitoring after treatment of convulsive status epilepticus.

Secondly, the differential diagnosis of hemiparesis or hemiplegia in patients with seizures should include structural lesions such as tumors, vascular events and encephalitis as well as functional abnormalities such as postictal Todd's paresis and ictal hemiparesis. While some authors proposed a highly variable duration of Todd's paresis lasting from several minutes to 36 hours,[2] in my experience Todd's paresis usually is much shorter, with a maximum duration of 15 minutes. In any case, a duration of several days for the hemiparesis in our patient would be a strong argument against a postictal phenomenon.

Thirdly, the true incidence of ictal paresis is unclear from the literature, owing to differences in definition. Some authors[3] have found a short ictal hemiparesis in up to 5 % of patients with temporal lobe seizures, which most probably represents a motor neglect rather then a true hemiparesis. On the contrary, a real paralysis caused by inhibitory motor seizures is an uncommon seizure symptom and most often occurs in patients with frontoparietal foci.[4]

Fourthly, this case may help to clarify the controversy about whether PLEDs represent a non-epileptiform or an epileptiform EEG abnormality and specifically whether PLEDs should be considered to be an interictal or an ictal phenomenon. PLEDs occur in a variety of disorders, most often in acute unilateral lesions such as ischemia, tumors or encephalitis. PLEDs are usually transient, and clinical seizures occur in approximately 70 % of patients with PLEDs.[5] The finding of a hyperperfusion of the entire right hemisphere on SPECT scanning during

193

hemiplegia as well as the appearance of a normal perfusion pattern after the resolution of the PLEDs and the resolution of hemiparesis represent strong evidence that, at least in this specific patient, PLEDs were an ictal phenomenon. This finding is in agreement with a positron emission tomographic study[6] that showed markedly increased mesiotemporal lobe metabolism in a case with PLEDs.

What did I learn from this case?

Apart from what I have outlined above, I was impressed by the existence of a long-lasting hemiplegia representing an ictal event. This case drew my attention towards non-convulsive status epilepticus as an important differential diagnosis in patients with unexplained mental obtundation, coma or focal neurological signs. I believe that EEG should be used more often in these patients. Finally, I think that SPECT can be used to distinguish between the interictal and the ictal state in patients with EEG patterns of unclear significance.

References

1. DeLorenzo RJ, Waterhouse E, Towne AR, *et al*. Persistent nonconvulsive status epilepticus after control of convulsive status epilepticus. *Epilepsia* 1998;**39**:833–40.

2. Rolak LA, Rutecki P, Ashizawa T, Harati Y. Clinical features of Todd's post-epileptic paralysis. *J Neurol Neurosurg Psychiat* 1992;**55**:63–4.

3. Oestreich LJ, Berg MJ, Bachmann DL, Burchfiel J, Erba G. Ictal contralateral paresis in complex partial seizures. *Epilepsia* 1995;**36**:671–5.

4. Smith RF, Devinsky O, Luciano D. Inhibitory motor status: two new cases and a review of the literature. *J Epilepsy* 1997;**10**:15–21.

5. Brenner RP, Schaul N. Periodic EEG patterns: classification, clinical correlation, and pathophysiology. *J Clin Neurophysiol* 1990;**7**:249–67.

6. Handforth A, Cheng JT, Mandelkern MA, Treiman DM. Markedly increased mesiotemporal lobe metabolism in a case with PLEDs: further evidence that PLEDs are a manifestation of partial status epilepticus. *Epilepsia* 1994;**35**:876–81.

Cases 49, 50 and 51

PERSISTENCE PAYS OFF

Mark D Bej

History

The first patient (case 49) was 17 years of age when she was first seen after having had several blackout spells. She also complained of severe fatigue and abdominal pains that had started after the death of her grandmother. The pains had no relationship to meals and were described as 'a weird sensation' and 'reminding me of something', although she denied *déjà vu* when specifically asked. Two blackouts occurred on the same day while she was visiting friends. Another event occurred later while she was on the phone: she suddenly stopped talking and appeared to be in a trance. There were no automatisms or convulsions. She had previously been seen for chronic fatigue.

The second patient (case 50) was seen when she was aged 35 years. She had had three episodes of loss of consciousness followed by some body jerking. A brain computed tomography (CT) scan was normal and she was placed on phenytoin. Another episode resulted in an emergency department evaluation, but the patient was discharged home. A third episode occurred in sleep. She also was having other episodes every couple of months, near the time of her menses. These episodes produced complaints of an unusual sensation without loss of consciousness. The only other significant history was that of being thrown out of the back of a truck at the age of 15 and suffering a wrist fracture (but no loss of consciousness). When she was evaluated, she had been, at different times, on phenytoin, carbamazepine, gabapentin, and phenobarbital, all of which had been stopped for various reasons. She had three EEGs; two were normal and one was read as demonstrating spike–wave activity. Despite the medications and consultations with several neurologists, the spells were not controlled.

The third patient (case 51) was aged 13 years when she first presented with focal seizures. She was placed on carbamazepine, and over subsequent years the dosage of this medication needed to be slowly increased. When she was aged 16 or 17, it became clear that the dose increases were proportionally greater than her normal peripubertal weight gain. Eventually the side effects of carbamazepine became intolerable and she was switched to another antiepileptic drug.

Examinations and investigations

In the first patient, examination was normal, as were a CT scan, routine EEG and a subsequent 72-hour ambulatory EEG during which seven of her episodes of abdominal pain were captured. A syncope clinic consultation with tilt table testing was sought; this revealed reduction of red cell mass and a marked hyperkinetic circulatory state in the supine position. She tolerated tilt for only 11 minutes, complaining of darkening vision. The test was terminated, owing to hypotension.

In the second patient, a 48-hour EEG ordered at a local academic center demonstrated an EEG seizure arising from the right temporal lobe. An epilepsy-protocol magnetic resonance imaging (MRI) scan was subsequently ordered and demonstrated a high-signal mass in the right hippocampus on fluid attenuation inversion recovery (FLAIR) and T2 weighting.

For the third patient, a thin-cut MRI scan was ordered. The scan demonstrated an area of focal cortical dysplasia in the right frontal lobe.

Diagnosis

Symptomatic partial epilepsy due to a low-grade glioma (Patient 1), and due to a hippocampal tumor (Patient 2) and cortical dysplasia (Patient 3).

Treatments and outcomes

The first patient was lost to follow-up until 2 years later when she presented to a local emergency department with a tonic–clonic seizure. Routine EEG was again normal but MRI scanning revealed a lesion in the right amygdalar area. The mass was excised and was felt to be a low-grade glioma with focal cortical dysplasia. Since surgery, the abdominal pains have resolved.

The second patient had appropriate ancillary testing of memory function, and her mass was then excised. The patient has been free of seizures since the surgery.

The third patient's seizures failed to respond to trials of three antiepileptic drugs over 2 years. After appropriate ancillary testing, she underwent an evaluation with subdural grid electrodes and ultimate excision of the dysplastic area of cortex, resulting in complete freedom from seizures.

196

Commentary

These three cases share a single common element: each patient was incompletely diagnosed during the early phases of their treatment. Definitive diagnosis was made only after a careful review of each patient's course; in two patients, the review occurred after referral or transfer to another neurologist.

It must be stated here that the simple fact that a diagnosis is not known with certainty is not of itself undesirable. This is true for more epileptic patients than any of us would like to admit. For medical, financial or social reasons, it is not always practical to do a thorough diagnostic evaluation on initial presentation.

However, these three cases demonstrate the need for vigilance with each follow-up visit. Significant changes in the patient's seizure history should prompt the neurologist to investigate further. The first patient had a change in the type of event – events that had not, up to that time, even been definitively diagnosed as seizures. The second patient's significant change (which had admittedly occurred previously) was intractability to several medications. The third patient's change was considerably subtler – increasing intractability to her first medication in the form of breakthrough seizures.

What did I learn from the cases?

The most valuable lesson for me is the need for continued vigilance and the utility of maintaining a seizure calendar. Only by reviewing the prior history well – in the case of the third patient, more than once   did it become obvious that the new or continuing seizures were evidence of something more than 'run-of-the-mill' epilepsy. Running a clinical practice often places significant pressures on one's time, and it is all too easy simply to increase dosages or add medications. One must watch for the 'red flags' and, when they appear, review the case again.

How did these cases alter my approach to the care and treatment of my epilepsy patients?

I try to review every case when a patient requires dosage increases or a new antiepileptic drug because of continuing seizures. If the epilepsy type has not been well defined, I order ambulatory EEG or inpatient video-EEG monitoring. If an epilepsy-protocol (thin-cut) MRI scan has not been done, then this is ordered. Ordering such studies has very often resulted in defining an etiology, defining the epilepsy syndrome and determining the best medications to use for the patient, even in cases where multiple routine EEGs were previously normal.

Case 52

DRUGS DID NOT WORK IN A LITTLE GIRL WITH ABSENCE SEIZURES

David B Bettis

History

J was a little girl with an angelic face and curly blonde hair. She was aged
2 years 8 months when her mother brought her to my office with a 6-month
history of staring spells. These attacks occurred one to four times a day and
consisted of a blank stare, eyelid fluttering, some jerking of the eyebrows and
rolling the eyes upwards. They lasted 5–20 seconds. During this time she was
motionless and unresponsive. The spells could not be interrupted. There was no
associated urinary incontinence, although some urinary urgency occurred after
the attacks. They were exacerbated by fatigue. Rarely, she had slight jerking
movements of her arms. These spells had never caused her to fall or lose
consciousness.

Her past medical history included being the product of an uncomplicated, full-
term pregnancy. Birth weight was 3.5 kg. Her development had been normal to
date. Her only medication was sulfasoxazole for prophylaxis of recurrent otitis
media. Her family medical history was negative for epilepsy, seizures or other
neurological disorders of significance. She had three healthy sisters.

Examination and investigations

Physical examination revealed a head circumference of 49.7 cm. General and
neurological physical examinations were entirely normal and age-appropriate.
Hyperventilation failed to elicit any events. Her EEG revealed multiple instances
of 3-Hz spike-and-slow wave generalized epileptiform discharges, sometimes
with a bifrontal predominance, which were slightly exacerbated by drowsiness.
Photic stimulation was unremarkable.

Diagnosis

Absence epilepsy.

Treatment and outcome

I counseled her mother on the typical benign prognosis of absence epilepsy, and started the patient on valproate. Her spells improved for a few weeks, but then relapsed. She was having three to 12 events a day. Ethosuximide was added; she again improved for a few weeks but then regressed again. She developed a sleep disturbance with restlessness, squirming and hallucinations. Ethosuximide was discontinued and her symptoms improved. A few months later, she was having dozens of seizures a day. A repeat trial of ethosuximide improved her symptoms but was associated with stomach upset and vomiting. She developed behavioral problems with uncharacteristically whiny and sometimes aggressive behavior. This improved when valproate was stopped and clonazepam was added. However, clonazepam was associated with behavioral side effects including crying and mood swings, and it was discontinued after a brief trial. She was having up to 20 absence spells a day.

A trial of amantadine improved her symptoms for 1 week, followed by yet another relapse. All medications were discontinued, and she improved, although she continued to have 20 seizures a day lasting 10–30 seconds. A repeat EEG revealed ongoing 3-Hz spike-and-wave generalized epileptiform discharges, but also some less frequent independent right and left parietal spike–wave discharges. A trial of phenytoin was not beneficial. This was followed by a trial of carbamazepine, which did not help. She was having up to 50 events per day, and was starting school.

Felbamate was initiated in September 1993, at a time when she was having 50 seizures a day. It did not help, and she was referred to a pediatric epileptologist at a major university. Review of several EEGs in the past confirmed typical changes for absence epilepsy. A trial of methsuximide was initiated and decreased the seizures frequency from 30 a day to 10 a day. This was the best seizure control that had been achieved in some time. Her family moved to a small town and she adjusted to her new school setting. Her seizures increased to 100 per day, and methsuximide was discontinued. She began having trouble in school. A trial of lamotrigine was discussed, but her mother was understandably hesitant to try a ninth medication. J continued to worsen and was having hundreds of events a day, associated with regression in school and occasional urinary incontinence.

In desperation, her mother asked about the ketogenic diet, a therapy that had

199

recently been resurrected following some attention in the national media. After some discussion, and shortly after the ketogenic diet became available at our center, J was hospitalized and underwent fasting. She was placed on the ketogenic diet at a 4:1 ratio of fat to carbohydrate and protein calories. Her seizures immediately decreased to only a few per day; she had a slight exacerbation associated with an episode of otitis media and fever. She then became seizure-free for the first time in years. As weeks went by, her cognitive abilities improved. Her mother observed that the changes were 'like taking a veil off of her brain'. She exhibited improved abilities in reading and mathematics in school.

The diet was not without side effects. J was observed to be hungry, tired and moody. She suffered a bout of renal stones after being on the diet for a little over 1 year. However, she continued to make vast progress in school, and became a straight A student. She won the 'most improved reader award'.

After being seizure-free for 20 months, the ratio of her ketogenic diet was gradually decreased and a weaning process was started. After being seizure-free for 2 years, the diet was discontinued. A follow-up EEG was normal. She has remained seizure-free since that time.

J and her family were deservedly given the 'winning kid with epilepsy award' from our local epilepsy foundation. Her mother shared this compelling story with a large audience.

Commentary

Absence epilepsy of childhood is typically a benign condition that responds well to medication in more than 90 % of cases. When a truly refractory case of absence epilepsy is encountered, effective treatment options are limited. Since this experience, I have become aware of at least one case of refractory absence epilepsy that responded well to a vagal nerve stimulator.

Although it is not possible to prove that the ketogenic diet was clearly responsible for curing this case of epilepsy, I cannot be convinced that her drastic improvement was mere coincidence after treating this child for more than 4 years with eight different anticonvulsant medications.

What did I learn from this case?

I once again learned a lesson that I had been taught in medical school and by my prior practice experience: the importance of remaining open-minded to unconventional therapies when standard therapy is clearly unsuccessful. Because the vast majority of cases of absence epilepsy are responsive to medication, I persisted with medication trials for a prolonged period, even though the patient had nothing but a succession of side effects to show for undergoing those treatments.

How did this case alter my approach to the care and treatment of my epilepsy patients?

I am happier now about thinking of non-medication options when a reasonable trial of at least a few appropriate medications has failed. Those options include epilepsy surgery, the ketogenic diet and the vagal nerve stimulator. I am haunted by the thought of how much sooner Justine would have improved had the ketogenic diet been tried earlier, and even more so by thoughts of other patients who have not been reached by non-medication therapies that could prove to be highly beneficial for their epilepsy.

Case 53

'ALTERNATIVE' THERAPY FOR PARTIAL EPILEPSY — WITH A TWIST

Nadir E Bharucha and Thomas Kuruvilla

History

A 20-year-old man presented with a 10-year history of partial seizures that had become generalized. A computed tomography scan of the brain, performed at the onset of the seizures, had shown a lesion, probably a tuberculous granuloma, in the right frontal cortex. He was started on antiepileptic drugs (carbamazepine and phenobarbital) and given a full course of antituberculous drugs. The seizures were well controlled and after about 5 years, anticonvulsants were discontinued.

About 1 year later, the seizures reappeared. Antiepileptic drugs were restarted but the seizures continued in spite of regular medication. This prompted the patient's relatives to consider alternative modes of therapy. The name of one doctor stood out prominently in this regard because he was widely advertised, even in leading newspapers, as a 'specialist in the treatment of epilepsy, having treated more than 25,000 patients over the last 15 years'. These claims were reinforced with highly favorable references from many prominent personalities. This was promising enough for a young man with uncontrolled epilepsy and he approached this doctor with hope of a cure. The antiepileptic drugs were discontinued and he was started on some tablets, which were to be taken daily. However, in spite of regular treatment, the seizures continued with a frequency of about one every month.

Examination and investigations

After several months, the patient came to Bombay Hospital for further advice. Clinical examination was normal. A magnetic resonance imaging scan of the brain showed a small cystic area in the right frontal cortex, probably representing the treated tuberculoma. His routine blood tests were normal. His blood was also sent for measurement of levels of the commonly used antiepileptic drugs. To our surprise, his serum phenytoin level was 13.1 μg/ml (which was in the

202

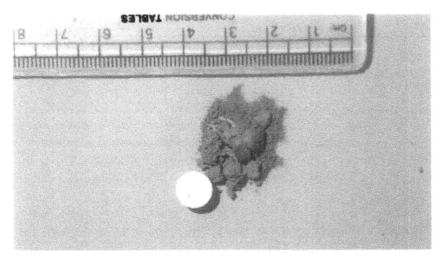

Figure 53.1: *The 'alternative' drugs that were given to the patient. The crushed, brown tablet contained a combination of phenytoin sodium and phenobarbital.*

therapeutic range) and his serum phenobarbital level was 14.8 μg/ml (slightly below the therapeutic level), even though he was supposedly not on either of these drugs! His medicines were then sent to an independent laboratory for analysis and one of the tablets was found to contain a combination of phenytoin sodium and phenobarbital (Fig. 53.1).

Diagnosis

Right frontal lobe epilepsy, probably due to a tuberculous granuloma.

Treatment and outcome

The 'traditional' medicines were discontinued and replaced with conventional antiepileptic drugs. With adjustment of doses and regular serum assays, optimal seizure control was achieved.

Commentary

Why did I choose this case?

Many patients have great faith in alternative systems of medicine. This is especially true in situations where modern medicine is considered to be either ineffectual or when the side effects of therapy are unacceptably severe. The merits of the alternative systems cannot be ignored, but it should be noted that the side effects of alternative drugs and drug interactions are often not clearly defined. Patients and even physicians tend to consider these medicines safe although there may be insufficient evidence to substantiate this claim. Similarly, most physicians do not consider prescription of non-allopathic drugs at the same time as 'conventional' drugs to be potentially harmful, and patients are rarely asked to discontinue 'alternative' drugs when conventional drugs are prescribed. In addition, as with conventional drugs, quality control may at times be suboptimal.

I chose this case because it illustrates the dangers of simultaneous prescription of allopathic and non-allopathic drugs, especially when the quality of drugs is not adequately monitored. With this patient, if conventional antiepileptic drugs had been started without discontinuing the 'alternative' ones, dangerous and even fatal toxic effects could have resulted.

What did I learn from this case?

The important lessons are:

- proper standardization and quality control are essential for all drugs, be they allopathic or non-allopathic;
- side effects and drug interactions of all drugs should be objectively studied and clearly defined;
- patients need to inform their physicians about other medications they may be taking;
- physicians should inform their patients that drug interactions may occur even between allopathic and non-allopathic medicines, and care needs to be exercised when such drugs are used in combination.

Further reading

Angell M, Kassirer JP. Alternative medicine, the risks of untested and unregulated remedies. *N Engl J Med* 1998;**339**:839–41.

Jonas WB. Alternative medicine: learning from the past, examining the present, advancing to the future. *JAMA* 1998;**280**:1616–18.

Psychology Treats Epilepsy (advertisement). *Times of India*. Mumbai; 14 June 1998:3.

Acknowledgment

This case has been reproduced with the kind permission of the publishers of the *Journal of the Royal College of Physicians of London*, in which it was first published as a scientific letter. (Bharucha NE, Kuruvilla T. Co-prescription of conventional and 'alternative medicines'. *J Roy Coll Phys Lon* 1999;**33**:285.)

205

Case 54

A 19-Year-Old Man With Epilepsy, Aphasia And Hemangioma Of The Cranial Vault

Paulo Rogério M de Bittencourt

History

I first met the patient in 1996 when he was 19 years old. He was having daily seizures, could not speak and was either hyperkinetic or autistic depending on the information that the mother chose to believe. He never slept well, never swallowed pills and always had trouble swallowing food. He received excellent attention from his parents and two sisters.

His mother's pregnancy had been normal and his birth had been by forceps. Cyanosis was noted. A laryngeal cyst was diagnosed. Despite esophageal dilatation procedures, he aspirated frequently. At the age of 2 months, the cyst was resected. Five hours after surgery he went into cardiac arrest and was resuscitated, requiring a tracheotomy.

He held up his head at age 3 months, sat at 4 months, made sounds at 8 months, walked at 2 years and controlled his sphincters at 4 years.

At 6 months of age, his sleep worsened. He did not sleep more than a few minutes at a time and was hyperkinetic during the day. When he was 4 years old, his physicians stopped treating him with sedatives because they made him more agitated.

At 5 years of age he developed absences, and Lennox–Gastaut syndrome was diagnosed. Soon after this, he developed drop attacks. At the age of 8 years, he began having tonic–clonic seizures. An eight-channel EEG showed bursts of generalized spike–waves, which were taken to be consistent with Lennox–Gastaut syndrome. An anesthetic accident that occurred during an attempted head computed tomography (CT) scan required resuscitation. Until he was 10 years of age, his buccal hygiene was poor because he would not allow contact with that area. He accepted only liquids and liquefied foods, and then only at the end of every second day. This situation remained until 1996, when he was 19.

206

Examination and investigations

On presentation in 1996 the patient had an expressive aphasia, making grunts and communicating by pointing out things with his eyes and hands. He understood most of what happened around him in spite of having brief absence seizures with eye blinking that occurred almost every minute. I estimated that his IQ, except for the aphasia, was in the 60s. He weighed 85 kg and was ataxic. There were no other physical or neurological abnormalities.

An EEG showed continuous slowing in the left frontocentral region, which frequently spread widely through the left hemisphere (Fig. 54.1) and eventually evolved to frequent absence seizures with blinking and generalized irregular spike–wave discharges. The seizures lasted 4–20 seconds and occurred every 10–30 seconds.

The mother refused to allow further investigations because of the anaesthetic accidents in childhood. Follow-up EEGs showed progressively less frequent abnormalities. Eventually, in late 1996, a waking background rhythm of 5–6 Hz was observed.

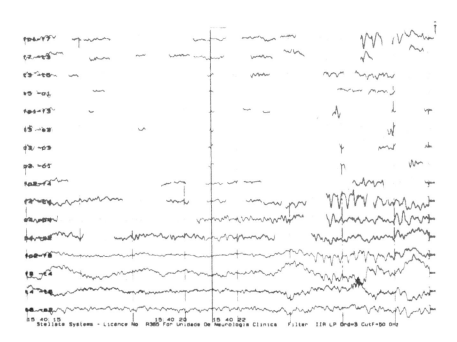

Figure 54.1: EEG showing continuous slowing in the left frontocentral region, which frequently spread widely through the left hemisphere.

A very old CT scan was reportedly normal. In mid-1999, a 99-technetium ECD cerebral single photon emission CT scan showed decreased perfusion in the left perisylvian region. A 2.0T magnetic resonance imaging (MRI) study showed a very large cranial vault hemangioma in the left parietal region. Five months later, a contrast MRI scan followed by a bone-density CT scan showed that the hemangioma was unchanged, had no intracranial extension and did not involve the meninges or cortex.

Diagnosis

A diagnosis of epilepsy with aphasia was made, which was felt to characterize the patient's neurological condition more accurately than either autism or hyperkinetic behaviour.

Treatment and outcome

On presentation in 1996 the patient was receiving valproate 2250 mg/day, carbamazepine 1800 mg/day and clonazepam 10mg/day. His therapy was slowly changed to oxcarbazepine 1600 mg/day and valproate 2000 mg/day. He lost 10 kg of excess weight and developed insomnia. He went into absence status epilepticus, vomiting profusely. Doses were changed to oxcarbazepine 1800 mg/day and valproate 1500 mg/day. In late 1997 he was having absences every few days. His drug regimen was changed to lamotrigine 150 mg/day and valproate 1000 mg/day.

Over the past 4 years, the patient has become a relatively docile and happy young man. He likes travelling by plane, riding cars and playing, but he does not sleep continously for more than 4 hours. He enjoys his family and understands most of what happens. Some of his noises have become objective. His swallowing problem ended in late 1998, allowing him to take tablets regularly and to eat everything. His seizures stopped in early 1999. His only word is *Mãe*, which is the word for Mum in Portuguese.

A thorough search of the literature and consultation with two expert neurosurgoens, including an uncle of the patient, as well as Dr Fred Andermann of Montreal, did not reveal any relationship between the bone malformation and the patient's epilepsy or aphasia. After the follow-up MRI scan showed that the lesion had not changed, everybody decided to leave it alone.

Commentary

This was a difficult case all around – the difficulties in successfully treating the seizures, the combination of seizures and aphasia, and the complex decision-making presented by the rare cranial vault hemangioma.

What did I learn from this case?

This case has reinforced my belief that benzodiazepines are as bad – or worse – than barbiturates. (One of my first publications dealt with this subject.) In my view, prescribing a benzodiazepine or a barbiturate to people with a chronic, long-standing disorder should only be a temporary maneuver. I also learned that Murphy's law applies to complex cases. Such patients may be victims of consecutive tragedies, rarities and mysterious undiagnosable conditions. One can only be humble and take things as they come, just as the families of these patients do.

Further reading

Bittencourt PRM, Richens A. Anticonvulsant-induced status epilepticus in Lennox–Gastaut syndrome: a case report. *Epilepsia* 1981;**22**:129 34.

Bittencourt PRM, Antoniuk AS, Bigarella MM, *et al*. Carbamazepine and phenytoin in epilepsies refractory to barbiturates: efficacy, toxicity and mental function. *Epilepsy Res* 1993;**16**:147–55.

Paillas JE, Grisoli F, Vincentelli F, Hassoun J. Hemangiomas of the cranial vault. Atypical forms: lacunar, pseudomeningiomatous, hyperostotic. *Neurochirurgie* 1977;**23**:475 90.

209

Case 55

SEVERE PSYCHIATRIC DISORDER IN AN 8-YEAR-OLD BOY WITH MYOCLONIC– ASTATIC SEIZURES

Cesare Maria Cornaggia, Alessandra Mascarini and Giuseppe Gobbi

History

This 8-year-old boy with epilepsy was initially diagnosed as autistic. Atypical absences had passed unobserved for a long time – consequently, epilepsy was not considered until he was 6 years old, when brief myoclonic–astatic seizures were recognised. The frequency of the seizures progressively increased until they were occurring more than once a day.

The initial EEG was performed when the patient was aged 6 years and 3 months. It showed background slowing and frequent diffuse spike–wave discharges. Frequent atypical absences were also recorded. Valproate alone and in combination with lamotrigine led to good control of the drop attacks but was associated with a rash and persistent myoclonic head drops. Complete seizure control was obtained for a short period of time with the combination of valproate and clobazam, but at the cost of worsening of the psychiatric and behavioural disturbances.

His behaviour problems were multiple. He jostled himself, avoided his parents and developed marked phobias against strong male figures. He also reported seeing monsters and hearing sudden noises. In addition, regression and disorganization of his language, with a loss of communicative content and an almost continuous use of the third person, were noted. His interests narrowed, and he scarcely involved himself in group activities and showed aggression towards his contemporaries, with little respect for group hierarchies and rules. Manual stereotypies were observed. At school, he subsequently developed marked learning difficulties in reading, writing and arithmetic. In addition, marked attention and concentration deficits were noted, to the extent that his scholastic performance was minimal and possibly non-existent.

His behaviour soon changed to almost continuous closure characterized by complete polarization of attention towards certain cartoon characters (Ninja turtles), which totally absorbed his interest, and the persistence of repetitive and stereotyped attitudes.

210

Examination and investigations

When he presented in November 1999, the patient's behaviour was characterized by impulsiveness with sudden changes in mood, little tolerance of frustration and thoughts that were concentrated on selective interests and motor hyperkinesia.

The neuropsychological assessment revealed markedly labile attention, deficits in concentration and learning (with no scholastic learning) and language atypias such as lexical impoverishment, a lack of relation to context and the use of the third person.

The results of neurological and neuroimaging assessments were normal. EEG examination showed slowing of background activity and frequent diffuse spike–wave discharges, which were more frequent during sleep (Figs 55.1 and 55.2).

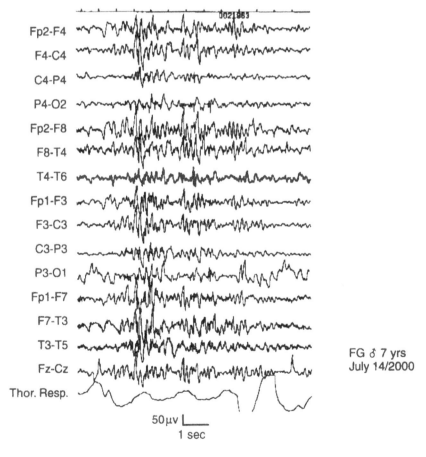

Figure 55.1: *Burst of diffuse spike-and-wave discharges, maximal in the anterior regions.*

211

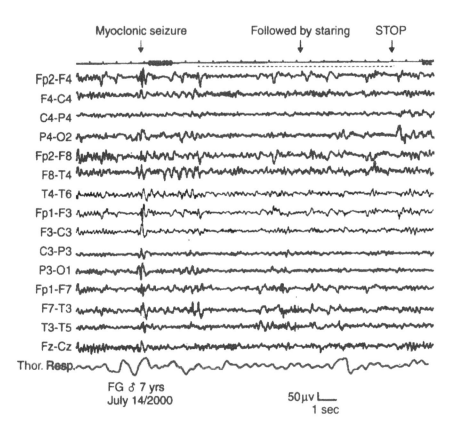

Figure 55.2: *The seizure starts with a myoclonic jerk concomitant with a generalized spike-and-wave discharge and is followed by staring lasting 14 seconds. During this phase, monomorphic theta activity interrupted by rapid rhythm appears bilaterally over the central regions.*

Diagnosis

Psychogenic disorder (DSM-IV 299.80) and 'mental retardation' (DSM-IV 319); epilepsy with myoclonic astatic seizures.

Treatment and outcome

Treatment with felbamate (45 mg/kg per day) and valproate (34.6 mg/kg per day) controlled the drop attacks and markedly decreased the other seizures (such as myoclonic head drops) without causing any severe unwanted psychiatric effects. The improvement in epilepsy was actually accompanied by modest behavioural improvement, although the cognitive difficulties persisted.

Commentary

Why did we choose this case?

We chose this case because it illustrates the interactions between epilepsy and psychiatric, cognitive and behavioural disturbances. Psychiatric, cognitive and behavioural disturbances can sometimes prevail over epileptic symptoms to the extent that the diagnosis of epilepsy is missed altogether for a number of years. Furthermore, in this case, the behavioural, relational and communicative disturbances were associated with a cognitive deficit.

A number of severe epileptic conditions, such as some frontal lobe epilepsies with subcontinuous specific EEG activity (including rapid activity lasting for 1–1.5 seconds) are associated with severe behavioural disturbances (sometimes with psychotic symptoms) or schizophrenia-like or autism-like syndromes. The literature also includes cases of selective cognitive disturbances associated with EEG anomalies, such as the Landau–Kleffner syndrome. There are also other cases in which an early disturbance of language function has led to a disturbance in communication and social interaction, such as the cases reported by Echenne et al.,[1] which others have included among the regressive autistic syndromes with epileptiform anomalies.[2] There are also extreme conditions involving severe and complex impairment of mental functions, such as the continuous spike–wave during sleep syndrome, in which cognitive deterioration (with deficits in attention, memory, problem solving, abstraction and learning) is associated with a behavioural and psychiatric disturbance characterized by hyperkinesia, impulsiveness, perseveration, personality alteration with autistic regression, and disintegrative psychosis. Roulet-Perez et al.[3] and Patry et al.[4] have proposed the hypothesis of an acquired epileptic frontal syndrome in these cases.

Clearly, our case is not as severe as that of the continuous spike–wave during sleep syndrome, and no EEG picture typical of the continuous spike–wave during sleep syndrome has ever been recorded. But is our case less serious because there are fewer EEG findings? And are interictal EEG abnormalities really just that, or could they be the expression of subtle seizures? The extent to which subtle seizures or epileptiform EEG activity affect learning and behaviour remains controversial. One wonders if some children who are diagnosed as having attention deficit disorders or autism may actually have undiagnosed manifestations of epilepsy.[5,6]

What did we learn from this case?

Cases such as this underline the need to clarify the causative role of epilepsy and non-convulsive EEG epileptiform discharges in childhood and adult behavioural problems. We believe that the use of EEG in children and adults with behavioural or learning disturbances should be carefully considered.[5] We similarly believe that it is worth reconsidering interventions aimed at ameliorating interictal EEG discharges, although we recognize that this requires particular prudence and has to be individually evaluated because antiepileptic drugs may, at least partly, disrupt cognitive processing.

We also believe that it is important to report cases such as this one because they are potential sources of serious diagnostic errors, such as the diagnosis of primary autism in this patient, in whom the psychiatric disturbance was probably secondary to the unrecognized epilepsy or secondary to epileptiform EEG discharges (not investigated) even in the absence of clinical seizures. The prognosis of a cognitive and behavioural disturbance of this type greatly depends on its duration, and so precious time may have been lost in this case as a result of the undiagnosed epilepsy.[7]

References

1.   Echenne B, Cheminal R, Rivier F, *et al*. Epileptic electroencephalographic abnormalities and developmental dysphasias: a study of 32 patients. *Brain Dev* 1992;14:216–25.

2.   Touchman R, Rapin I. Regression in pervasive developmental disorders: seizures and EEG correlates. *Pediatrics* 1997;99:560–6.

3.   Roulet-Perez E, Davidiff V, Despland PA, Deonna T. Mental and behavioural deterioration of children with epilepsy and CWCS: acquired epileptic frontal syndrome. *Dev Med Child Neurol* 1993;35:661–74.

4.   Patry G, Lyagoubi S, Tassinari CA. Subclinical 'electrical status epilepticus' induced by sleep in children. *Arch Neurol* 1971;24:242–52.

5.   Cornaggia CM, Gobbi G. Learning disability in epilepsy: definitions and classification. *Epilepsia* 2001;42(suppl 1):2–5.

6.   Hughes JR, DeLeo AJ, Melyn MA. The electroencephalogram in attention deficit disorder: emphasis on epileptiform discharges. *Epilepsy Behav* 2000;1:271–7.

7.   Besag FMC. Epilepsy, learning, and behaviour in childhood. *Epilepsia* 1995;36(suppl 1):58–63.

Case 56

A GIRL WITH TWO EPILEPSY SYNDROMES

Marie-José Penniello, Isabelle Jambaqué, Perrine Plouin and Olivier Dulac

History

The patient is a right-handed girl who was born at full term after a normal pregnancy and delivery. She had two healthy siblings and no familial antecedents of epilepsy. Psychomotor development was initially normal. At the age of 41 months, she had her first febrile convulsion, which consisted of loss of consciousness, trismus and limb hypertonia with massive jerks, mydriasis and cyanosis around the mouth. The convulsion lasted over 30 minutes, but because the onset was not noticed, the precise duration could not be determined. It was followed by right hemiparesis that lasted for several hours. Carbamazepine treatment was started.

At the age of 47 months, a second long-lasting but non-febrile seizure was also followed by transient weakness of the right arm and leg. After recovery from the transient postictal paresis, neurological examination failed to demonstrate any motor defect or pyramidal signs, but there was lack of speech, including very poor comprehension and no expression. The child seemed to react to a few familiar noises, including those produced by some animals, and to very high-pitched sounds, but she did not react to speech. Indeed, during the child's third year of life, the parents had noticed the insidious regression of speech abilities with aggressive behavior and poor interpersonal communication resulting in schooling difficulties. However, they did not seek medical advice for these troubles until the occurrence of the convulsions.

After the second seizure, an EEG showed paroxysmal focal spike–wave activity predominating in the left temporal area, becoming diffuse and continuous in sleep (Fig. 56.1). Transmission deafness could be excluded, and brainstem evoked potentials were normal. Brain magnetic resonance imaging (MRI) disclosed no abnormality (Fig. 56.2).

Landau–Kleffner syndrome was diagnosed and carbamazepine was replaced with the combination of valproate and diazepam. Within 3 months, the EEG tracings returned to normal and the child showed major improvement in speech (both perception and expression). She started to read at the age of 7.5 years.

215

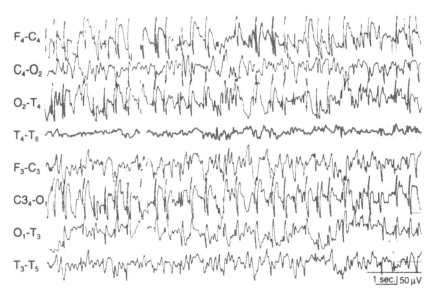

Figure 56.1: *Sleep EEG recording at the age of 4 years, showing interictal paroxysmal spike–wave activity that is continuous and diffuse, although it predominates in the left temporal area.*

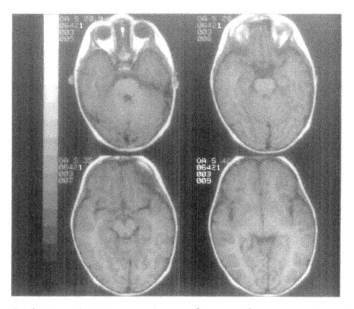

Figure 56.2: *Normal MRI scan at the age of 4 years after the second episode of long-lasting unilateral convulsive seizure. There is no evidence of mesial temporal abnormality.*

216

Sodium valproate was gradually tapered at the age of 7.75 years, and diazepam was stopped 8 months later.

After cessation of treatment, the child remained seizure-free for the next 2.5 years, but at the age of 10.25 years, a new type of seizure occurred. It consisted of an arrest of activity and speech with fixed gaze, bilateral mydriasis and head shaking that seemed to be automatic. When the child resumed normal activity, she complained of epigastric heaviness, and there was complete amnesia of the ictal event. These seizures lasted 30 60 seconds and occurred twice a week.

Investigations

On neuropsychological investigation, the child proved to have good attention. The Wechsler Intelligence Scale for Children (version III) disclosed clear dissociation between verbal abilities (a score of 56) and non-verbal abilities (a score of 90). There were phonological defects and articulation troubles. The Chevrie–Muller test revealed major difficulties in repetition of simple words as well as dyssyntaxia. Naming remained difficult, with phonemic paraphasias. In addition, memory for both verbal and non-verbal items was affected. While these neuropsychological findings are consistent with the Landau–Kleffner syndrome, the patient's persistent speech abnormalities meant that it was not possible to determine whether she was affected by additional cognitive dysfunction consistent with mesial temporal sclerosis.

Ictal EEG recording showed that most discharges affected the left temporal area, although a single seizure affected the right temporal area (Fig. 56.3). An MRI scan showed left mesial temporal atrophy (Fig. 56.4).

Diagnosis

Mesial temporal lobe epilepsy with mesial temporal sclerosis.

Treatment and outcome

Treatment with valproate, gabapentin and vigabatrin failed to control the seizures.

Commentary

Because epilepsy in childhood demonstrates such great variability, the use of epilepsy syndromes to categorize patients considerably helps the clinician to

217

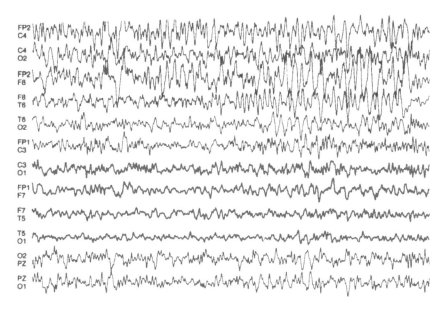

Figure 56.3: Ictal EEG recording at the age of 12 years, showing a right temporal focal seizure discharge. There was no concomitant clinical manifestation.

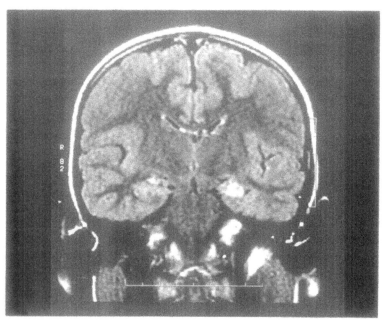

Figure 56.4: FLAIR MRI sequence at the age of 12 years, showing bilateral mesial temporal atrophy, predominating on the left, with hypersignal on this side.

218

approach diagnosis in a pragmatic fashion[1,2] and to select optimal treatment.[3] However, the situation may be complicated when a patient seems to combine two epilepsy syndromes, as in this case.

To our knowledge, this is the first reported case combining Landau–Kleffner syndrome with mesial temporal epilepsy. Although both of these types of epilepsy affect the temporal lobe, they are clearly distinct from each other. One exhibits no evidence of a brain lesion and mainly affects the neocortex during the course of development of speech, while the other results from focal atrophy and affects the mesial temporal lobe after speech is fully acquired. In this patient, both types of epilepsy were separated by a silent period of over 2 years.

The first signs of epilepsy in this case very probably consisted of speech deterioration, although the parents considered this concern as a possible neurological disorder only when the child experienced convulsive seizures. Thus, features of Landau–Kleffner syndrome were the first to appear. EEG abnormalities and speech troubles were controlled when carbamazepine was stopped and replaced by valproate and a benzodiazepine. Corticosteroids are usually advocated to control continuous spike–wave activity in patients with Landau–Kleffner syndrome,[4] but this was not necessary in the present case. Carbamazepine is known to increase spike–wave activity and to eventually trigger the development of continuous spike–waves in slow sleep and its psychomotor correlates.[5] Stopping this drug is therefore a prerequisite for the treatment of this condition.

The other major and very unusual event in the history of this child was the occurrence of two long-lasting, focal motor seizures followed by transient motor deficit. When she presented with mesial temporal epilepsy, the MRI scan showed atrophy that predominated on the side contralateral to the transient postictal motor deficit. This finding was not present on the first MRI scan, which was performed when Landau–Kleffner syndrome was diagnosed.

As in this case, long-lasting seizures followed by motor deficits are known to precede mesial temporal atrophy by several years in a number of patients.[6] The fact that her MRI scan was normal just after the initial episode of status epilepticus suggests that atrophy did not precede this event but rather that it may have been a consequence of it.

In this case, complex partial seizures occurred over a period of 4 years after the disappearance of the continuous spike–waves in slow sleep. Ictal recording showed that these new seizures originated from the left temporal lobe, the site of the hippocampal sclerosis that was disclosed on MRI.

What did we learn from this case?

The relationship between Landau–Kleffner syndrome and mesial temporal sclerosis is difficult to establish. Mesial temporal sclerosis is not a usual finding in patients with Landau–Kleffner syndrome, in which the MRI scan is most often normal,[7] as was the case in this child when the syndrome was identified. In an attempt to improve speech in patients with Landau–Kleffner syndrome, temporal lobectomies have been performed, but without success.[8] The most striking characteristic of Landau–Kleffner syndrome is, in fact, the scarcity of ictal discharges. The animal model of continuous spike–wave activity developed by Barbarosie and Avoli[9] demonstrated the difficulty in eliciting tonic discharges, which are the hallmark of convulsive status epilepticus, as if continuous spike–wave activity could prevent tonic discharges.

Therefore, any cause-and-effect relationship between Landau–Kleffner syndrome and mesial temporal sclerosis in this case is most unlikely. However, both the epilepsy syndromes exhibited by this patient could in fact have resulted from a common predisposition to epilepsy that produced both status epilepticus and major spike–wave activity. Pre-existing anatomical anomalies that were not disclosed on either MRI scan, such as microdysgenesis, cannot be ruled out.

There is growing evidence that cognitive functions are affected differently in different epilepsy syndromes.[10] In this patient, the cognitive troubles were those of Landau–Kleffner syndrome, but memory disturbances related to mesial temporal sclerosis could not be identified because of the limited language function.[11] Therefore, this case taught us that the impact of continuous spike–wave activity on developing speech during childhood is so striking that it masks the later effects of hippocampal sclerosis and mesial temporal epilepsy.

References

1. Roger J, Bureau M, Dravet C, Dreifuss F, Perret A, Wolf P. *Epileptic syndromes in infancy, childhood and adolescence*. London: John Libbey; 1991.

2. Commission on Classification and Terminology of the International League against Epilepsy. Proposal for revised classification of epilepsies and epileptic syndromes. *Epilepsia* 1989;30:389–99.

3. Dulac O, Leppik I. Initiating and discontinuation treatment. In: Engel J, Pedley J, eds. *Epilepsy: a comprehensive textbook*. New York: Lippincott–Raven; 1998;1237–46.

4. Lerman P, Lerman-Sagie T, Kivity S. Effects of early corticosteroid therapy for Landau–Kleffner syndrome. *Dev Med Child Neurol* 1991;33:257–60.

5. Perucca E, Gram L, Avanzini G, Dulac O. Antiepileptic drugs as a cause of worsening seizures. *Epilepsia* 1998;39:5–17.

6. Cendes F, Andermann F, Dubeau F, *et al*. Early childhood prolonged febrile convulsions, atrophy and sclerosis of mesial structures, and temporal lobe epilepsy: an MRI volumetric study. *Neurology* 1993;43:1083–7.

7. O'Regan ME, Brown JK, Goodwin GM, Clarke M. Epileptic aphasia: a consequence of regional hypometabolic encephalopathy? *Dev Med Child Neurol* 1998;**40**:508–16.

8. Cole AJ, Andermann F, Taylor L, *et al*. The Landau–Kleffner syndrome of acquired epileptic aphasia: unusual clinical outcome, surgical experience, and absence of encephalitis. *Neurology* 1988;**38**:31 8.

9. Barbarosie M, Avoli M. CA3-driven hippocampal–entorhinal loop controls rather than sustains *in vitro* limbic seizures. *J Neurosci* 1997;**17**:9308–14.

10. Dulac O. Mechanisms, classification and management of seizures and epilepsies. In: Jambaqué I, Lassonde M, Dulac O, eds. *Neuropsychology of epilepsy in childhood*. (in press).

11. Jambaqué I, Dellatolas G, Dulac O, Ponsot G, Signoret JL. Verbal and visual memory impairment in children with epilepsy. *Neuropsychologia* 1993;**31**:1321–37.

Addendum

We have just learned that the patient whose story is reported here was shown to have neuropathologically hippocampal sclerosis and nodular heterotopias, discovered following surgery.

THE OBVIOUS CAUSE OF SEIZURES MAY NOT BE THE UNDERLYING CAUSE

Keith R Edwards

History

The patient is a 48-year-old man with a previous history of alcohol and drug abuse. He presented to the emergency department following a generalized tonic–clonic seizure. He had no history of seizures and no history of head trauma, but he did have a recent history of alcohol abuse with decreasing amounts over the last several days, although he had not totally stopped drinking.

Examination and investigations

In the emergency department, the patient was initially postictal but without focal findings. A cranial computed tomography (CT) scan without contrast was unremarkable, and the patient quickly regained orientation. He was not started on any anticonvulsant therapy. Outpatient follow-up with EEG was scheduled in 1–2 weeks.

However, 48 hours later, the patient returned in status epilepticus. He responded to lorazepam 2 mg intravenously. He was then given phenytoin 1g intravenously without further seizures, but he had a prolonged postictal state that required careful observation. He aspirated and was treated for pneumonia. Repeat cranial CT with and without contrast was unremarkable. The patient could not co-operate for a magnetic resonance imaging (MRI) scan. EEG showed generalized slowing but no seizure activity.

Initial diagnosis

Seizures related to alcohol abuse and past history of head trauma (the patient had had numerous falls).

Treatment and outcome

Following the episode of status epilepticus, it was determined that long-term phenytoin was necessary. He was therefore discharged on phenytoin 300 mg daily and did well for the next 3 months. He attended Alcoholics Anonymous and remained free of further seizure activity. On two office visits 6 weeks apart, the patient had a normal examination, including a normal cognitive status.

The patient then began having right arm tremor associated with an altered state of consciousness and loss of speech lasting 5–10 minutes. He was seen in the emergency department and found to have undetectable phenytoin levels. He was given 500 mg phenytoin intravenously. He was felt to be non-compliant.

However, over the next 2 weeks, the patient continued to have intermittent complex partial seizures with a therapeutic phenytoin level.

The EEG was repeated, showing focal slowing in the left frontal region. Cranial MRI showed a neoplasm in the left frontal lobe. Craniotomy revealed high-grade malignancy consistent with glioblastoma multiforme.

Commentary

The patient had an all-too-familiar seizure presentation associated with alcohol. However, when the seizure pattern changed to multiple complex partial seizures, further imaging was done with MRI scanning. The underlying neoplasm was found in a reasonably timely fashion but there was still considered to be a delay, owing to the multifactorial aspect of the patient's seizure etiology.

What did I learn from this case?

In this case, timely follow-up with the patient and listening to his complaints and those of his family saved the patient from a delayed diagnosis, from which there may have been more disastrous results. I learned that patients may have multiple etiologies for seizures and to reconsider the underlying cause if the seizure type or frequency changes.

How did this case alter my approach to the care and treatment of my epilepsy patients?

Although alcohol abuse is a common cause of seizures, I am more alert to patients' breakthrough seizures, particularly with any focal type of symptomatology. The presentation of status epilepticus just 2 days after a first seizure, even with alcohol, should have prompted me to follow up with an MRI scan sooner than was done in this case, once the patient was stable and able to co-operate. The fact that he had continued seizures long after he was alcohol-free should have altered my thinking away from the patient's alcohol as a precipitating factor of his seizure to other etiologies.

Case 58

ABSENCE SEIZURES IN AN ADULT

Edward Faught

History

The patient is a 53-year-old woman with a history of seizures beginning at the age of 5 years. The seizures occurred several times daily when she was a young child. Witnesses described a sudden blank stare, sometimes accompanied by humming or picking at her clothes. Occasionally she walked around during the episodes but she never fell down. Urinary incontinence occurred with some of the seizures up until the age of 12. Although she never had a warning or an aura, she usually knew when she had a seizure because she recalled a sensation 'as if daydreaming'. She specifically described this as not merely a loss of time but as a definite feeling. She has had only four generalized tonic–clonic seizures in her life, each proceeded by an odd feeling of 'going down a tunnel.'

Precipitating factors included the premenstrual state and 'stress'. As a car passenger, she noted that sunlight flickering through the trees made her feel as if she were going to have a seizure.

Previous treatments had included phenobarbital, ethosuximide, phenytoin, primidone and acetazolamide. She had a previous EEG that was abnormal, but she reported that her doctors couldn't decide whether she had 'petit mal' or 'frontal' seizures. When I first saw her, she was 42 years old and was taking carbamazepine 1400 mg/day. She was having up to 20 seizures each day, and she stated that she had never gone more than 3 days in her life without seizures. Despite this, she had 13 years of education, was married with children and had a supervisory job.

Examination and investigations

General and neurological examinations were normal. The patient appeared to be of above-average intelligence. An EEG demonstrated hyperventilation-induced three-per-second spike–wave discharges with a generalized distribution and a bifrontal voltage maximum. One of these discharges lasted 14 seconds and was

225

accompanied by staring, lip smacking and patting the thigh with the right hand. No photosensitivity was detected. A magnetic resonance imaging scan was normal.

Diagnosis

Childhood-onset absence epilepsy persisting into adult life.

Treatment and outcome

Valproate was begun and gradually increased to 30 mg/kg per day, and carbamazepine was stopped. The patient improved immediately, but she still had one or two seizures each day. Over the next 5 years, addition of ethosuximide or felbamate to valproate was of little help. At the age of 47, a lamotrigine–ethosuximide combination rendered her seizure-free. After 3 years without seizures, at her request, and after a normal 24-hour ambulatory EEG, first ethosuximide then lamotrigine was tapered and stopped, during a 6-month driving restriction. She has remained free of seizures, off all medications, for 3 years. A recent 24-hour ambulatory EEG recording was normal.

Commentary

This patient was treated with carbamazepine because she was thought to have complex partial seizures. This error could have been avoided by recognizing that:

- automatisms occur in 38–63 % of absence seizures;[1,2]
- in adults, generalized spike–wave discharges usually have a frontal voltage predominance, and may be asymmetrical;[3] and
- that patients with generalized epilepsies may have prodromal sensations and unusual perceptions.[4]

Nevertheless, differentiation of absence from frontal lobe complex partial seizures can be quite difficult. Bancaud et al.[3] demonstrated experimentally that stimulation of mesial frontal structures can produce symmetrical spike–wave discharges, and it is clear that this happens clinically. This EEG phenomenon is called 'secondary bilateral synchrony.' The assumption that adults with staring spells have complex partial seizures should be examined in each case.

Carbamazepine often worsens absence seizures,[5] so that this distinction is important. Eventual complete control of seizures in this patient required a prolonged, determined quest culminating in an exotic combination of medications – ethosuximide and lamotrigine.

Because 92 % of patients with late persistent absences have generalized tonic–clonic seizures as well,[6] ethosuximide alone should not be relied on for therapy; it should be combined with valproate or a sodium channel blocking agent. Of the sodium channel blockers, lamotrigine may also have some antiabsence action, and phenytoin may be less likely to exacerbate absence than carbamazepine or oxcarbazepine. If valproate is unsatisfactory as monotherapy, another broad-spectrum drug such as lamotrigine, topiramate, zonisamide or eventually felbamate may be considered.

Perhaps the most surprising feature of this case was the occurrence of a terminal remission of seizures after 49 years, including 42 years of therapeutic futility. Gastaut *et al.*[6] studied the course of primary generalized epilepsy with absences persisting after the age of 30 up to the age of 61 and found that remission was rare, although the frequency of seizures tended to diminish with time. Although it is not wise to raise false hopes, it is comforting to know that remissions may occur even after half a century of troubles.

What did I learn from this case?

A diagnosis of seizure type requires careful consideration of age of onset, seizure semiology, patient report, EEG pattern and response to therapy – and is not always simple. Patients with generalized epilepsies may report experiential phenomena that are easy to interpret as aurae of partial-onset seizures.

Not all absence epilepsies are easily treated, but one should never give up. I found an odd but surprisingly effective medication combination, so an empirical trial of an unreported polytherapy may be worthwhile.

How did this case alter my approach to the care and treatment of my epilepsy patients?

I am less smug when informing patients with a new diagnosis of absence epilepsy that they have an easily treatable syndrome. I look more carefully at my patients with diagnoses of frontal lobe complex partial seizures to consider whether they might have a primary generalized disorder. I do not dismiss out of hand a patient's request to try a medication taper after years of absence seizures, but I do carefully negotiate the conditions of the discontinuation, including restrictions on driving. I also routinely obtain a 24–48 hour EEG recording before beginning the process and again before removing activity restrictions at the end.

227

References

1. Penry JK, Porter RJ, Dreifuss FE. Simultaneous recording of absence seizures with videotape and EEG. *Brain* 1975;**98**:427–40.

2. Stefan H, Burr W, Hildenbrand K, Penin H. Computer-supported documentation in the video analysis of absences; preictal–ictal phenomena: polygraphic findings. In: Dam M, Gram L, Penry JK, eds. *Advances in epileptology: the XIIIth Epilepsy International Symposium.* New York: Raven Press, 1981.

3. Bancaud J, Talairach J, Morel P, *et al.* 'Generalized' epileptic seizures elicited by electrical stimulation of the frontal lobe in man. *Electroencephalogr Clin Neurophysiol* 1974;**37**:275–82.

4. Faught E, Falgout J, Nidiffer FD, Dreifuss FE. Self-induced photosensitive absence seizures with ictal pleasure. *Arch Neurol* 1986;**43**:408–10.

5. Snead OC, Hosey LC. Exacerbation of seizures in children by carbamazepine. *N Engl J Med* 1985;**313**:916–21.

6. Gastaut H, Zifkin BG, Mariana E, Pulg JS. The long-term course of primary generalized epilepsy with persisting absences. *Neurology* 1986;**36**:1021–8.

Case 59

A CASE SOLVED BY SEIZURES DURING SLEEP

Jacqueline A French

History

The patient was an 18-year-old right-handed woman who had seizures dating back to the age of 2 years. These initially consisted of staring, picking at clothes, automatisms and pacing the room. She was treated through her childhood with phenobarbital, carbamazepine, phenytoin and primidone. By her adolescence, the patient's seizures had changed in character. They were now described as thrashing, rocking back and forth, at times striking out in a seemingly purposeful way, and injuring herself, with resultant ecchymoses of the elbow and forehead. Seizures also increased in frequency, so that she was having multiple seizures each day, preventing her from attending school. Medication included primidone, valproate and phenytoin.

The patient had a significant family history. Her maternal great-grandfather and first cousin had generalized tonic–clonic convulsions and her brother may have had a partial seizure. Her mother was institutionalized with schizophrenia.

Examination and investigations

Physical and neurologic examinations were normal, as were magnetic resonance imaging scan and EEG.

The patient was admitted for video-EEG monitoring. Standard and sphenoidal electrodes were placed. Background EEG was entirely normal. Eight typical events were recorded, consisting of clenching her teeth, clenching her fist and shaking in a rhythmical fashion. She would frequently utter sentences or fragments of sentences that might include obscenities. There was no apparent alteration of consciousness, and the patient was able to respond to commands to move extremities during the event. She seemed anxious and upset during these events, and she had full recollection of them afterwards. During the events there was no discernible electrographic discharge. Because of this, a diagnosis of psychogenic seizures was made.

The patient continued to have frequent events and was therefore transferred to a psychiatric unit. After discharge, daytime events decreased markedly in frequency for several months. However, the patient presented again after about 6 months. Her father reported that he had witnessed no daytime events but that episodes were occurring nightly during sleep.

The patient was readmitted for video-EEG monitoring. Multiple nocturnal events were recorded. These events had identical clinical characteristics as had been seen during the first monitoring session and, again, no ictal or interictal EEG changes were noted. However, some events occurred directly out of stage 2 sleep, and the patient returned directly to sleep afterwards. This prompted subsequent intracranial EEG monitoring, which confirmed that both the diurnal and nocturnal events were frontal lobe complex partial seizures.

Diagnosis

Frontal lobe complex partial seizures.

Treatment and outcome

A right mesial frontal resection was performed. Pathology revealed microdysgenesis and gliosis.

Commentary

This patient had many characteristics that led to a diagnosis of psychogenic seizures:

- a family history of psychiatric disease;
- a change in seizure semiology from her childhood seizures;
- events with no loss of awareness, purposeful movements, and full recall; and
- normal ictal and interictal EEGs.

In fact, she was having frontal lobe complex partial seizures. Several characteristics of her seizures might have raised suspicion of this diagnosis, including the fact that the events were brief and stereotyped, with rapid return to normal function. Another clue was the occurrence of stereotyped events

230

in sleep, without awakening. These characteristics have been identified in several articles on frontal lobe epilepsy.[1] [3] These articles also report characteristic seizure manifestations in patients with frontal lobe complex partial seizures, including:

* bilateral movements and complex automatisms, which are often bizarre;
* vocalizations; and
* a high seizure frequency.

The absence of an ictal or interictal correlate, although rare, may be seen in patients with frontal lobe foci.[1,2]

It is important to distinguish patients with frontal lobe complex partial seizures from those with non-epileptic seizures. Usually, diagnosis requires admission to a video-EEG monitoring unit and withdrawal of any antiepileptic drugs. Such withdrawal may increase seizure spread, causing identifiable EEG ictal changes. Inpatient monitoring may allow recognition of seizures beginning directly out of stage 2 sleep, as in this case. Such findings are rarely or never seen in patients with psychogenic events.[3]

If a diagnosis of frontal lobe complex partial seizures is confirmed and the patient has been demonstrated to be refractory to antiepileptic drug therapy, referral for surgical management should be considered. Up to 67 % of patients with an identified frontal focus may become seizure-free after surgical resection.[1]

What did I learn from this case?

I learned that there is a great deal of overlap between the characteristics of pseudoseizures and those of frontal lobe complex partial seizures. Both may cause events that are bizarre in appearance. The presence or absence of an ictal discharge does not absolutely distinguish between the two. Patients may be responsive throughout a bizarre ictal event that is physiological in nature.

How did this case alter my approach to the care and treatment of my epilepsy patients?

I am always very aware of the characteristics that may indicate frontal lobe complex partial seizures. I am careful to ask family members about nocturnal events that mimic events seen during the day. I will not rush to a diagnosis of psychogenic seizures based on one or two brief events seen in the monitoring unit if these events have any characteristics of frontal lobe complex partial seizures. In these patients, I will withdraw antiepileptic drugs while continuing monitoring. Also, I feel that some patients who have received a diagnosis of psychogenic seizures deserve a second evaluation if seizures do not remit.

231

References

1. Laskowitz DT, Sperling MR, French JA, O'Connor MJ. The syndrome of frontal lobe epilepsy: Characteristics and surgical management. *Neurology* 1995;**45**:780–7.

2. Williamson PD, Spencer DD, Spencer SS, Novelly RA, Mattson RH. Complex partial seizures of frontal lobe origin. *Ann Neurol* 1985;**18**:497–504.

3. Saygi S, Katz A, Marks DA, Spencer SS. Frontal lobe partial seizures and psychogenic seizures: comparison of clinical and ictal characteristics. *Neurology* 1992;**42**:1274–7.

Case 60

ALTERNATIVE PSYCHOSIS IN AN ADOLESCENT GIRL?

Andres M Kanner

History

The patient is a 17-year-old adolescent girl with a history of partial epilepsy of unknown etiology. Her seizures began at 17 months of age and have consisted primarily of complex partial seizures and less frequently of secondarily generalized tonic–clonic seizures. The semiology of her seizures and her ictal recordings are suggestive of frontal lobe epilepsy.

Examination and investigations

Prolonged video-EEG monitoring studies with scalp and intracranial electrodes failed to identify the exact location of the ictal onset. No abnormalities were identified with high-resolution brain magnetic imaging resonance scans. Testing revealed an IQ in the mild mentally retarded range.

Diagnosis

Probable frontal lobe onset seizures.

Treatment and outcome

The patient's seizures had failed to respond to multiple trials of antiepileptic drugs and to vagal nerve stimulation. At the age of 15 years, after being started on clonazepam (in combination with carbamazepine) and reaching a dose of 1.5 mg/day, her seizures stopped completely.

After being seizure-free for a period of 6 weeks, her parents noted a change in her behavior – she became irritable and refused to use the toilet to urinate. The patient claimed that 'she was a baby' and she therefore insisted on wearing diapers. She refused to go to the bathroom when she had the urge to urinate and would often hold the urine until she would become incontinent. Treatment with sertraline (selective serotonin reuptake inhibitor) and behavioral strategies were unsuccessful.

After several weeks, her behavior became increasingly more erratic. She seemed to be responding to auditory hallucinations and a thought disorder became apparent. Sertraline was discontinued and she was started on haloperidol. Failure to respond to neuroleptic medication led me to taper clonazepam off at a rate of 0.25 mg/week. Her psychiatric symptoms disappeared 2 days after she experienced a generalized tonic–clonic seizure that occurred upon reaching a daily dose of clonazepam of 0.25 mg/day.

In the past 2 years, this patient has had two additional prolonged seizure-free periods. The first period, while she was on a combination of valproate and lamotrigine, lasted for 4 months; the second period (while she was on levetiracetam, valproate and lamotrigine), has so far lasted 9 months. In the course of these seizure-free periods, the patient has not had a recurrence of psychotic symptoms, despite the fact that she had been restarted on clonazepam after the seizures recurred while on valproate and lamotrigine. She does experience frequent episodes of increased irritability and poor frustration tolerance that have occasionally been associated with short bouts of aggressive behavior. This cluster of symptoms has been controlled to a certain degree with two selective serotonin reuptake inhibitors (sertraline and paroxetine).

During a recent attempt to taper off valproate, the patient developed insomnia, pressured speech and increased energy. Sertraline was discontinued but these symptoms disappeared only after she was placed back on higher doses of valproate.

Commentary

I chose this case because it exemplifies the complex relationship between epilepsy and psychiatric disorders. The psychotic episode that followed a complete cessation of seizure activity could be an example of the phenomenon of 'alternative psychosis'.[1] At first I could not exclude the possibility that clonazepam may have been the culprit for this patient's psychiatric symptoms. Yet a significant reduction of its dose failed to yield any improvement in her psychiatric symptoms, which remitted only after she experienced a generalized tonic–clonic seizure. Furthermore, a subsequent reintroduction of clonazepam was not associated with recurrence of these symptoms.

The concept of alternative psychosis was developed from observations by

234

Landolt in 1953 of an inverse relationship between control of seizures and occurrence of psychotic symptoms.[2] In fact, Landolt described a 'normalization' of EEG recordings with the appearance of psychiatric symptoms and coined the term 'forced normalization'. Wolf and Trimble suggested the term 'paradoxical normalization' while Tellenbach proposed the term of 'alternative psychosis'.[1]

This phenomenon is rare. Landolt reported 47 cases between 1951 and 1958. Single case studies were reported by others,[3] and in 1988, Schmitz estimated the prevalence of alternative psychosis to be of 1 % among 697 patients followed at a university epilepsy center.[4]

Forced normalization has been reported in patients with temporal lobe epilepsy and generalized epilepsy. The psychotic manifestations were identified after a relatively long duration of the seizure disorder. Wolf reported a 15-year history of epilepsy in 23 patients.[5] Both Landolt and Wolf reported a pleomorphic clinical presentation, with a paranoid psychosis without clouding of consciousness being the most frequent manifestation. As with other types of psychosis in epilepsy, a richness of affective symptoms is a characteristic finding.

As stated above, although the psychotic episodes in this patient could be construed as an expression of an 'alternative psychosis' phenomenon, subsequent prolonged seizure-free periods have not resulted in a recurrence of psychotic symptoms or bizarre behavior. In fact, after 9 months of being seizure-free on levetiracetam, valproate and lamotrigine and a low dose (5 mg/day) of paroxetine, the patient is attending school on a daily basis. With the exception of occasional outbursts of anger and irritability, she is functioning well. This may, in fact, be one of the unusual features of this case: namely, that it exemplifies that the phenomenon of 'alternative psychosis' need not be a chronic process but can occur as an isolated event. On the other hand, I cannot exclude the possibility that the mood-stabilizing properties of valproate and lamotrigine[6] are 'protecting' this patient from subsequent psychotic episodes.

What did I learn from this case? How did this case alter my approach to the care and treatment of my epilepsy patients?

This case highlights the multiple variables that can operate in the psychiatric comorbidity of patients with epilepsy. I am now more careful to perform a thorough assessment of the role of negative and positive psychotropic properties of antiepileptic drugs, the patient's risk factors for psychopathology (i.e. past personal and familial psychiatric history) and the actual impact of seizure occurrence versus seizure control as determinants of psychopathology.

References

1. Tellenbach H. Epilepsie als Anfallseiden und als Psychosen. Über alternative psychosen paranoider Pragung bei 'forcierter Normalisierung' (Landoldt) des Elektroencephalogramms Epileptischer. *Nervenarzt* 1965;**36**:190.

2. Landoldt H. Some clinical electroencephalographical correlations in epileptic psychosis (twilight states)[abstract]. *Electroencephalogr Clin Neurophysiol* 1953;**5**:121.

3. Ried S, Mothersill IW. Forced normalization: the clinical neurologist's view. In: Trimble MR Schmitz B, eds. *Forced Normalization and alternative psychoses of epilepsy*. Petersfield: Wrightson Biomedical Publishing; 1998:77 94.

4. Schmitz B. Psychosen bei Epilepsie. Eine epidemiologische Untersuchung. PhD Thesis, West Berlin.

5. Wolf P. The prevention of alternative psychosis in outpatients. In: Janz D, ed. *Epileptology*, Stuttgart: Thieme; 1976:75–9.

6. Kanner AM, Palac S. Depression in epilepsy: A common but often unrecognized comorbid malady. *Epilepsy Behav* 2000;**1**:37–51.

Case 61

EXACERBATION OF SEIZURES IN A YOUNG WOMAN

Pavel Klein

History

A 31-year-old woman suffered head trauma with transient coma at the age of 3 years and developed seizures at the age of 16. The seizures consisted of feeling strange and vertiginous, with a feeling of impending doom, word-finding difficulties, speech perseveration and inability to focus her thoughts. They lasted 4–5 minutes and were followed by drowsiness. They occurred once or twice a month, mostly 2–3 days after the onset of menstruation or at the time of ovulation. Rarely (five or six times during 15 years), the patient had secondary generalization. Over the past 2–3 years, her seizures became more frequent – three or four times a month – and the perimenstrual worsening became less apparent, although the patient still felt that the seizures and her menses were related.

She was treated with phenytoin 300 mg at bedtime. Past treatments had included carbamazepine, phenobarbital and valproate.

Past medical history was positive for recent gingivectomy. Family history was significant for hypothyroidism and anxiety but negative for epilepsy. The patient's menarche had occurred at the age of 13, with initially regular menses that had become irregular, every 5–10 weeks, 3 years earlier. She had developed hirsutism during the past 3 years.

Examination and investigations

The patient was mildly overweight and mildly hirsute (on the face, arms and legs). The rest of the general and neurological examinations were normal.

Evaluations included an EEG, which showed occasional left anterior spike discharges and theta slowing, and a normal magnetic resonance imaging scan.

Reproductive endocrine evaluations showed mild hyperandrogenism (free testosterone level 0.3 ng/dl, normal <0.2 ng/dl), elevated ratio of luteinizing hormone to follicular stimulating hormone (menstrual cycle day 3 luteinizing hormone 12.4 IU, follicular stimulating hormone 4.7 IU; normal LH:FSH ratio <2.5), and the presence of anovulatory menstrual cycles with impaired luteal ovarian progesterone secretion (menstrual cycle day 22 estradiol level 182 pg/ml, normal 50–270 pg/ml), progesterone 1.2 ng/ml (normal >6 ng/ml). These findings were consistent with the diagnosis of polycystic ovarian syndrome with mild hyperandrogenism. An ovarian ultrasound showed a couple of ovarian cysts bilaterally.

Trough phenytoin level was 21.4 µg/ml on menstrual cycle day 22 and 16.1 µg/ml on menstrual cycle day 1. Triphasil, an estrogen-containing oral contraceptive preparation, was started by the patient's gynecologist for the treatment of the polycystic ovarian syndrome. Seizures worsened so that they were occurring five or six times a month, and the patient had three secondarily generalized seizures in 2 months. Repeated estradiol level on triphasil was 661 pg/ml.

Diagnoses

Polycystic ovarian syndrome and anovulatory menstrual cycles. Seizure exacerbation related to polycystic ovarian syndrome and to estrogen-containing therapy.

Treatment and outcome

An increase of phenytoin dose to 400 mg at bedtime produced mild somnolence and diplopia with a level of 24.0 µg/ml. The dose was reduced back to 300 mg at bedtime. Oral progesterone was added at 600 mg/day in three divided doses on days 1 to 12 of each calendar month, with taper over days 13 to 15. After three menstrual cycles, the menses became more regular – every 30–35 days – and the progesterone administration was changed to days 15 to 28 of each menstrual cycle. Seizure frequency decreased to one seizure every 2 months, often at the time of progesterone withdrawal, which was improved further by a slow taper over 4 days. On menstrual cycle day 22, the estradiol level was 89 pg/ml and the progesterone level was 28 ng/ml. The patient experienced mild breast discomfort and feeling of fullness and a 3 kg weight gain. The mastalgia improved with progesterone dose reduction to 500 mg/day in three divided doses (200 mg, 100 mg, 200 mg).

Commentary

This patient had partial complex seizures with perimenstrual and periovulatory exacerbation of seizures (catamenial epilepsy type 1 and 2).[1] Twelve years after the onset of seizures, she developed a reproductive endocrine disorder (polycystic ovarian syndrome), with concomitant exacerbation of her seizures. The customary gynecological treatment of this condition further exacerbated her seizures. Treatment with natural progesterone improved both the seizures and the polycystic ovarian syndrome.

Temporal lobe epilepsy is associated with increased risk of reproductive endocrine disorders.[2] Left-sided temporal lobe epilepsy is associated with an increased incidence of polycystic ovarian syndrome, while right-sided temporal lobe epilepsy may be associated with hypothalamic hypogonadism.[2,3] In either case, the reproductive endocrine consequence is the development of anovulatory cycles.[4] During anovulatory cycles, the ovary continues to secrete estrogen, but secretion of progesterone is minimal. Estrogens have proconvulsant properties whereas progesterone has potent anticonvulsant properties.[4] Thus, the development of reproductive endocrine disorders such as polycystic ovarian syndrome or hypothalamic hypogonadism in women with temporal lobe epilepsy may lead to exacerbation of seizures, as occurred in this case. Progesterone is a potent inhibitor of neuronal excitation because of its potentiating effect on gamma-aminobutyric acid A receptors. This effect is exerted indirectly, via allopregnanolone, a metabolite of progesterone, but it is very potent, equal to the most potent of benzodiazepines.[4,5] Progesterone may thus be used as an adjunct anticonvulsant and has been shown to be effective in several open label studies in women with temporal lobe epilepsy, refractory seizures and reproductive endocrine disorders.[6]

In women with perimenstrual seizure exacerbation, reduced serum levels of phenytoin and possibly of other antiepileptic drugs that induce hepatic enzymes may also be associated with perimenstrual seizure exacerbation, as may have occurred in the present case. When menses are predictable, increase in the dose of the antiepileptic drug 7–10 days before expected menstruation may be an effective treatment. Because this patient's menses were irregular, it was not feasible to adjust the phenytoin dose perimenstrually. Adjunct treatment with natural progesterone may be beneficial in such cases, as it was here.[7]

What did I learn from this case?

I learned that chronic temporal lobe epilepsy can lead to the development of a reproductive endocrine disorder, and that the development of such a reproductive endocrine disorder may be associated with worsening of previously stable seizures. I also learned how important it is to pay attention to the hormonal treatment of a reproductive endocrine disorder – one treatment (an estrogen-containing oral contraceptive) exacerbated the patient's seizures, whereas another treatment (progesterone) improved both the reproductive endocrine disorder and the seizures.

239

How did this case alter my approach to the care and treatment of my epilepsy patients?

I pay attention to reproductive history in women with epilepsy. I include a history of hormonal factors in my evaluation of possible exacerbating factors of a seizure disorder. In my female patients with temporal lobe epilepsy, I look for clinical evidence of anovulatory cycles, such as menstrual cycles that are too short (under 23 days) or too long (over 35 days), and also for other evidence of reproductive endocrine dysfunction, such as hirsutism. I work closely with my gynecological colleagues to decide on the most appropriate hormonal treatment for patients with epilepsy and reproductive endocrine dysfunction. I also keep in my mind the possibility of hormonal therapy as adjunct treatment for seizures in women with refractory epilepsy and reproductive endocrine dysfunction.

References

1. Herzog AG, Klein P, Ransil BJ. Three patterns of catamenial epilepsy. *Epilepsia* 1997;**38**:1082–8.

2. Herzog AG, Seibel MM, Schomer DL, et al. Reproductive endocrine disorders in women with partial seizures of temporal lobe origin. *Arch Neurol* 1986;**43**:341–6.

3. Drislane FW, Coleman AE, Schomer DL, et al. Altered pulsatile secretion of luteinizing hormone in women with epilepsy. *Neurology* 1994;**44**:306–10.

4. Klein P, Herzog AG. Hormonal effects on epilepsy in women. *Epilepsia* 1998;**39(suppl 8)**:S9–S16.

5. Paul SM, Purdy RH. Neuroactive steroids. *FASEB J* 1992;**6**:2311–22.

6. Herzog AG. Progesterone therapy in women with complex partial and secondary generalized seizures. *Neurology* 1995;**45**:1660–2.

7. Roscizewska D, Buntner B, Guz I, et al. Ovarian hormones, anticonvulsant drugs and seizures during the menstrual cycle in women with epilepsy. *J Neurol Neurosurg Psychiatry* 1986;**49**:47–51.

Case 62

Genetic Counseling In A Woman With A Family History Of Refractory Myoclonic Epilepsy

Dick Lindhout

History

A woman with therapy-resistant epilepsy was referred for genetic counseling. Her first male child had moderate mental retardation. The patient wanted to know the cause of her epilepsy while hoping that this would lead to a better treatment resulting in seizure freedom. Her husband was more concerned about the risk of epilepsy and mental retardation to subsequent offspring.

At the age of 10 years, the patient had her first generalized tonic–clonic seizure while watching television. Subsequently, myoclonic seizures developed, initially during the morning shortly after awakening but gradually more evenly distributed over the day. The seizures predominantly affected the trunk and the proximal extremities. Generalized tonic–clonic seizures continued infrequently.

The patient's past medication history consisted of an extensive list of different antiepileptic drugs used singly and in combinations, including 6 years of phenytoin. However, the myoclonic seizures had persisted. During the past treatment with phenytoin, her mental performance had deteriorated progressively and signs of ataxia had developed. Her son with mental retardation had been exposed to phenytoin throughout the entire pregnancy.

At the time of referral, the patient was on valproate 2000 mg/day and clonazepam.

The patient had a mildly affected sister who was treated with valproate and ethosuximide. This sister had finished high school. The patient also had an affected brother who had a severe and progressive course of disease and who had been on long-term phenytoin medication. He had died of aspiration pneumonia during a period of phenobarbital intoxication. The patient's parents were healthy, non-consanguinous and native Dutch.

Examination and investigations

Physical examination of the patient confirmed the myoclonus of the trunk and proximal extremities, and signs of ataxia. She was mentally subnormal. The EEG showed generalized polyspike–waves and photosensitivity.

The patient's son was confirmed to be mentally retarded, and he showed hypertelorism, a depressed nasal bridge and distal phalangeal hypoplasia.

Mutation analysis of the cystatin B gene in the mother showed only an expanded dodecamer repeat and no normal-sized allele. Subsequently, the same DNA result was obtained in her affected sister. The parents were not available for DNA analysis.

Diagnosis

Progressive myoclonus epilepsy of Unverricht–Lundborg in the mother.
Fetal hydantoin syndrome in her son.

Treatment and outcome

The patient's medication was adjusted by dividing the total daily dose of valproate of 2000 mg in four equal dosages of 500 mg each. Clonazepam was discontinued and low-dose folic acid supplementation (0.5 mg/day) was started.

The patient was informed about the following risks to future offspring above standard population risks:

- risk of recurrence of epilepsy: less than 1 %;
- risk of recurrence of the fetal hydantoin syndrome: zero, provided that phenytoin is not used; and
- risk of teratogenesis from valproate use: 5 % risk of congenital abnormalities, including a 1–2 % risk of neural tube defects.

The patient was offered prenatal diagnosis of congenital abnormalities in the fetus by means of amniotic fluid analysis (alpha-1-fetoprotein level) and structural ultrasound examination.

Commentary

To the patient and her husband, the risk of recurrence of epilepsy in their children was unexpectedly low. This can be explained by the autosomal-recessive mode of inheritance of progressive myoclonus epilepsy of Unverricht–Lundborg.

242

Each child of a patient will inherit one of the two abnormal genes from the patient. However, the disease may only occur if the other parent is a carrier (heterozygous) for the same disease. This chance is low when the other parent has no family history of epilepsy and is not related to the patient. In addition, one may offer carrier detection to the healthy partner for currently known mutations in the cystatin B gene. A normal result (the most likely outcome) would further decrease the risk to the offspring, whereas the finding of a mutation (the less likely outcome) would increase the risk towards 50 %.

Adjustment of the dosage scheme for valproate was made in order to reduce peak levels that are possibly related to the risk of teratogenesis. Clonazepam was discontinued in view of reports that suggest potentiation of teratogenic risks with the combination of valproate and clonazepam.

Low-dose folic acid supplementation was prescribed according to the guidelines of the Dutch Health Council. High-dose folic acid supplementation is reserved for women with a previous child with an open neural tube defect. Effectiveness as well as safety of the high-dose folic acid is proven only in women at increased risk because of a previous child with a neural tube defect, but not in women at increased risk because of other risk factors such as maternal use of antiepileptic drugs.

This case was chosen in order to outline the complex issues that may be encountered when dealing with maternal epilepsy and maternal use of antiepileptic drugs. Genetic counseling in epilepsy should always explore and address three main questions:

- what is the etiology and recurrence risk of epilepsy;
- can seizures during pregnancy damage the mother or the unborn child; and
- what is known about the effects of maternal antiepileptic drugs on the developing embryo and fetus?

What did I learn from this case?

Until this case, progressive myoclonus epilepsy of Unverricht–Lundborg existed for me only in the textbooks. The discovery of the cystatin B gene currently provides an efficient and specific diagnostic tool. Some reports suggest that the course of the disease is less severe and the prognosis is favorable when valproate is used and phenytoin and carbamazepine are avoided.

Since this case, I have diagnosed seven other cases in a short period of time. Many of these patients were initially diagnosed as juvenile myoclonus epilepsy. The clinical presentation of progressive myoclonus epilepsy of Unverricht–Lundborg may show considerable overlap with juvenile myoclonus epilepsy, especially at onset. Atypical occurrence of myoclonias, therapy-resistant myoclonias, progression of the disease, development of ataxia or mental

243

regression, parental consanguinity or parental origin from the Baltic, the Mediterranean or the Middle East should suggest the diagnosis and lead to DNA analysis of the cystatin B gene.

This case underscores the importance of early diagnosis for better prognosis and optimal genetic counseling, and it illustrates one of the many new benefits of genetic research.

Further reading

Berkovic SF, Cochius J, Andermann E, Andermann F. Progressive myoclonus epilepsies: clinical and genetic aspects. *Epilepsia* 1993; **34(suppl 3)**:S19–S30.

Eldridge R, Iivanainen M, Stern R, Koerber T, Wilder BJ. 'Baltic' myoclonus epilepsy: hereditary disorder of childhood made worse by phenytoin. *Lancet* 1983;2:838–42.

Laegreid L, Kyllerman M, Hedner T, Hagberg B, Viggedahl G. Benzodiazepine amplification of valproate teratogenic effects in children of mothers with absence epilepsy. *Neuropediatrics* 1993;24:88–92.

Lehesjoki AE, Koskiniemi M. Progressive myoclonus epilepsy of Unverricht–Lundborg type. *Epilepsia* 1999;**40(suppl 3)**:23–8.

Lindhout D, Omtzigt JGC. Latest report on teratogenic effects of antiepileptic drugs: implications for the management of epilepsy in women of childbearing age. *Epilepsia* 1994;**35(suppl 4)**:19–28.

Samrén EB, van Duijn CM, Christiaens GC, Hofman A, Lindhout D. Antiepileptic drug regimens and major congenital abnormalities in the offspring. *Ann Neurol* 1999;**46**:739–46.

Note:

This case history has been modified for privacy reasons and educational purposes and should not be included in any kind of meta-analysis without prior consultation of the author.

Case 63

'FUNNY JERKS' RUN IN THE FAMILY

Heinz-Joachim Meencke

History

A 21-year-old right-handed woman was seen in the outpatient department of an epilepsy centre 1 week after a generalized tonic–clonic-seizure.

The report from the emergency room described tongue biting, and I got an unequivocal description of a generalized tonic–clonic seizure from the patient's mother. The seizure happened 1 hour after awakening. She had not slept adequately for several days because she was studying for an examination.

I asked them about a previous history of other seizures and epilepsy, which both she and her mother denied strongly. Then I discussed specific signs and symptoms of seizures. When I demonstrated jerks with my arms and shoulders, the patient told me that this was very familiar to her and that she often had similar jerks in the morning, dating back to when she was aged 12 or 13.

However, these jerks, in her mind, had nothing to do with her seizure. To her, they were just a personal mode of behaviour. Her mother admitted to having the same problem beginning in her school years, which she described as 'funny jerks'. She strongly denied having any 'blackouts'. Doctors, she noted, had explained the jerks as just tics. She had been satisfied with this explanation, because her aunt was also reported to have these 'funny jerks'. It seemed that in this family, to some extent, jerks were acceptable behaviour in the women.

Examination and investigations

Physical and neurological examinations were normal. A magnetic resonance imaging scan showed slight frontoparietal parasaggital atrophy. The routine EEG showed increased generalized intermittant rhythmic slowing that was excessive for her age. With sleep deprivation, bilateral polyspike-and-wave complexes were seen, which were intermittently accompanied by bilateral myoclonic jerks of the upper extremities.

An EEG of the mother was obtained, which showed increased generalized intermittent rhythmic slowing but no epileptiform potentials, even after sleep deprivation.

Diagnosis

Juvenile myoclonic epilepsy (impulsive petit mal, Janz Syndrome, generalized idiopathic epilepsy).

Treatment and outcome

It was very difficult to explain to the patient and her familiy that the myoclonic jerks were, in fact, a feature of generalized epilepsy. We counselled her about seizure-provoking factors, especially sleep deprivation, and started monotherapy with valproate 1500 mg/day. At 1-year follow-up, the myoclonic jerks had stopped and she had had no more tonic–clonic seizures. She did not return for a further appointment.

Commentary

What did I learn from this case?

First, I learned that what initially appears to be a first seizure is very often not, in fact, the first seizure. This case taught me that it is absolutely necessary to ask carefully for other signs and symptoms of seizures and that it is mandatory to demonstrate signs and symptoms of different seizure types. Very subtle ictal behavioural changes might be misinterpreted as 'personal' or idiosyncratic behaviour. In this case, earlier initiation of appropriate antiepileptic drug therapy together with adequate lifestyle counselling may have avoided the development of generalized tonic–clonic seizures.

Second, this case shows that the phenotypic expression of idiopathic generalized epilepsies may be very mild over many generations and may be manifested only as myoclonic jerks that may never be identified as epilepsy. The psychological and social consequences of epilepsies are strongly influenced by the type of epilepsy syndrome.

Third, this case highlights the problem of underdiagnosing juvenile myoclonic epilepsy, a syndrome that responds very favourably to appropriate treatment.

Bearing these lessons in mind will positively influence my strategy for choosing an appropriate therapy after a so-called first seizure.

Case 64

SIDE EFFECTS THAT IMITATE SEIZURES

George Lee Morris III

History

The patient is a 41-year-old woman who developed seizures in her early teens. Her seizures consisted of premonitory sensations for a day before the events and an aura of language difficulties   she understood that speech was occurring but could not determine what was being said to her. Episodes of loss of consciousness with or without preceding auras occurred several times a month. Auras without subsequent loss of consciousness occurred rarely.

Her past medical history included minor surgeries, two uneventful pregnancies with normal children, and the occasional treatment of depression with tricyclic antidepressants. There was no history of head trauma, febrile seizures or previous hospitalization. Prior medications included divalproex, phenytoin, felbamate, gabapentin and lamotrigine. Each was unsuccessful in stopping her seizures and several had significant cognitive effects.

She used low-estrogen oral contraceptives and daily multivitamins. She was married with two children of elementary-school age, and she had worked as a nurse before her second child. She did not drink alcohol or smoke tobacco. Her health was currently good and she reported a positive mood. Her current medication for seizures was carbamazepine 1400 mg/day in three divided doses.

Examination and investigations

The patient's general appearance, physical examination and neurological examination were normal.

She had a routine EEG that showed left mid-temporal spike-and slow-wave discharges and intermittent slowing in the left temporal lobe. Cranial magnetic imaging resonance scanning was normal and showed symmetric hippocampal structures.

Diagnoses

Complex partial seizures, with and without preceding simple partial seizures. Intractable, cryptogenic left temporal lobe localization-related epilepsy.

Treatment and outcome

The patient was presented with the options of further medication trials, vagus nerve stimulation or hospitalization for seizure confirmation via video-EEG monitoring for a potential surgical epilepsy treatment. The patient elected to try an additional medication. She reviewed the benefits and risks of each of the available medications, including commercially available and investigational drugs, and she chose tiagabine. A gradual titration over 6 weeks to 32 mg/day in three divided doses was begun.

Three weeks later the patient called to report her auras were occurring early in the morning, after her children went to school, but she was without further complex partial seizures and no side effects had appeared. In several additional phone calls over the following weeks the patient expressed concern over lengthy morning auras that were stronger. No loss of consciousness occurred but she was having more trouble speaking.

She then had a complex partial seizure. Because she was currently taking tiagabine 32 mg/day, her carbamazepine dose was lowered in the hope of raising the tiagabine level. However, the patient was now reporting daily auras for 30 minutes or more. She requested video-EEG monitoring.

The patient was hospitalized and her medications were tapered over three days. EEGs over 7 days showed occasional left mid-temporal epileptiform discharges but no seizures. Sleep-deprivation, hourly hyperventilation and light stimulation were performed and the patient requested discharge so that she could return to caring for her children. Both medications were started again at their prehospital doses. The patient's discharge was planned for the following morning.

The following morning the patient motioned to the technician to come in her room. She was unable to speak and could not read. She appeared sedated and motioned that she felt dizzy. The patient's EEG was reviewed and found to be unchanged during the episode.

Commentary

The paroxysmal nature of epilepsy vexes a physician's diagnosis in several ways. The variable presentation of medication side effects is a particularly difficult area.

248

Whereas a transient side effect from an antiepileptic drug can be readily attributed to rapidly escalating or high plasma concentrations, ictal symptoms are generally differentiated by their longer duration. Indeed, antiepileptic drugs produce a variety of clinical symptoms that may be similar to a seizure phenomenon. The unusual or 'indescribable' feeling of limbic seizures begins as undefinable by the patient, making it difficult for a patient to separate these sensations from a drug-induced sensation. Dizziness, paresthesias, vision alteration and various cognitive difficulties may all overlap and be paroxysmally related to peak concentration of these medications.

On further questioning, this patient related that these 'seizures' occurred only on school days and that her breakfast was limited to tea because she was busy getting her children ready for school. The rapid absorption of tiagabine produced by administration on an empty stomach led to these transient symptoms that were similar to her habitual auras.

What did I learn from this case?

An issue that I raise constantly with patients is the need to confirm that events they experience are seizures. Direct confirmation by video-EEG recordings is invaluable in patient management. The correct diagnosis may be suspected before monitoring but the outcome that was seen in this case is always a possibility.

How did this case alter my approach to the care and treatment of my epilepsy patients?

In my daily practice I use such illustrative cases with my patients. Describing to them the various potential outcomes from monitoring educates them as to the many benefits of disease confirmation and makes the process of managing patients who have been unresponsive to medications much easier. This patient's outcome is one that I use frequently when describing how patients may benefit from hospitalization for video-EEG monitoring.

Case 65

An Unusual Application Of Epilepsy Surgery

Mark Quigg, Edward H Bertram and Jaideep Kapur

History

The patient is a 57-year-old, right-handed woman who has two kinds of seizures. The first type occurs primarily during the day and consists of *déjà vu* followed by staring, confusion, orofacial automatisms and dystonic posturing of the left hand. The second type consists of distressing nocturnal episodes of abrupt arousal from sleep followed by severe pain in the left hand and arm accompanied by bilateral arm movement, incomprehensible screams, a frightened look on the face, and brief confusion.

Seizures started at the age of 43 without a clear history of febrile convulsions, head trauma or central nervous system infection. Her seizures were not reliably triggered by any particular events, but she did note that seizures recurred periodically two or three times each month in clusters. Her anticonvulsant was topiramate 400 mg/day in two divided doses. Carbamazepine, valproate, phenytoin and gabapentin administered in various combinations did not control her seizures. Lamotrigine was discontinued because of a rash. Other medications were estrogen–progesterone for prevention of osteoporosis and propranolol for poorly documented 'palpitations'.

She had no significant past medical history. There is no history of epilepsy in the family. Her mother died from carcinoma of the stomach, and father from lung carcinoma. She is married and has four healthy children. She has stopped working as a receptionist as a result of her epilepsy.

Examination and investigations

Physical and neurological examinations were unremarkable. The patient was admitted for video-EEG monitoring with scalp electrodes for two reasons:

- to evaluate medically intractable seizures; and
- to establish that the nocturnal painful episodes were epileptic seizures.

250

The seizures with staring and lip smacking were associated with electrographic seizures over the right mid-temporal region. EEG activity during the episodes of nocturnal left arm pain were partially obscured by muscle and movement artifact, although there were some changes that suggested a right hemispheric onset. These spells were considered epileptic on the basis of their stereotyped nature and their occurrence during sleep.

A magnetic resonance imaging (MRI) scan of the brain disclosed dual pathology of right hippocampal atrophy and a subtle right parietal cortical malformation. Neuropsychological testing revealed mild generalized cognitive dysfunction and no clear lateralization of deficits. Psychological assessment revealed a significant level of depression and anxiety.

Since scalp EEG monitoring was insufficient to localize the site of origin of painful seizures, intracranial monitoring was performed using subdural strip electrodes and bilateral, occipitally inserted intrahippocampal-depth electrodes. Intracranial EEG disclosed two distinct seizure foci – a right temporal focus corresponding to the complex partial seizures and a right parietal focus corresponding to the nocturnal ictal pain.

Diagnosis

Symptomatic localization-related epilepsy with independent right temporal and right parietal epileptic foci.

Treatment and outcome

The right parietal focus was resected following cortical mapping with a subsequently implanted subdural grid. Microscopic evaluation of the samples taken from the right parietal lobe revealed focal cortical dysplasia with gliosis.

Since surgery, the frequency and intensity of nocturnal ictal pain continues to decline. Currently, these episodes occur about once every 2 months and cause tingling but no disabling pain or disorientation. The patient continues to have daytime complex partial seizures.

Commentary

This case demonstrates that two types of seizures in a patient can arise from two different seizure foci and that seizures arising from two different regions of the brain are differentially susceptible to circadian modulation.

Patients with partial epilepsy commonly have two or more types of seizures arising from a single focus. A common example of this phenomenon is the patient who has simple partial, complex partial and secondarily generalized tonic–clonic seizures, all arising from a single mesial temporal focus. In addition, some patients have two distinct types of events, one epileptic and the other non-epileptic.[1]

Several clinical features, however, suggested that this patient had two distinct seizure foci causing two different seizure types. The clinical features of the daytime seizures – *déjà vu*, orofacial automatisms and arm dystonia – suggested a temporal lobe origin. None of these features was present in the nocturnal spells, the dominant clinical feature of which was distressing pain. The brain MRI scan and the scalp and intracranial EEG monitoring further supported the association of two seizure types with two distinct seizure foci. The fact that resection of the dysplastic area in the parietal cortex reduced the intensity and frequency of the nocturnal spells further suggests that these seizures originated in the parietal lobe and that the daytime seizures were arising from the temporal lobe.

The present case also illustrates that the endogenous circadian clock modulates seizure recurrence depending on the location of seizure foci. Seizures that involve the limbic system may be especially sensitive to circadian modulation as mediated by the hypothalamus, since the limbic system and the hypothalamus share anatomic and functional interconnections.[2,3] Cortically based seizures that spare the limbic system may be more susceptible to mediators of cortical excitation, such as the rhythm of the sleep–wake cycle. Furthermore, the sleep–wake cycle may contribute to both limbic and non-limbic seizure patterns, with limbic seizure facilitated by wakefulness (or resistant to effects of sleep) and extralimbic seizures promoted by sleep (or inhibited by the waking state). Transition states are particularly seizure-provoking for a variety of epileptic syndromes and may be a strong factor independent of syndrome.

There are two possible mechanisms by which two seizure foci developed in this patient. It is possible that focal cortical dysplasias are present in both the hippocampus and the parietal cortex, each independently serving as a seizure focus. Focal cortical dysplasia is a rare disorder characterized by histological features of disturbed cortical lamination, large abnormal neurons and the presence of large balloon cells with glassy eosinophilic cytoplasm and eccentric nuclei.[4] Alternately, the dysplastic parietal cortex may have served as a primary focus that 'kindled' another secondary focus in the right temporal lobe.[5] (Kindling refers to a phenomenon in experimental animals whereby repeated focal application of initially subconvulsive electrical stimulations results in intense partial and secondarily generalized seizures. Limbic structures are particularly susceptible to kindling.)

What did we learn from this case?

We learned that two distinct seizure types can result from two separate seizure foci in a single patient. We also learned that some patients can significantly improve their lives despite the lack of a seizure-free outcome after epilepsy surgery when their predominantly disabling symptoms have resolved. This patient, for example, was satisfied by the resolution of severe ictal pain despite the persistence of other seizures.

How did this case alter our approach to the care and treatment of our epilepsy patients?

When patients have two types of seizures with distinct signs and symptoms, we carefully evaluate them for evidence of two seizure foci. In addition, we take a careful history of the patterns of recurrence of seizures. If there is a diurnal pattern of recurrence of seizures, we may adjust the timing of daily activities and anticonvulsant administration with the aim of best helping the patient.

References

1. Henry TR, Drury I. Non-epileptic seizures in temporal lobectomy candidates with medically refractory seizures. *Neurology* 1997;**48**:1374–82.

2. Quigg M, Clayburn H, Straurne M, Menaker M, Bertram EH. Hypothalamic neuronal loss and altered circadian rhythm of temperature in a rat model of mesial temporal lobe epilepsy. *Epilepsia* 1999;**40**:1688–96.

3. Quigg M, Clayburn H, Straurne M, Menaker M, Bertram EH. Effects of circadian regulation and rest–activity state on spontaneous seizures in a rat model of limbic epilepsy. *Epilepsia* 2000;**41**:502 9.

4. Cotter DR, Honavar M, Everall I. Focal cortical dysplasia: a neuropathological and development perspective. *Epilepsy Res* 1999;**36**:155–64.

5. Majkowski J. Kindling: clinical relevance for epileptogenicity in humans. *Adv Neurol* 1999;**81**:105 13.

Case 66

EPILEPSY, MIGRAINE AND CEREBRAL CALCIFICATIONS

Willy O Renier

History

When the patient was 5 years old, he suffered two events while at school that were characterized by nausea, sweating and confusion. Examination at that time was normal, as was blood and urine screening, except for a mild anaemia. The EEG was described as normal for age but with some sharp theta-wave activity over the left temporo-occipital region. An EEG after sleep deprivation did not contribute further to the diagnosis. The events were interpreted as non-specific vegetative reactions, and iron supplementation was prescribed.

Six months later, another event occurred during the holidays. After a flight of 22 hours, the boy awoke in his hotel room in a confused state, complained of visual hallucinations ('moving walls') and had verbal dyspraxia. One hour later, left-sided hemiclonic jerks occurred for 2 minutes. After two similar seizures within 1 hour, the boy was transfered to a hospital.

General examination was again normal. EEG showed irregular sharp theta-waves over both posterior regions. A computed tomography (CT) scan (Fig. 66.1) showed bilateral parieto-occipital calcifications with a garland pattern. Laboratory investigations revealed a microcytic anaemia. The boy was administered diazepam 5 mg and the parents were advised to contact a neurologist.

Two uneventful weeks later, the neurological examination was normal. It was concluded that the seizures had been provoked by fatigue. Over the following months, the patient suffered two additional episodes of nausea – one at the end of a 4-day sport meeting and the other during an episode of flu. He was referred to my department for a second opinion.

When the history was explored in greater detail with the patient's mother, she expressed her feeling that her son was having migraines. Migraine was well known in her family because she herself, her sister, her brother and the younger brother of the patient regularly suffered from migraine headaches. When the general medical history was taken, she reported that her son had mild chronic intestinal problems and had regularly taken ferrous salts for anaemia since the age of 3.

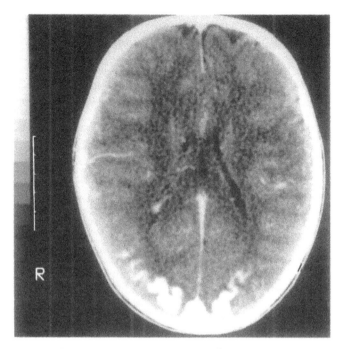

Figure 66.1 *Cerebral CT scan with typical calcifications in the parieto-occipital lobes*

Examination

The patient was a hyperactive but otherwise normal child.

Diagnosis and further investigations

Coeliac disease with epilepsy. Further laboratory investigations confirmed the diagnosis of coeliac disease (Table 66.1).

Treatment and outcome

The boy was treated with a gluten-free diet and carbamazepine 100 mg at bedtime. Three months later, the mother described her son as 'a completely new child'. He was more alert, more pleasant, and had better school performance. The EEG was normal. After having been seizure-free for 1 year, carbamazepine

255

Table 66.1 Laboratory investigations confirming the diagnosis of coeliac disease (glutenenteropathy). In addition, duodenal biopsy showed villous atrophy.

Test	Result before therapy	Result 8 months after therapy	Normal values
Hb (mmol/l)	6.4	6.8	6.0–9.0
Iron (μmol/l)	7	17	10–25
Iron binding capacity (μmol/l)	68	54	45–75
Folic acid (nmol/l)	3.3	21	5.5–40
Anti-gliadine IgG (U/ml)	49	negative	<12
Anti-gliadine IgA (U/ml)	5	negative	<4
Anti-reticuline IgA (U/ml)	+++	±	
Anti-endomysium IgA (U/ml)	+++	+	

was stopped. Four years later, the boy is still doing well without seizure recurrence on a gluten-free diet.

Commentary

Migraine-like seizures have been described in occipital lobe epilepsy[1] and in this case could have been related to the occipital calcifications. The association of migraine-like seizures, parieto-occipital calcifications, and intestinal complaints with chronic anaemia are pathognomonic for coeliac disease with epilepsy (Table 66.2).[2,3]

The case illustrates the pitfalls in the diagnosis of epilepsy. The final diagnosis was based on the description of the seizure pattern, a detailed history of all body systems and the typical appearance of the cerebral calcifications.

Visual auras followed by hemisensory or hemiconvulsive attacks (or both) have been described in benign epilepsy of childhood with occipital paroxysms. The varied manifestations of occipital lobe epilepsy resulting from multiple spread patterns to the temporal, frontal, supplementary motor or parietal regions are a source of diagnostic error. Interictal surface EEG is helpful in localizing the seizure focus in only approximately 20 % of cases.

Another confounding factor is the family history of migraine. The mother was

Table 66.2 The syndrome of the parieto-occipital calcifications with coeliac disease and epilepsy[2,3]

Clinical characteristics

Epilepsy

* In most cases, partial seizures with the characteristics of occipital paroxysms (migraine-like headache, nausea, visual complaints); cognitive disturbances and deterioration (with great individual variability)

Coeliac disease

* First signs and symptoms in infancy, toddler age or childhood (dysphoric episodes, dystrophic habitus, loss of appetite, growth retardation, puffed belly, malabsorption)

* Frequent association with HLA-B8 and HLA-DW3

Neuropathology

* Calcifications at the corticomedullary junction

* 'Patchy' glial angiomatosis ('Sturge–Weber' without cutaneous angiomas)

Possible mechanisms of pathogenesis:

* Chronic iron and folic acid deficiency ?

* HLA related auto-immune pathology ?[4]

Evolution

* Can lead to severe encephalopathy in cases without treatment

Treatment

* Start as early as possible with a gluten-free diet and iron and folic acid; continue the gluten-free diet

* Anti-epileptic drugs when seizures recur

familiar with signs and symptoms of migraine and, therefore, was not aware of the possibility of epileptic events. In families of children with benign epilepsy of childhood with occipital paroxysms, a history of epilepsy is present in 30 % and a history of migraine is present in 15 %.

Paroxysmal neurovegetative events, a normal neurological examination and non-specific EEGs do not necessarily exclude the diagnosis of epilepsy or signify a non-lesional epilepsy. In parietal and occipital lobe epilepsy, there is frequently a poor correlation between clinical and EEG features.

Chronic gastrointestinal complaints and anaemia are common complaints in children, particularly in hyperactive children, but they can also be the expression of coeliac disease. The typical garland configuration of parieto-occipital calcifications should alert the physician to this diagnosis.

What did I learn from this case?

The case illustrates that the diagnosis of epilepsy is primarily a clinical one and that clinical epileptology is based on experience, knowledge of the literature and good visual memory. Once you have seen the typical calcifications on CT scans in cases of coeliac disease, you remember the picture.

Taking a history from patients with seizures and their family members should be as complete as possible and not restricted to the description of the seizure pattern, though the information has to be interpreted with caution. The brain is not an isolated organ. Therefore, attention should be paid to complaints other than neurological ones. Developing knowledge about metabolic disorders should be part of the training of neurologists. In symptomatic epilepsy, treating the underlying cause at an early stage can prevent further deterioration and, in some cases, avoid antiepileptic drug treatment.

Further reading

1. Gastaut H. Benign epilepsy of childhood with occipital paroxysms. In: Roger J, Bureau M, Dravet Ch, Dreifuss FE, Perret A, Wolf P, eds. *Epileptic syndromes in infancy, childhood and adolescence*, 2nd ed. London: John Libbey; 1992:201–17.

2. Gobbi G, Sorrenti G, Santucci M, *et al.* Epilepsy with bilateral occipital calcifications: a benign onset with progressive severity. *Neurology* 1988;38:913–20.

3. Gobbi G, Bouquet F, Greco I, *et al.* Coeliac disease, epilepsy, and cerebral calcifications. *Lancet* 1992;340:439–43.

258

Case 67

ALL IS NOT WHAT IT SEEMS

William E Rosenfeld and Susan M Lippmann

History

The patient is a 35-five-year old white man referred for evaluation of an increased number of seizures. He is the manager of a pediatric practice.

Eleven years before referral, in May 1989, the patient was moving furniture and hit his head in the right temporal region on a steel beam and a dresser. He fell, with loss of consciousness that lasted several minutes. A few days later he had jerking of the left lower extremity and was told he had post-traumatic seizures. He was placed on divalproex sodium.

In June 1996, the patient reported sustaining a right hemispheric stroke, resulting in a visual field cut, left hemiparesis and left hemianesthesia. The stroke was felt to be cardioembolic–aortic valvular in etiology and was non-hemorrhagic on brain computed tomography (CT) scanning.

Six months later, the patient was seen for increased expressive aphasia and left-sided weakness. A stroke was suspected and a CT scan was negative. Shortly after this, he was admitted again with increased left upper extremity weakness and numbness as well as slurred speech. Again there was the impression that the patient had had a right cerebral infarction of possible embolic etiology. The possibility of a conversion reaction was also suspected.

In July 1997, the patient was admitted with severe anemia, which was thought to be secondary to low-grade hemolysis caused by his artificial heart valve. At this time, he had his 'first major motor seizure' and was treated with phenytoin. He remembers having an 'aura' of a sensation of smelling a grapefruit and then losing consciousness.

One year later, the patient suddenly fell. In the emergency department, his phenytoin level was undetectable. He left the hospital against medical advice. Subsequently, he had three traffic violations, possibly related to seizures.

In the month before coming to our office, the patient recorded up to one seizure a day. He reported his aura as consisting of a 'citrus smell, weird feelings, and then I don't remember'. He noted that his room-mates heard him 'flopping around'. He reported biting his tongue, occasionally chipping his teeth and occasionally being incontinent of urine.

When we first saw the patient, he reported being under treatment for a brain tumor. He stated that his brain magnetic resonance imaging (MRI) scan showed a tumor the size of a walnut and that a biopsy approximately 2 weeks earlier had revealed a grade IV astrocytoma. He reported participating in a 'phase I chemotherapy trial' and receiving intramuscular chemotherapy. He stated that another 'phase I procedure' was tried. He said that a craniotomy was performed and that 'the tumor was zapped twice with a laser', resulting in 95 % tumor eradication. He could not give us the names of the neurologist, neurosurgeon or oncologist who had treated him. He stated that he did not want us to look at previous records because he was afraid that this would interfere with his work.

The patient's past medical history was notable for a diagnosis of presumptive connective tissue disorder, which had eventually led to aortic valve replacement in October 1994. He also has a history of supraventricular tachycardia.

Examination and investigations

The patient appeared in our office with 10 bottles of 'study drugs'. These included phenytoin, clonazepam, phenobarbital, primidone, alprazolam, amitriptyline, temazepam, omeprazole, atenolol and warfarin.

On examination, the patient had a scalp incision with staples in the right posterior parietal region. His motor examination was inconsistent. Strength in the left upper and lower extremities was at least 4/5. On gait examination the patient occasionally dragged his left lower extremity but did not circumduct it. His heart examination revealed a holosystolic murmur that was greater over the aorta. In his extremities there was mild pitting edema.

Previous studies included a brain MRI scan from August 1998 that was normal. A brain CT scan from September 1998 was similarly negative, as was a follow-up MRI.

On the day that the patient was to be hospitalized in the epilepsy monitoring unit (in September 1998), he appeared in the emergency department after falling. His prothrombin time was 81.3 sec and his international normalized ratio was 8.5.

On admission to the epilepsy monitoring unit, he underwent Minnesota Multiphasic Personality Inventory testing, which showed increased scales for hysteria, depression and histrionics. Phenytoin, primidone, phenobarbital and clonazepam were withheld. EEGs over the next 5 days showed no evidence of interictal or ictal abnormalities. He then had a generalized tonic–clonic seizure that was documented on video-EEG, and he was reloaded with phenytoin.

Diagnoses

Four diagnoses were made:

*   Munchausen's syndrome with regard to the history of tumor (pseudoglioblastoma multiforme);
*   generalized tonic–clonic seizure documented by a physiological seizure in the epilepsy monitoring unit;
*   a history of supraventricular tachycardia with ablation and subsequent aortic valve replacement;
*   warfarin toxicity from an overdose.

Commentary

The patient has an obvious psychiatric disturbance that manifested as Munchausen's disorder with regard to 'the tumor' and, possibly, the history of 'strokes'. His presentation may also have included conversion reactions and non-epileptic episodes. Nonetheless, his testing confirmed that he also did have truly epileptic generalized tonic–clonic seizures.

What did we learn from the case?

We learned that psychological disorders can manifest in many different ways, including self-mutilation (incision and surgical staples). Secondly, this case demonstrated that patients with Munchausen's syndrome, conversion disorder and non-epileptic episodes could still have physiological seizures. Therefore, such patients must be carefully monitored so that appropriate therapies can be instituted.

How did this case alter our approach to the care and treatment of our epilepsy patients?

We are careful to evaluate a patient's episodes thoroughly before jumping to conclusions. Too often, patients receive a diagnosis of non-epileptic episodes without undergoing thorough video-EEG monitoring.

Further reading

Wyllie E, Glazer JP, Benbadis S, Kotagal P, Wolgamuth B. Psychiatric features of children and adolescents with pseudoseizures. *Arch Pediatr Adolesc Med* 1999;153:244–8.

261

Kalogjera-Sackellares D, Sackellares JC. Intellectual and neuropsychological features of patients with psychogenic pseudoseizures. *Psychiatry Res* 1999;**86**:73–84.

Torta R, Keller R. Behavioral, psychotic, and anxiety disorders in epilepsy: etiology, clinical features, and therapeutic implications. *Epilepsia* 1999;**40(suppl 10)**:S2–S20.

Barry E, Krumholz A, Bergey GK, Chatha H, Alemayehu S, Grattan L. Nonepileptic posttraumatic seizures. *Epilepsia* 1998;**39**:427–31.

Sigurdardottir KR, Olafsson E. Incidence of psychogenic seizures in adults: a population-based study in Iceland. *Epilepsia* 1998;**39**:749–52.

Devinsky O. Nonepileptic psychogenic seizures: quagmires of pathophysiology, diagnosis and treatment. *Epilepsia* 1998;**39**:458–62.

Scheepers B, Clough P, Pickles C. The misdiagnosis of epilepsy: findings of a population study. *Seizure* 1998;**7**:403–6.

Bowman ES. Pseudoseizures. *Psychiatr Clin North Am* 1998;**21**:649–57.

Westbrook LE, Devinsky O, Geocadin R. Nonepileptic seizures after head injury. *Epilepsia* 1998;**39**:978–82.

Davard G, Andermann F, Teitelbaum J. Epileptic Munchausen's syndrome: a form of pseudoseizures distinct from hysteria and malingering. *Neurology* 1998;**38**:1628–9.

262

Case 68

A Patient Whose Epilepsy Diagnosis Changed Three Times Over Twenty Years

Masakazu Seino and Yushi Inoue

History

A 42-year-old, right-handed housewife had a cerebral contusion from a fall at the age of 4 years. At the age of 18, she experienced her first seizure, with loss of consciousness followed by a convulsion. Subsequently, she repeatedly had seizures consisting of right-sided hemifacial spasms and slight turning of the head and eyes toward the right; these seizures occurred several times a day. Seizures with impairment of consciousness lasting 20–30 minutes preceded by an indiscernible aura and accompanied by automatisms were also observed.

During a follow-up of more than 20 years, absence-like seizures characterized by momentary loss of consciousness were often observed, in addition to the focal motor seizures and long-lasting impairment of consciousness with automatisms mentioned above, each occurring independently. At 38 years of age, she had an episode of convulsive status epilepticus as a result of taking her antiepileptic drugs irregularly.

Examination and investigations

Because her seizures were resistant to drug treatment, the patient was hospitalized at our centre four times over a period of 20 years and investigations were carried out.

At 19 years of age, short bursts of bisynchronous spike-and-wave or polyspike-and-wave activity slightly slower than 3 Hz were observed (Fig. 68.1). Coincident with the generalized and diffuse spike-and-wave discharges was a brief arrest of motion, which was documented by video–EEG monitoring. The bursts of bisynchronous and diffuse discharges persisted into the patient's 20s and 30s although spike-and-wave formation became less discrete, transforming to high-voltage slow wave rhythms (Fig. 68.2). Immediately after the cessation of discharges, she could sometimes recognize an interruption of awareness/or difficulty speaking. Ictal EEGs that were associated with a slight deviation of head and eyes showed flattening of background activities followed by a gradual build-

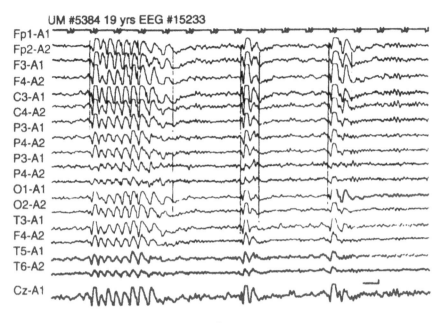

Figure 68.1 Awake EEG at 19 years of age.

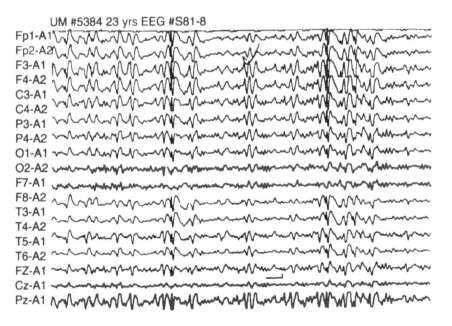

Figure 68.2 Awake EEG at 23 years of age.

up of spike-wave rhythms without focal findings. In other words, these two seizure events were electro-clinically independent.

Magnetoencephalography demonstrated that the localization of estimated dipoles of the spike component of the spike–waves clustered diffusely in the left frontal lobe (Fig. 68.3). Magnetic resonance imaging of the brain revealed a wedge-shaped, T2-weighted, high signal lesion in the left frontal lobe (Fig. 68.4).

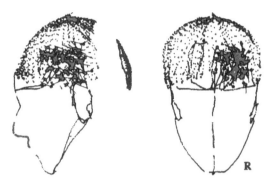

Figure 68.3 *Magneto-encephalography (BTi, Magnes, 74 ch)*

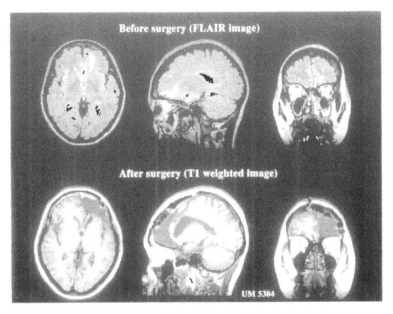

Figure 68.4 *MRI; pre- and post-surgery*

An ictal technetium-99 ECD revealed an area of hyperperfusion in the mesial basal part in the left frontal lobe.

The patient's IQs as measured by the Wechsler Adult Intelligence Scale (Revised) were within a subnormal range, with a comparatively lower IQ in the verbal domain. On the Wisconsin Card Sorting Test, categories achieved were 6. A Wada test showed that speech and memory dominance were on the left.

Diagnosis

Frontal lobe epilepsy with focal motor seizures, occasionally secondarily generalized, and absence-like seizures.

Treatment and outcome

Phenytoin, carbamazepine and valproate, often in combination, were administered at maximal dosage with insufficient control of seizures. The seizures occurred on a daily to weekly basis.

The patient underwent a left frontal resection at the age of 41. Scar tissue was found at surgery in the antero-inferior portion of the left frontal lobe. Seizures subsided for 6 months, but then simple and complex focal seizures recurred, although they were obviously less frequent and not as disabling as before.

Commentary

The diagnosis of this patient during more than 20 years of follow-up has changed twice, with three different diagnoses – idiopathic generalized epilepsy with absences, symptomatic generalized epilepsy with atypical absences, and frontal lobe epilepsy with simple and complex focal seizures. Once subtle but definite focal motor and dysphasic seizure manifestations became evident, there was no doubt that her seizures were of frontal lobe origin. Furthermore, the outcome of her surgery supports this diagnosis.

However, at least in her 20s, episodes of brief and abrupt loss or impairment of consciousness accompanied by bisynchronous spike-and-wave rhythms, both interictally and ictally, were interpreted as absence seizures, even though they were atypical in terms of EEG expression. Since the epileptogenic zone was proven to localize in the frontal lobe, the episode of impairment of consciousness was, by definition, complex focal seizures rather than absence.

266

What did I learn from this case?

A time-honoured term, secondary bilateral synchrony, was first described by Jasper *et al*., nearly half a century ago, as bursts of high-amplitude synchronous slow spike-and-wave complexes that are more or less symmetrical over both hemispheres and are caused by a unilateral epileptogenic lesion of the mesial surface of the frontal or temporal lobe. The term originally referred to an interictal EEG expression and not to an ictal manifestation. For the past two decades, it has been reported that patients having focal seizures with secondary bilateral synchrony may have non-convulsive seizures that mimic absences, especially when an epileptogenic focus is localized in the frontal lobe.

Differentiation between idiopathic generalized epilepsy and frontal lobe epilepsy, or between symptomatic generalized epilepsy of the Lennox–Gastaut type and symptomatic partial epilepsy with secondary bilateral synchrony, has been a subject of controversy. It can be difficult to differentiate absence seizures from complex focal seizures of frontal origin. The choice of drug treatment, the evaluation for surgical interventions and the prognosis of the disorder considerably differ between these two conditions.

This patient showed that secondary bilateral synchrony might be associated with ictal phenomena that mimic absences. This case also teaches us that long-term follow-up may be necessary to define an epileptic syndrome, whether focal or generalized.

Further reading

Blume W. Lennox –Gastaut syndrome and secondary bilateral synchrony: a comparison. In: Wolf P, ed. *Epileptic seizures and syndromes*. London: John Libby; 1994:285–97.

Holthausen H. Lennox–Gastaut Syndrom vs. sekundäre bilaterale Synchronie. In: Fröscher W, Kramer G, Ried S, Vassella F, eds. *Das Lennox-Gastaut Syndrom*. Berlin: Blackwell; 1998:65–102.

Gastaut H, Zifkin B, Maggauda A, *et al*. Symptomatic partial epilepsies with secondary bilateral synchrony: differentiation from symptomatic generalized epilepsies of the Lennox-Gastaut type. In: Wieser HG, Elger CE, eds. *Presurgical evaluation of epileptics*. Berlin: Springer-Verlag; 1987:308–17.

Kudo T, Sato K, Yagi K, *et al*. Can absence status epilepticus be of frontal lobe origin? *Acta Neurol Scand* 1995;**92**:472–7.

Lombroso CT. Consistent EEG focalities detected in subjects with primary generalized epilepsies monitored for two decades. *Epilepsia* 1997;**38**:797–812.

Roger J, Bureau M. Distinctive characteristics of frontal lobe epilepsy versus idiopathic generalized epilepsy. In: Chauvel P, Delgado-Escueta AV, eds. *Advances in neurology* vol 57. New York: Raven; 1992:399–410.

Yagi K. Evolution of Lennox-Gastaut Syndrome: a long-term longitudinal study. *Epilepsia* 1996;**37(suppl 3)**:48–51.

Case 69

IF YOU DON'T SUCCEED, INVESTIGATE

Michael R Sperling

History

A woman first came to the epilepsy center at the age of 28 years for management of uncontrolled seizures. Her seizures had begun at the age of 7, immediately after a bout of measles with high fever. She had previously been in good health and had no antecedent risk factors for epilepsy. The seizures were characterized by staring and unresponsiveness that started without warning and lasted for less than 1 minute. At the age of 12 she began to experience tonic–clonic seizures, which began with a feeling of restlessness and the urge to defecate. Next, she lost her ability to speak, blinked her eyes and paced back and forth for half a minute, and her head would then turn to the left. This was followed by generalized tonic–clonic activity. She was confused for several hours after each seizure and was sleepy for the remainder of the day.

Until the age of 28, she had one seizure at the start of each menstrual period approximately 10 times per year. At the age of 28, the seizures became more frequent. She reported between three and 10 seizures separated by 15–60 minutes in a single day at the onset of menses. She had been treated with phenytoin, phenobarbital, carbamazepine, mephenytoin, trimethadione, primidone, acetazolamide and chlorazepate in the past without benefit.

At the time of her initial evaluation, she was taking phenytoin, carbamazepine and chlorazepate. A maternal second cousin and paternal aunt had a history of seizures, but the patient could not provide any details about their condition. She was married and had two healthy children. She had formerly worked as a keypunch operator but had lost her job on account of the seizures. She also complained of poor memory.

Examination and investigations

The general physical examination was normal. She weighed 72 kg and had normal vital signs. Her neurological examination was remarkable for moderately

269

impaired long-term memory and nystagmus on horizontal gaze in either direction. The remainder of the examination was normal. A magnetic resonance imaging scan showed two small, high-signal intensity lesions in the left centrum semiovale. Her first EEG showed intermittent left temporal theta activity and the second EEG showed left mid-temporal sharp waves in sleep. Neuropsychological testing revealed a full-scale IQ of 84, mild to moderate impairment of verbal and visuospatial memory, and markedly impaired naming, phonemic verbal fluency and repetition.

She was given a provisional diagnosis of catamenial partial epilepsy, with monthly bouts of status epilepticus. She expressed a decided lack of interest in having an inpatient evaluation, and elected to continue to try medical therapy. Her drug regimen was changed to carbamazepine and acetazolamide without benefit. A combination of phenytoin and carbamazepine was then used, but she continued to experience monthly episodes of tonic–clonic status epilepticus. Another further interictal EEG again showed left temporal sharp waves.

She was admitted to the hospital during a bout of status epilepticus and had video-EEG monitoring. The EEG showed generalized, frontally predominant spike–wave discharges during her 'interictal' confusional period and generalized spikes followed by muscle artifact during the tonic–clonic activity. When the cluster of seizures ended, the EEG showed diffuse background theta and delta waves for several days without interictal spikes. Her serum carbamazepine level was subtherapeutic, and she was discharged on increasing doses of carbamazepine and phenytoin.

Her monthly clusters of status epilepticus continued. She was instructed to discontinue carbamazepine, and valproate was prescribed at doses sufficient to produce a therapeutic level. The seizures persisted on a combination of phenytoin and valproate, although they diminished in frequency to one a month. Eight months later, phenytoin was discontinued and the seizures stopped.

Diagnosis

Based on the observed ictal behavior, EEG findings of a generalized spike–wave pattern, the remarkable response to valproate and the strong family history of epilepsy, the patient was given a diagnosis of generalized epilepsy. The etiology remains uncertain, with weak evidence for an underlying static encephalopathy, although an idiopathic generalized epilepsy is possible in light of her response to valproate. A unilateral neocortical focus with secondary bilateral synchrony in the EEG is also possible but unproven.

Treatment and outcome

She had no seizures for the subsequent 12 years while taking valproate 1250 mg/day. Her serum levels have ranged between 55 and 70 mg/l. Her weight increased to 107 kg in the first 6 months after beginning valproate, and she then stabilized at 113 kg. She experienced a single recurrent seizure in late 1999, and has remained free of seizures since then on a dose of valproate 1500 mg/day. While somewhat dissatisfied with her weight gain, the patient finds it preferable to recurrent bouts of status epilepticus.

Commentary

This patient had uncontrolled tonic–clonic seizures that were refractory to a variety of antiepileptic drugs. Her condition worsened over time despite therapy, so that she experienced monthly bouts of status epilepticus with its attendant risks before her condition was controlled. This happened in part because of an incorrect diagnosis and, as a result, treatment for presumed partial epilepsy without knowledge and, later, attention to the generalized spike–wave findings on EEG.

Several features in the history and EEG were misleading. The seizures began after a bout of measles, which is often associated with encephalitis and consequent focal brain injury. The childhood seizures, which were probably absence attacks, lasted longer than usual and complex partial seizures were suspected. Moreover, the tonic–clonic seizures began with what resembled an aura, and the late head turning also suggested the possibility of a focal process. Her early interictal EEGs suggested a focal disturbance, with left temporal sharp waves noted on two occasions.

Only after ictal recording was performed did the generalized nature of her epilepsy begin to reveal itself. Her condition began to improve only when she was treated with valproate for generalized epilepsy. Combining phenytoin and valproate did not completely stop the seizures, and it was necessary to use valproate in monotherapy to abolish her seizures. The favorable response to valproate helped to establish the diagnosis and confirm the clinical impression.

This case history demonstrates the importance of accurately diagnosing the seizure type and epilepsy syndrome. Accurate diagnosis leads to appropriate therapy, which offers the best chance of a successful result. Although other antiepileptic drugs are sometimes effective in idiopathic generalized epilepsy, many patients with generalized spike–wave discharges respond only to valproate.[1,2] Older antiepileptic drugs such as phenobarbital, phenytoin and carbamazepine are often less effective than valproate or produce only a partial response. Rarely, antiepileptic drugs other than valproate exacerbate some types of generalized seizures. For example, carbamazepine may exacerbate absence seizures.[3] Several of the newer antiepileptic drugs such as topiramate and lamotrigine are also beneficial in treating generalized epilepsy; others such as zonisamide and levetiracetam are promising for these conditions as well.[4,5] There are no published studies comparing the efficacy of different antiepileptic drugs in the generalized epilepsies, and such trials are desirable. At present, valproate remains the first-line choice for most patients after due consideration of its potential side effects.

These side effects should also be mentioned, however briefly. Valproate is associated with many potential adverse reactions. These include fatigue, tremor, hair loss, teratogenic effects, polycystic ovarian disease, idiosyncratic liver and hematopoetic reactions, and weight gain.[6] The patient in this case experienced serious weight gain. Her weight quickly ballooned by more than 30 kg and has not diminished over the succeeding decade. Nonetheless, her sensible opinion is that the benefits of seizure control far outweigh the detriment of obesity. Usually this decision must be made by the patient, who ultimately bears the burden both of the illness and the treatment.

What did I learn from this case?

I learned that it is important to question the diagnosis early when the treatment is not working. In retrospect, I used ineffective therapy for too long and should have insisted on obtaining an ictal EEG recording sooner. In addition, therapy for generalized epilepsy should have been instituted earlier rather than continuing to use carbamazepine. This case history also reinforces the importance of using valproate as monotherapy in generalized epilepsy and in patients whose EEG shows generalized spike–wave discharges when the etiology is uncertain. Valproate is often most effective when used alone. This case history demonstrates the value of using valproate in monotherapy despite the lack of seizure control at the same serum levels when used in conjunction with another agent.

How did this case alter my approach to the care and treatment of my epilepsy patients?

I question my original diagnosis more readily if seizures do not respond to therapy, and I advise video-EEG or ambulatory EEG monitoring early if seizures remain uncontrolled. I spend more time verifying the seizure history and family history during follow-up office visits, and have somewhat less faith in the interictal EEG as a guide for therapy.

272

References

1. Davis R, Peters DH, McTavish D. Valproic acid: a reappraisal of its pharmacological properties and clinical efficacy in epilepsy. *Drugs* 1994;**47**:332–72.

2. Simon D, Penry JK. Sodium di-n-propylacetate (DPA) in the treatment of epilepsy: a review. *Epilepsia* 1975;**22**:1701–8.

3. Liporace JL, Sperling, MR, Dichter MA. Absence seizures and carbamazepine in adults. *Epilepsia* 1994;**35**:1026–8.

4. Matsuo F. Lamotrigine. *Epilepsia* 1999;**40(suppl 5)**:S30–S36.

5. Glauser TA. Topiramate. *Epilepsia* 1999; **40(suppl 5)**:S71–S80.

6. Dreifuss FE, Langer DH. Side effects of valproate. *Am J Med* 1988;**84**:34–41.

IV

Unforeseen Complications and Problems

A 35-YEAR-OLD MAN WITH POOR SURGICAL OUTCOME AFTER TEMPORAL LOBE SURGERY

Gus A Baker

History

The patient is a 35-year-old man with a long-standing history of temporal lobe epilepsy.

Despite intractable seizures, he had managed to attend mainstream schooling and obtain his school certificates in six subjects. He left school at the age of 16 years and worked for 4 years as a television salesman. Unfortunately his seizures became more frequent and as a consequence he was forced to give up work in 1983. He tried a combination of antiepileptic drugs but was unable to obtain satisfactory control.

He lived at home with his parents and had never been in a romantic relationship. His family was reluctant to explore the possibility of surgery for the control of his seizures because they were fearful that he might be left disabled by the operation. However, after his father died suddenly from a cardiovascular disorder, the patient decided to reconsider the surgical option. He underwent a number of investigations and was considered a good candidate for surgery.

Examination and investigations

Results from the surgical assessment (EEG, brain magnetic imaging, intracarotid sodium amytal test [ICSA], neuropsychology) confirmed that right mesial temporal sclerosis was responsible for his seizures.

Diagnosis

Right mesial temporal sclerosis with nocturnal seizures and occasional daytime seizures.

276

Treatment and outcome

A right anterior temporal lobectomy was carried out in 1997. The operation was complicated by a right third nerve palsy and mild expressive dysphasia. No significant changes in neuropsychological functioning from the pre-operative baseline were noted.

Initially there was a reduction in the frequency and severity of his nocturnal seizures. However, at a 12-month assessment, his seizures had returned to their pre-operative status.

Commentary

I chose this case for several reasons. First, despite the impressive results obtained from epilepsy surgery programmes in the USA and Europe, not all patients fare well. In this case, a young man who underwent a right temporal lobectomy did not have a good surgical outcome. While there was an initial reduction in the frequency of seizures, within 6 months his seizures returned to the level that existed before his surgery.

Second, the patient had a number of expectations of the surgery, the most important being that he would become more independent as a result of being rendered seizure-free. At the time of the operation he was heavily reliant on his mother, who was in her late 70s and not in good health. He had two siblings who lived away from the family home. His family was naturally concerned about his future, particularly if his mother's health deteriorated further.

Third, he showed great courage in going for the surgery, particularly as both he and his family were concerned about the risk of something awful going wrong during the surgery and of him being left severely disabled.

Fourth, despite the failure of the surgery to meet his expectations, the patient did not suffer any significant psychosocial consequences. This may have been because he felt that had he not gone for the surgical option, he would always have regretted not knowing whether or not it would have worked.

What did I learn from this case?

It is important to recognize that, for many patients and their families, the idea of brain surgery may create a number of anxieties. It is important for the epilepsy surgery team to be sure that the patient and the patient's family have a clear conception about what surgery will entail. Furthermore, there should be discussion about the relative risks and benefits associated with the procedure. In my practice, it is not uncommon to put prospective candidates in touch with others who have been through the surgery programme.

This case highlights the importance of spending time with patients and their families to discuss their expectation of surgery. Patients will undoubtedly have varying expectations of the surgery. The way they react to the outcome of such a radical intervention is influenced by a number of factors, including whether they are rendered seizure-free or not, their own and their family's expectations of surgery, whether there are any emotional changes associated with the surgery, their premorbid psychological and neuropsychological functioning, and the level of social support they have both before and after surgery.

Clinical experience from my own surgical series suggests that even when surgery is successful it is not always accompanied by an improved quality of life. Equally, as in this case, the failure to render a patient seizure-free does not necessarily lead to a reduction in quality of life. This patient was grateful for the opportunity at least to see if surgery could help with the management of his seizures.

Further reading

Engel J, ed. *Surgical treatment of the epilepsies*, 2nd ed. New York: Raven; 1993.

Hermann BP, Seidenberg M, Wendt G, Bell B. Neuropsychology and epilepsy surgery: optimising the timing of surgery, minimising cognitive morbidity and maximising functional status. In: Schmidt D, Schachter S, eds. *Epilepsy: problem solving in clinical practice*. London: Martin Dunitz; 2000, 279–90.

Wilson S, Saling MM, Kincade P, Bladin PF. Patient expectations of temporal lobe surgery. *Epilepsia* 1998;**39**:167–74.

Case 71

WHEN MORE IS LESS

Carl W Bazil

History

A 42-year-old woman was admitted because of exacerbation of her chronic seizure disorder. Her pertinent history began at the age of 13 years, when she began to experience frequent seizures consisting of head dropping, eye blinking, and eye deviation, sometimes with loss of awareness. She occasionally sustained injury during the head drops as a result of suddenly falling to the floor. She also had very rare secondarily generalized seizures.

The patient was found to have aqueductal stenosis and hydrocephalus. A ventricular shunt was placed; however, her course was complicated by multiple shunt revisions and infections. She had been treated with virtually all antiepileptic drugs, often in combination, including bromides and mephenytoin. She was placed on vigabatrin 5 years ago, which resulted in excellent seizure control. However, she developed visual symptoms over the following 2 years and was found to have vigabatrin-related visual field loss. Topiramate treatment resulted in severe word-finding difficulty, and the initial dose had to be decreased.

Two years before admission, she developed a new seizure type, which consisted of sudden unresponsiveness with eyes closed and all limbs limp. She was evaluated with video-EEG monitoring, and these episodes were found to be non-epileptic. They resolved with psychotherapy, including training in self-hypnosis. Tiagabine was also started at this time, resulting in improved seizure control. Over the 2 weeks before admission, however, she began to have prolonged episodes of confusion, which were sometimes associated with violent behavior. These episodes were described by her family as being unlike all previous seizure episodes – longer (lasting several hours) and usually associated with some purposeful behavior. Oral diazepam led to resolution of some of these episodes within seconds or minutes. However, owing to the increasing frequency of seizures, she was admitted for monitoring and further treatment.

Medications on admission were:

- extended-release carbamazepine 800 mg three times a day;

279

- topiramate 25 mg three times a day;
- tiagabine 20 mg in the morning and 16mg twice a day;
- zolpidem 5 mg at bedtime as needed;
- folic acid 1 mg once daily.

Examination and investigations

The general and neurological examinations were normal. The patient was admitted to the epilepsy monitoring unit for video-EEG monitoring. On the day after admission she had a 3-hour episode of prolonged confusion with staring and irregular movements. The EEG during this time showed an irregular, generalized spike–wave discharge that was more pronounced on the right at times (Fig. 71.1). Diazepam was administered, initially rectally then (after 30 minutes) intravenously. She began to improve 10 minutes after the intravenous administration, although nearly 2 hours passed before there was complete resolution of the clinical symptoms and the EEG changes. Figure 71.2 shows her EEG 10 hours later.

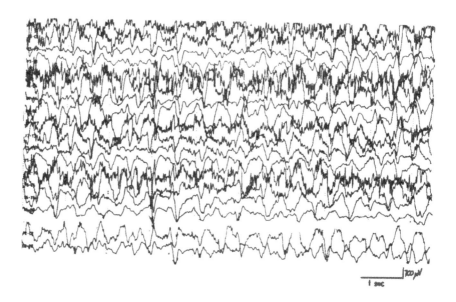

Figure 71.1: *EEG from the patient during an episode of confusion and irregular movements. A diffuse, irregular spike–wave discharge was seen most prominently in the anterior region.*

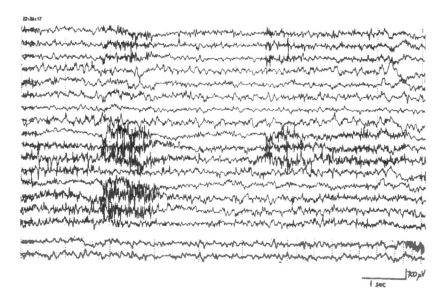

Figure 71.2: *EEG from the same patient 10 hours later, after resolution of the symptoms. There is mild diffuse slowing, probably caused by benzodiazepines.*

Diagnosis

The diagnosis was non-convulsive status epilepticus.

Treatment and outcome

Non-convulsive status epilepticus has been described as an unusual complication of tiagabine. However, this patient had responded well to tiagabine for control of her other seizures. Tiagabine was, therefore, decreased to a total of 28 mg/day. She had another, briefer episode of confusion associated with irregular spike–wave discharges during the taper. She has remained now on this dose of tiagabine for 18 months, with no recurrence of non-convulsive status epilepticus.

Commentary

It is well known that epileptic and non-epileptic seizures frequently coexist. For this reason, both diagnoses must be considered in any patient with epilepsy who develops a new seizure type. As clinicians, we always operate at a disadvantage since we are unable to observe the symptom (the seizure) directly. The history is necessarily biased, and any caregiver (no matter how experienced and knowledgeable about epilepsy) can inadvertently give misleading information.

My initial thought in this patient was that she was experiencing a new type of non-epileptic event. From the history, the episodes had a number of characteristics that would be unusual for epileptic seizures. First, they were variable in quality and duration. Second, she was reported to be unresponsive and yet able to perform purposeful tasks during the episodes. Third, although the episodes resolved with benzodiazepines, even though this was described as occurring within seconds to minutes of an oral dose – not enough time for absorption of oral diazepam and therefore suggestive of a placebo effect. Finally, most of the episodes lasted several hours whereas typical complex partial seizures last no more than 2 minutes.

On the other hand, I have been humbled a number of times when attempting to make such a diagnosis by history alone. Furthermore, this patient was already known to suffer both epileptic and non-epileptic seizures. It was fortunately my standard to admit such complicated patients for definitive diagnosis using video-EEG monitoring. It was also fortunate that her seizures were frequent enough for this to be feasible.

What did I learn from this case?

This case illustrates the possibility of new seizure types induced by medication changes. Most commonly, partial seizures change somewhat in quality; for example, a psychic aura may appear when none was present before, or nonsensical speech may occur as a result of a change in the pattern of spread. Rarely (as in this case) a totally new seizure type can emerge. The most common example is myoclonus induced by phenytoin, carbamazepine or gabapentin, which can occur in patients with no history of myoclonus. These patients probably have an underlying susceptibility to such seizures and most would have a typical spike–wave or polyspike–wave discharge on EEG. Tiagabine has been described as inducing non-convulsive status epilepticus in a few patients.

How did this case alter my approach to the care and treatment of my epilepsy patients?

I now recognize the need for healthy skepticism with patients who have complicated epilepsy. Whenever the treatment does not work as expected or the described event does not make neurological sense in the context of the patient's known disease, I consider alternative explanations. Although, in a few cases, it might be appropriate to treat empirically first (e.g. with an increase in medication dosage), I now realize that most such patients will require video-EEG monitoring.

282

Case 72

Change Of Antiepileptic Drug Treatment For Fear Of Side Effects In A 45-Year-Old Seizure-Free Patient

Elinor Ben-Menachem

History

The patient, born in 1956, was healthy until the age of 12 years, when he began to have seizures. First he had some jerks accompanied by short periods of unconsciousness and then had a few generalized tonic–clonic seizures. The diagnosis of juvenile myoclonic epilepsy was made.

The seizures slowly increased in frequency; by the time he was 16, he was in and out of hospital with repeated episodes of status epilepticus. He was treated with combinations of carbamazepine, phenobarbital, phenytoin and valproate, but he had daily seizures in spite of adequate serum concentrations.

Examination and investigations

The patient had a normal neurological and psychiatric examination. Video-EEG monitoring showed evidence of bifrontal epilepsy.

Diagnosis

Partial seizures of bifrontal lobe onset, with occasional secondary generalization and status epilepticus.

Treatment and outcome

In 1987, at the age of 31, the patient weighed 120 kg, mainly because of previous valproate therapy that caused a large weight increase. He was prescribed vigabatrin 50 mg/kg per day (6 g/day) and instantly became seizure-free. Phenobarbital was titrated down and stopped in 1989 and he remained on carbamazepine and vigabatrin. After becoming seizure-free, the patient began full-time work, learned to drive, and established a family with a wife and 2 children. He has lived, in other words, a normal life.

During the last few years, there has been a lively discussion of the appropriateness of vigabatrin therapy in the light of its association with irreversible visual field defects in up to 40 % of patients, even though most patients are asymptomatic. On the other hand, 60–80 % of patients on vigabatrin do not experience this side effect. When our patient heard of the possibility of visual field defects, although he had normal visual field testing, he was reluctant to continue on vigabatrin. Moreover, he was found to have anemia, which can be caused by vigabatrin, so the decision was made to slowly down-titrate the drug and replace it with topiramate.

Over 4 months, vigabatrin was titrated down to 1 g/day and topiramate up to 400 mg/day. His dose of carbamazepine stayed the same. At a vigabatrin dose of 4 g/day the patient began to have myoclonic jerks and occasional generalized tonic–clonic seizures again. He had to stop driving and often stayed home from work. His children were in a state of shock to see their father have seizures because they had not witnessed them before. The patient's anemia resolved with iron replacement therapy and was thought to be due to a low iron content in his diet – an extensive investigation found no other cause.

The patient lost weight on topiramate, became extremely irritable and had trouble expressing himself. Finally the situation deteriorated with such frequent generalized tonic–clonic seizures that he was hospitalized in March 2000. Topiramate was stopped and vigabatrin was reinstated at a dose of 5 g/day. He immediately became seizure-free again and regained his usual personality. His hemoglobin count and visual fields are being regularly monitored.

Commentary

This case illustrates the dilemma that patients and doctors find themselves in concerning vigabatrin. It is still a very effective antiepileptic drug and not all patients experience side effects. This drug has changed the lives of many patients with refractory epilepsy for the better, and changes in this medication should be made with the greatest caution.

What did I learn from this case?

Overly enthusiastic elimination of vigabatrin from a patient's therapy may ruin his or her life, as happened with my patient until vigabatrin was started again. Both the pros and cons of discontinuing any treatment must be discussed with the patient in detail before it is stopped.

Case 73

Personality And Mood Changes In A Teenager

Ahmad Beydoun, Ekrem Kutluay and Erasmo Passaro

History

The patient is a 17-year-old woman whose present medical illness started in February 2000 when she was diagnosed with a left frontal abscess complicating a pansinusitis. She underwent a left frontal craniotomy with an evacuation of the left frontal brain abscess and her sinuses. Perioperatively, she was treated with antibiotics and put on phenytoin prophylaxis for 3 weeks. She remained seizure free and was discharged home with no apparent neurological sequelae.

She remained asymptomatic until early July 2000, when she experienced two generalized tonic–clonic seizures and multiple complex partial seizures that were characterized by staring and unresponsiveness. She was treated with intravenous lorazepam and loaded with phenytoin.

Over the next few days, she had two brief staring spells and developed personality changes, which were characterized by an unusual amount of energy, racing thoughts, inappropriate laughter, irritability, and a reduced attention span. However, she remained fully alert, oriented and conversant. The phenytoin level was 19 mg/l.

Examination and investigations

She was admitted to the hospital for an evaluation. During the 3 days of monitoring, her awake EEG revealed well-modulated posterior 8–9 Hz activity, a left frontal breach rhythm, continuous slowing over the left frontal region and intermittent bifrontal spike–wave activity, which occurred occasionally in bursts of up to 5 seconds. In addition, a total of five electrographic partial seizures without clinical accompaniment were recorded. The seizures consisted of rhythmic 5–7 Hz sharp wave activity lasting for 15–45 seconds over the left frontal and frontopolar regions with a maximal field at the F7 electrode site (Fig. 73.1).

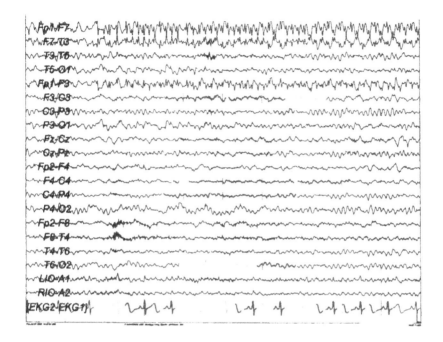

Figure 73.1: *Ictal EEG during one of the patient's typical electrographic seizures, showing rhythmic 6–7 Hz sharp wave activity over the left frontal electrode sites.*

Diagnosis

Simple partial seizures of frontal lobe origin.

Treatment and outcome

The patient was discharged home on carbamazepine and then converted to levetiracetam monotherapy because of a rash. Approximately 2 weeks later, during a 30-minute outpatient EEG, she had more than 20 electrographic seizures of left frontal origin and was diagnosed with non-convulsive status epilepticus.

She was readmitted for video-EEG monitoring. She was alert and oriented but had persistent personality changes. Her short-term and long-term memory were intact, she could spell appropriately, she could calculate and she could follow three-step commands without difficulty. Her general neurological examination

287

was normal. During the 24 hours of monitoring, 32 subclinical electrographic seizures originating from the left frontal region were recorded. During these electrographic seizures, her examination and cognitive abilities did not differ from baseline: she was able to carry on a conversation, was fully alert and oriented, and was totally unaware of the seizures when they occurred. The only detectable clinical correlate was subtle hesitancy while performing complex calculations.

On the insistence of the patient and her mother, she was discharged home the next day on levetiracetam 1500 mg/day and divalproex 1250 mg/day. A brain magnetic imaging resonance scan showed an area of encephalomalacia in the left frontal lobe at the site of her known previous abscess. Several weeks later, nine electrographic seizures originating from the left frontal region lasting 10–144 seconds were recorded over a period of 82 minutes. The doses of levetiracetam and divalproex sodium were gradually increased. In spite of this, she remained in electrographic partial status epilepticus and a subtraction ictal single photon emission computed tomography showed increased perfusion in the left orbitofrontal region, adjacent to the area of encephalomalacia (Fig. 73.2).

On the combination of levetiracetam 3000 mg/day and divalproex 1500 mg/day she was seizure-free on prolonged EEG monitoring and her personality returned to baseline.

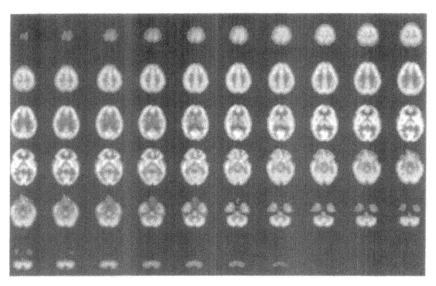

Figure 73.2: Subtraction ictal SPECT study showing increased uptake in the left frontal and frontopolar regions.

Commentary

The interesting feature of this case was the dissociation between the electrographic findings and the clinical manifestations. Status epilepticus is a medical emergency that requires immediate and aggressive treatment in order to prevent mortality or significant morbidity. Non-convulsive status epilepticus is usually suspected when there is a sudden and persistent change in mental status or behavior and confirmed by EEG.

Based on the ictal EEG findings, non-convulsive status epilepticus is divided into two categories:

- generalized non-convulsive status epilepticus; and
- partial non-convulsive status epilepticus.

Although the majority of cases of partial non-convulsive status epilepticus originate from the temporal lobes, extratemporal non-convulsive status epilepticus is usually of frontal lobe origin, as in this case.

The fascinating feature of this case is how subtle the clinical manifestations were. Even during her electrographic seizures, she was fully aware of her environment and cognitively unimpaired except for minimal hesitancy during calculations. The behavioral abnormalities were perceived by her mother but were unimpressive to her examiners except for occasional inappropriate comments and irritability that could normally be observed in any teenager.

As illustrated by this patient, non-convulsive status epilepticus of frontal lobe origin frequently occurs without alteration in the level of awareness, in contrast to non-convulsive status epilepticus of temporal lobe origin. When this is the case, as in our patient, a diagnosis of simple partial non-convulsive status epilepticus should be made. Since mood disturbances are a frequent clinical manifestation, it is not uncommon for patients with non-convulsive status epilepticus of frontal lobe origin to be initially diagnosed with hypomania or hysteria. This indicates that non-convulsive status epilepticus should be considered if a patient has an unexplained subacute change in behavior.

What did we learn from this case?

Although the patient was functioning well, we were concerned about the potential cognitive morbidity that could be caused by prolonged partial non-convulsive status epilepticus. At various times, we considered aggressive medical treatment, including drug-induced coma or surgical intervention. Both the patient and her mother were understandably concerned about our recommendations for aggressive interventions since she was otherwise performing well. After numerous discussions with the family, we decided to maximize dual therapy with levetiracetam and divalproex, titrated to tolerability. If this had failed to abort the non-convulsive status epilepticus, she would have had surgical resection of the encephalomalacia with electrocorticography to guide the margins of the resection.

Her long-term prognosis remains uncertain. Data from the largest series to date on non-convulsive status epilepticus of frontal lobe origin suggest that recurrence of status epilepticus is uncommon in this patient population. Despite being in non-convulsive status epilepticus for more than 1 month, this patient did not have detectable cognitive sequelae, although formal neuropsychological testing was not done.

How did this case alter our approach to the care and treatment of our epilepsy patients?

We now approach the treatment of simple partial non-convulsive status epilepticus of frontal lobe origin conservatively before more aggressive interventions are considered. Our case illustrates that non-convulsive status epilepticus of frontal lobe origin may present with behavioral changes not associated with impairment of awareness. In fact, had our patient not had video-EEG monitoring, the diagnosis would have been unrecognized. Our case underscores the pleomorphic clinical features of non-convulsive status epilepticus for which a high index of suspicion is necessary for prompt diagnosis and management.

Further reading

Thomas P, Zifkin B, Migneco O, et al. Nonconvulsive status epilepticus of frontal origin. Neurology 1999;52:1174–83.

Thomas P. Status epilepticus with confusional symptomatology. Neurophysiol Clin 2000;30:147–54.

Kaplan PW. Assessing the outcomes in patients with nonconvulsive status epilepticus: nonconvulsive status epilepticus is underdiagnosed, potentially overtreated, and confounded by comorbidity. J Clin Neurophysiol 1999;16:341–52.

Krumholz A, Sung GY, Fisher RS, et al. Complex partial status epilepticus accompanied by serious morbidity and mortality. Neurology 1995;45:1499–504.

Case 74

Monitoring Patients May Be More Important Than Their Laboratory Tests

Jane Boggs

History

The patient is a 56-year-old white woman with a 3-year history of seizures, presumably due to known cerebrovascular disease. Her moderately demented husband brought her to the emergency department for evaluation because she had remained lethargic on the kitchen floor (for 3 days) after a single witnessed seizure. Although she was treated with phenytoin, her compliance was suspect because her home situation was somewhat unsupervised.

A neurologist had never previously seen her. Her first known seizure occurred 8–12 months after having a stroke that caused right-sided weakness and difficult-to-understand speech. A computed tomography (CT) scan reportedly showed a 'stroke' but was unavailable for review. The patient's husband could not remember the name of the hospital where it was performed.

The patient's family described the initial seizure as 'grand mal', and phenytoin 300 mg at bedtime was the only antiepileptic drug ever prescribed. Refills had been generated by rotating clinic physicians and by episodic visits to local emergency departments for 'occasional' seizures. No EEG, repeat neuroimaging or laboratory investigations had been done as far as the patient's husband could remember.

The patient's past medical history was significant for diabetes mellitus, mild congestive heart failure following three-vessel coronary artery bypass graft surgery 4 years previously, chronic obstructive pulmonary disease, depression, rheumatoid arthritis and colostomy for resected colon cancer. Medications included phenytoin as above, insulin (Humulin 70/30) 20 units subcutaneously in the morning and 10 units in the evening, clopidogrel 75 mg/day, amitriptyline 25 mg/day at bedtime and sertraline 100 mg/day in two divided doses. Her only known allergy was to penicillin. She had a previous history of smoking, no history of alcohol or drug abuse and a strong family history of diabetes and coronary artery disease in middle age.

291

Examination and investigations

Vital signs on presentation were blood pressure 110/68 mmHg, pulse 96 beats/minute, regular respirations 16 per minute and unlabored, and rectal temperature 37.3°C. Her general examination was remarkable for the following: mild diabetic retinal changes; dependent decubitus stage IV ulcers over her left hip, sacrum, arm and lower face with mildly purulent oozing; dry oral mucosa; and a clean colostomy with heme-negative contents in the colostomy bag.

Her neurological examination revealed normal cranial nerve function, but assessment of cranial nerves I, XI and XII was not possible. She had increased tone on passive movement of the right arm and leg, with a mild flexion contracture of the right elbow. There were no spontaneous movements and withdrawal to pain was better on the left side than on the right. Reflexes were minimally brisker on the right side than on the left, and ankle jerks were absent. Plantar responses were bilaterally extensor. She moaned with uncomfortable parts of the examination, but was otherwise unresponsive and followed no commands. She was intubated because of failure to protect her airway adequately.

A CT scan of the head revealed multiple old lacunae bilaterally. A lumbar puncture documented mildly elevated cerebrospinal fluid protein of 75 mg/dl, but otherwise normal studies and no growth on cultures. Phenytoin level was 9.8 μg/ml with a normal level serum albumin of 3.0 g/dl and a creatinine level of 1.6 mg/dl. Serum ammonia was 98 μmol/l. Blood chemistry, liver function tests and blood counts were otherwise surprisingly normal, but urinalysis and culture indicated a pseudomonal urinary tract infection. Wound cultures also grew *Pseudomonas* spp. Troponin levels and electrocardiography suggested a subacute subendocardial myocardial infarction.

The neurology team was consulted after the patient's mental status remained unimproved after 24 hours of antibiotics and gentle hydration. An EEG revealed diffuse slowing with superimposed 2–3 Hz, rhythmic, sharply contoured biphasic and triphasic waveforms maximally expressed in the left frontotemporal region. This activity did not change with painful, auditory or visual stimulation, but was replaced within 2 minutes by irregular, reactive theta activity after a total of 10 mg of intravenous diazepam. The patient was treated with intravenous fosphenytoin, which raised her phenytoin level to 16 μg/ml.

Her mental status and EEG still did not improve, and occasional myoclonic jerks of the right arm were noted, with concomitant spiking seen at electrode F7; this spiking persisted after administering clinically effective paralytics. This activity persisted despite a total of 20 mg of intravenous diazepam, which resulted in a 20 mmHg drop in mean arterial pressure. The activity was stopped by valproate 500 mg intravenously, and the patient was placed immediately on maintenance intravenous fosphenytoin and valproate. The EEG improved to generalized theta waves, left slower than right (but non-rhythmic and reactive to stimulation). Within 24 hours she had spontaneous limb movements and opened her eyes to auditory stimulation. Within 1 week she was extubated and was able to answer yes–no questions appropriately.

For an unclear reason, her serum ammonia was repeated at this point and was found to be 150 μmol/l. The medical team abruptly discontinued the valproate. Three days later she answered questions more hesitantly and inappropriately. The EEG revealed recurrence of her previous left hemispheric ictal pattern. Raising her phenytoin dose to achieve a free level of 3.0 μg/ml failed to resolve the recurrent complex partial status epilepticus. Phenobarbital, gabapentin and topiramate were also tried without success.

After much discussion, the medical team agreed to resume valproate, and the EEG ictal pattern resolved. Within 24 hours she again showed clinical improvement, but required 2 weeks to regain her previous verbal skills. Serial serum ammonia levels remained between 200 μmol/l and 300 μmol/l.

Diagnosis

Recurrent left complex partial status epilepticus responsive to valproate. Asymptomatic hyperammonemia secondary to valproate.

Treatment and outcome

Six months later, the patient was brought to the emergency department again for altered mental status. The nursing home physician had discontinued oral generic valproate about 3 months previously because of gastrointestinal distress, and so she was receiving only oral phenytoin. Once again, the EEG showed ictal left patterns, which were responsive to intravenous valproate. She was discharged on phenytoin and divalproex after 3 weeks. Because she maintained a clinically improving picture, measurement of serum ammonia levels was not repeated.

Commentary

This patient had the typical clinical presentation of complex partial status epilepticus, which in her case came from the left frontotemporal region. Although no specific cerebrovascular lesion was identified as the culprit, remote stroke or new-onset cortical stroke were the most likely inciting events. Because she had been left on the kitchen floor for 3 days, the documentation of a new,

293

small cerebral lesion would have required more detailed neuroimaging (e.g. magnetic resonance imaging scans with Fluid Attenuated Inversion Recovery [FLAIR] images), which was unfortunately difficult to perform in such an unstable patient.

Her initial outpatient management with phenytoin, although a reasonable choice, appeared to have been incompletely successful and upward adjustment of the dose or consideration of another antiepileptic drug should have been considered before the subsequent acute events. Other factors that probably contributed to lowering the seizure threshold in this patient were infection, non-antiepileptic medications (particularly antibiotics) and possible chronic hypoxia.

Clearly, however, phenytoin appeared insufficient to abort non-convulsive status epilepticus in this patient. Increasing the serum level was an appropriate first attempt at treatment, although this patient's slightly decreased creatinine clearance and the concomitant use of other competitive protein-bound drugs probably raised the free fraction of phenytoin anyway.

Even so, the most common error in the early treatment of status epilepticus is administering too little of the initial antiepileptic drug. Adding a second agent is necessary when higher doses of the first drug are ineffective. All parenteral antiepileptic drugs other than valproate have some potential for causing cardiovascular instability. The relatively inert cardiovascular profile of valproate makes it an appropriate choice in any patient who has cardiac disease or who has had documented hypotensive responses to other antiepileptic drugs. In the unstable patient who requires urgent treatment, even rapid intravenous infusions of valproate have not caused significant hypotension.[1] Although valproate is not licensed in the USA for the treatment of status epilepticus, recent studies have documented success in this indication.[2,3]

Hyperammonemia is a well-known metabolic cause of altered mental status. Valproate formulations are among the drugs that may result in elevated serum ammonia levels, especially in patients with defects in the urea cycle.[4] Asymptomatic hyperammonemia should not routinely prompt discontinuation of an effective medication.[5] This patient's clinical improvement despite the higher level of ammonia after addition of valproate is supportive of an incidental laboratory finding with no evidence of clinical toxicity. It is, however, prudent to monitor steadily increasing ammonia levels in any patient with altered mental status. The risk of precipitating recurrent status epilepticus should be balanced against the risks of continuing all components of the medication regimen that aborted the seizures. Perhaps a more logical medication to consider discontinuing in this case was phenytoin, since it had failed to control both individual seizures and status epilepticus without the addition of another agent.

294

What did I learn from this case?

I learned that elevations in serum ammonia concentrations could occur with short-term use of valproate. The elevation may be as high as those that usually cause altered mental status. In an asymptomatic – indeed improving – patient, discontinuation of valproate may risk recurrent seizures. Ongoing neurologic consultation is often helpful to non-neurologists in such complex patients, even after seizures are controlled.

How did this case alter my approach to the care and treatment of my epilepsy patients?

I am now more insistent that the neurology service remain involved in the care of inpatients after the neurological crisis has seemingly ended. Although this can create a large list of 'inactive' patients, it is far easier to remedy a problem acutely than after the fact. I also make sure that I mention in my consult notes that ammonia levels need not necessarily be measured in the absence of related clinical symptoms.

References

1. Venkataraman V, Wheeless JW. Safety of rapid intravenous infusion of valproate loading doses in epilepsy patients. *Epilepsy Res* 1999;**35**:147–53.

2. Kaplan PW. Intravenous valproate treatment of generalized nonconvulsive status epilepticus. *Clin Electroencephalogr* 1999;**30**:1–4.

3. Chez MG, Hammer MS, Loeffel M, Nowinski C, Bagan BT. Clinical experience of three pediatric and one adult case of spike-and-wave status epilepticus treated with injectable valproic acid. *J Child Neurol* 1999;**14**:239–42.

4. Murphy JV, Marquardt K. Asymptomatic hyperammonemia in patients receiving valproic acid. *Arch Neurol* 1982;**39**:591–2.

5. Wyllie E, Wyllie R, Rothner AD, Erenberg G, Cruse RP. Valproate-induced hyperammonemia in asymptomatic children. *Cleveland Clin Q* 1983;**50**:275–7.

Case 75

Depression In A Student With Juvenile Myoclonic Epilepsy

Enrique J Carrazana

History

The patient is a 19-year-old man who had his first convulsion at the age of 18 during a week of intense studying for his college final examinations. The event occurred during his chemistry examination, and witnesses' accounts were suggestive of a generalized tonic–clonic seizure. The patient was seen at a local hospital, loaded with 1 g of fosphenytoin and then started on phenytoin 300 mg at bedtime. A brain computed tomography scan was unremarkable.

His second convulsion occurred 6 months later at his fraternity house, the day after a night of heavy drinking with friends. Urinary incontinence and a violent postictal phase were noted in the paramedics' report. His phenytoin level was therapeutic at 17 mg/l. The seizure was attributed to alcohol withdrawal; nevertheless, a neurological evaluation was requested.

In review of the patient's history, it was noted he had frequent 'morning jerks' and that these were more frequent during anxiety-provoking situations, at times of sleep deprivation and on the morning after heavy alcohol consumption.

Examination and investigations

The patient's physical and neurological examinations were unremarkable.

An EEG revealed frequent brief generalized bursts of 3–4 Hz polyspike–wave complexes that lasted from less than 1 second to 2 seconds. These complexes were superimposed over a normal background. Hyperventilation induced the occurrence of the discharges accompanied by bilateral arrhythmic myoclonic jerks of the arm and facial musculature.

Diagnosis

Juvenile myoclonic epilepsy.

296

Treatment and outcome

The antiepileptic drug regimen was changed to valproate. At a follow-up visit
2 months later, the patient reported being seizure-free and was no longer
experiencing myoclonic jerks. The valproate level was 105 mg/l and his EEG had
normalized.

Two months later, a psychologist at the patient's college contacted me with
concerns about the patient. Following his second seizure, he had become more
withdrawn and isolated. He moved out of the fraternity house to a small studio
apartment somewhat distant from the campus. His grades were less than optimal,
which he blamed on poor concentration. He dropped out of intramural softball,
which he had not only enjoyed in the past but was also quite good at. He
expressed feelings of hopelessness, frustration and inferiority. He had a fear of
having another seizure in front of his classmates and verbalized concerns about
becoming the subject of cruel jokes and gossip.

Depression was diagnosed, and treatment was initiated with citalopram
20 mg/day together with weekly psychotherapy sessions. The patient had a positive
response to the psychiatric intervention with gradual lifting of his depression.

He has remained seizure-free on valproate monotherapy and has commented
that excellent seizure control was important to him in establishing his self-
confidence and calming his fears. He is currently completing a doctorate program
and is in a committed serious relationship.

Commentary

Depression is an important concomitant of epilepsy. Community-based studies
have reported depression in 20–30 % of patients with epilepsy. The importance of
diagnosing depression is highlighted when the frequency of suicide in the epileptic
population is considered, especially in patients with temporal lobe epilepsy.

While the definition of depression may be quite obvious, the condition is often
underdiagnosed in epileptic patients. Thus, it is important to review the
presentation and diagnosis of depression.

Patients with depression will often present with:

- feelings of worthlessness, guilt, discouragement, hopelessness or sadness;
- significant loss of interest in pleasurable activities;
- feelings of being overwhelmed by ordinary, everyday situations;
- insomnia or hypersomnia;
- anxiety, panic attacks (pseudoseizures), obsessive–compulsive traits or
  irritability;

297

- abnormal appetite and weight change;
- sexual dysfunction; and
- suicidal ideation.

According to the DSM-IV diagnostic criteria, at least five symptoms (including depressed mood or anhedonia) that significantly interfere with the patient's life need to be present for over 2 weeks in order to establish a diagnosis of major depression.

Because the etiology of depression is often multifaceted, the treatment approach towards the depressed patient with epilepsy should encompass several factors. Initially, a clinical assessment of the severity of the depression should be made because of the increased risk of suicide. In addition, seizure frequency and type, antiepileptic drug regimen and psychosocial variables need to be examined. Other medical causes for a depression should be considered, such as structural brain lesions, hypothyroidism, vitamin B12 deficiency and substance abuse.

Antidepressants should be chosen carefully. Safety, tolerability, efficacy, cost and simplicity of dosing need to be considered. While tricyclic antidepressants such as amitryptiline and desipramine are relatively inexpensive, side effects such as sedation, memory impairment, constipation and weight gain are common. Cardiac arrhythmias are of concern at higher doses. Monoamine oxidase inhibitors are problematic in patients with epilepsy. Of the atypical antidepressants, bupropion should be used with caution because of the increased risk of seizures.

Selective serotonin reuptake inhibitors are generally well tolerated and safe in this setting, as was the case with my patient. Common side effects of the selective serotonin reuptake inhibitors include nausea, sleep disturbance and sexual dysfunction, although these tend to occur in a small minority of patients.

Seizure control needs to be optimized. Although loss of seizure control may certainly lead to a depressed state; the reverse is possible as well. A change in sleep patterns or the loss of compliance with the antiepileptic drug regimen may lead to an increase in seizure frequency.

Psychotherapy is of paramount importance in the management of depressed patients with epilepsy. Psychologists and social workers can be particularly beneficial for helping the patient establish a support system. A reactive depression as a result of discrimination, loss of driving privileges, loss of employment and unfounded fears can often be managed by psychotherapy alone or by psychotherapy together with patient education.

What did I learn from this case?

I was reminded that depression commonly occurs in patients with epilepsy and that it is frequently unrecognized and undertreated. As physicians, we need to encourage our patients to discuss their feelings and troubles openly and we need to respond by diagnosing and treating depression and other mood disorders appropriately.

How did this case alter my approach to the care and treatment of my epilepsy patients?

I am careful to inquire about symptoms that could be suggestive of an underlying depression and refer patients for psychiatric consultation and treatment when indicated.

Further reading

Barraclough B. Suicide and epilepsy. In: Reynolds ER, Trimble MR, eds. *Epilepsy and psychiatry*. Edinburgh: Churchill Livingstone; 1981:72–6.

Diagnostic and statistical manual of mental disorders, *4th ed text revision (DSM-IV-TR)*. *Washington DC: American Psychiatric Association; 2000*.

Kanner AM, Palac S. Depression in epilepsy: A common but often unrecognized comorbid malady. *Epilepsy Behav* 2000;1:37–51.

Mendez MF, Cummings JL, Benson F. Depression in epilepsy: significance and phenomenology. *Arch Neurol* 1986;43:766–70.

Robertson MM, Trimble MR. The treatment of depression in patients with epilepsy. A double-blind trial. *J Affect Disord* 1985;9:127–36.

Case 76

OSTEOMALACIA IN A PATIENT TREATED WITH MULTIPLE ANTICONVULSANTS

Joost PH Drenth, Gerlach FFM Pieters and Ad RMM Hermus

History

A 67-year-old farmer was admitted because of suspicion of osteomalacia. His medical history revealed epilepsy caused by cerebral trauma in 1947, an implanted dynamic hip screw for a right femur neck fracture in 1991 and a fracture of the left humerus in 1996.

He complained of progressive difficulty of walking because of generalized weakness, but he denied bone pain. He had a limited walking span that prevented him from going out but he enjoyed adequate sun exposure. Three weeks before admission he fractured his left femur neck after a fall, necessitating a total hip prosthesis. Further, he had noticed diarrhoea after fatty meals but denied any other abdominal symptoms.

Despite an impressive daily regimen of carbamazepine (600 mg), valproate (2100 mg), phenytoin (250 mg), vigabatrin (100 mg) and acetazolamide (250 mg), the patient experienced repetitive absence seizures.

Examination and investigations

When we first saw him in February 1998 the patient had a waddling gait. On admission in March 1998, both hips showed signs of the surgical procedures but muscle atrophy was absent. There was no apparent muscular dysfunction, and neurological testing was normal.

Laboratory testing revealed reduced serum calcium (1.86 mmol/l) and phosphate (0.77 mmol/l), high alkaline phosphatase (378 U/l), high parathyroid hormone (45 pmol/l, normal below 6.5 pmol/l), and low levels of 25-hydroxy vitamin D_3 (5 nmol/l, normal 25–72.5 nmol/l) and 1,25-dihydroxy vitamin D_3 (37 pmol/l, normal 80–200 pmol/l).

Lumbar bone mineral density was 3.2 standard deviations below the mean value of a reference group of 30-year old males (T-score). A bone biopsy specimen demonstrated osteomalacia and signs of secondary hyperparathyroidism. These findings led to a presumptive diagnosis of osteomalacia and secondary hyperparathyroidism due to hypovitaminosis D.

Because dietary intake of vitamin D and calcium in our patient was normal, malabsorption of vitamin D remained as a possibility. We therefore embarked on a search for a cause of malabsorption of vitamin D. Liver disease was absent and a small bowel enema yielded normal results. A biopsy specimen of the proximal jejunum showed only minor atrophy of villi. Anti-endomysium and anti-gliadin antibodies were absent, ruling out a gluten-sensitive enteropathy. A 24-hour stool specimen contained 34 g fat (normal below 7.2 g). Skeletal X-rays showed chalky depositions in the pancreas, suggesting that the steatorrhoea could be caused by chronic pancreatitis. This was surprising because our patient had never had significant abdominal symptoms. A specific cause for the chronic pancreatitis was not found.

Diagnoses

Osteomalacia due to anticonvulsant therapy and vitamin D deficiency; malabsorption due to chronic pancreatitis with exocrine dysfunction.

Treatment and outcome

The patient was treated with high dosages of vitamin D, calcium and pancreatic enzymes. After 1 year this treatment resulted in complete disappearance of clinical symptoms, increased weight (by 13.5 kg), increased lumbar bone density (T score of -1.4) and normalization of biochemical parameters (Fig. 76.1).

Commentary

Vitamin D is made available to the body by photogenesis in the skin and by absorption from the intestine. It is hydroxylated in the liver to 25-hydroxy vitamin D_3 and further in the kidney to 1,25-dihydroxy vitamin D_3. Anticonvulsants impair bone metabolism by induction of hepatic microsomal enzymes, resulting in increased catabolism of 25-hydroxy vitamin D_3 and perhaps through inhibition of intestinal transport of calcium. Although clinical and biochemical findings in our patient could be explained by the long-term use of anticonvulsants, osteomalacia is rare in these patients when they are well nourished and normally active. Almost invariably, other factors must be present before the complete clinical picture develops.

Anticonvulsant-related osteomalacia is an insidious disorder that may lead to

301

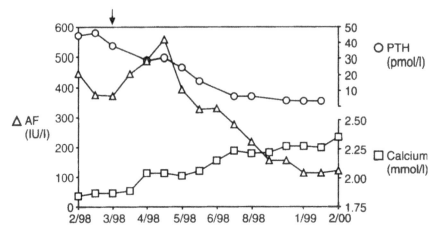

Figure 76.1: *Treatment with 300,000 IU cholecalciferol intramuscularly was commenced in March 1998 (arrow) and repeated every 6 months. Effects on serum alkaline phosphatase (AF, left axis), serum calcium (right lower axis), and parathyroid hormone concentrations (right upper axis) are shown.*

considerable morbidity if not detected at an early stage. Our case shows the need for monitoring vitamin D levels in patients using anticonvulsants.

Supplementation of vitamin D in our patient led to an impressive improvement of clinical symptoms. It reminds us that vitamin D therapy should be considered in patients who are taking multiple antiepileptic drugs and who are at the greatest risk of developing osteomalacia, such as those with malabsorption, as in this case, or reduced sun exposure or poor dietary intake.

What did we learn from this case?

We knew that antiepileptic drugs could cause hypovitaminosis D. This case taught us that additional factors such as malabsorption or inadequate sun exposure need to be present for osteomalacia to develop. Because our patient was normally active and his dietary intake of calcium and vitamin D was normal, we suspected an additional factor and searched for other causes. We learnt that a systematic analysis of the metabolic pathway of vitamin D in these cases will be needed in order to yield the eventual diagnosis.

Further reading

Hahn TJ. Drug-induced disorders of vitamin D and mineral metabolism. *Clin Endocrinol Metab* 1980;9:107–29.

Hahn TJ, Birge SJ, Scharp CR, Avioli LV. Phenobarbital-induced alteration in vitamin D metabolism. *J Clin Invest* 1972;**51**:741–8.

Shafer RB, Buttall FQ. Calcium and folic acid absorption in patients taking anticonvulsant drugs. *J Clin Endocrinol Metab* 1975;**41**:1125–9.

Francis RM, Selby PL. Osteomalacia. *Baillieres Clin Endocrinol Metab* 1997;**11**:145–63.

Acknowledgement

Published in and copyright by *The Lancet* 2000;**355**:1882. Adapted and reprinted here with permission.

Case 77

PARKINSONISM AND COGNITIVE DECLINE IN A 64-YEAR-OLD WOMAN WITH EPILEPSY

Manuel Eglau, Peter Hopp and Hermann Stefan

History

A 64-year-old woman with symptomatic epilepsy caused by perinatal brain damage was admitted to hospital because of progressive deterioration of her general health over the preceding 2 weeks, intermittent clouding of consciousness, dizziness and nausea. Parkinsonism had been diagnosed recently on the basis of tremor and motor slowing. Current complaints were constant whole body tremor and a mostly frontal headache.

Her seizures, which were complex partial and secondary generalized tonic–clonic, had been well controlled over the years with valproate 3000 mg/day and lamotrigine 200 mg/day, a regimen that the patient had tolerated well until 2 weeks before admission. No apparent cause for her deterioration, such as infection or dehydration, was found.

Examination and investigations

On neurological examination, the patient was awake but disoriented. Her psychomotor performance was impaired. A remarkable resting tremor of the whole body was found, as well as increased muscle tone and impaired motor coordination with bilateral bradykinesia and severe limb ataxia. Standing or walking was impossible. The other neurological and general physical findings were normal.

The initial EEG revealed background slowing in the theta range with bilaterally synchronous high-voltage slow wave activity. No epileptiform activity was recorded.

Laboratory studies showed elevated levels of blood urea nitrogen (35 mg/dl, normal range 8–20 mg/dl) and ammonia (123 µg/dl, normal range 19–82 µg/dl). The serum concentration of valproate was 134.6 mg/l (normal

304

range 50–100 mg/l), and the serum concentration of lamotrigine was 19.9 mg/l. No other abnormalities were found, including on liver function tests. An abdominal ultrasound was normal except for liver steatosis.

Diagnosis

Valproate-induced encephalopathy.

Treatment and outcome

As the valproate dose was reduced, her physical and cognitive condition improved significantly. Valproate was then completely withdrawn, resulting in complete remission of both the cognitive impairment and the parkinsonian syndrome. Subsequently, the EEG showed normalization of the background activity and resolution of the generalized epileptiform activity.

Commentary

What did we learn from this case?

First, we learned that although valproate may be well tolerated over many years, changes in alertness, disorientation, a worsened general health condition and impairment of motor co-ordination can occur without any obvious underlying cause as manifestations of valproate-induced encephalopathy.

In addition, this case shows that treatment with valproate may cause a syndrome that imitates Parkinson's disease. The insidious onset of valproate-associated movement disorder – after months or years of otherwise well-tolerated treatment with valproate – increases the probability that these symptoms may be mistaken for a neurodegenerative disease.[1,2,5]

In this case, clinical symptoms, hyperammonemia and EEG findings led to the diagnosis of valproate-induced encephalopathy. It should be noted that the serum valproate concentration was only moderately elevated above the therapeutic range. This observation is consistent with several reports that valproate-induced parkinsonism is independent of valproate serum concentrations.[3]

Different pathophysiological mechanisms underlying valproate encephalopathy have been proposed.[4] A crucial factor seems to be hyperammonemia, which interferes with excitatory and inhibitory neurotransmission and causes deficits in cerebral energy metabolism. Consequently, ammonia concentrations should be measured in cases of suspected valproate encephalopathy.

305

References

1. Armon C, Shin C, Miller P, *et al*. Reversible parkinsonism and cognitive impairment with chronic valproate use. *Neurology* 1996;**47**:626–35.

2. Nouzeilles M, Garcia M, Rabinovicz A, Merello M. Prospective evaluation of parkinsonism and tremor in patients treated with valproate. *Parkinsonism Rel Disord* 1999;**5**:67–8.

3. Butterworth RF. Effects of hyperammonaemia on brain function. *J Inherit Metab Dis* 1998:**21(suppl 1)**:6–20.

4. Göbel R, Görtzen A, Bräunig P. Enzephalopathien durch Valproat. *Fortschr Neurol Psychiatr* 1999;**67**:7–11.

Further reading

Onofrj M, Thomas A, Paci C. Reversible parkinsonism induced by prolonged treatment with valproate. *J Neurol* 1998;**245**:794–6.

Case 78

PROBLEMS IN MANAGING EPILEPSY DURING AND AFTER PREGNANCY

Cynthia L Harden

History

The patient is a 30-year-old woman with a history of epilepsy since the age of 13. Her epilepsy began with myoclonic jerks of the hands and arms, occasionally associated with falling down. She also developed brief staring spells associated with thought interruptions, and she had extremely rare convulsions.

She underwent trials of valproate, carbamazepine, ethosuximide and phenytoin, but had difficulty with side effects from each medicine.

At the age of 17, she was diagnosed with pseudoseizures after seeking a second opinion. Consequently, she was taken off antiseizure medicines and continued to have myoclonus, with menstrual exacerbations. After having an escalation of myoclonus associated with falls at the age of 23, just before her marriage, she was restarted on valproate on the assumption that her seizures were epileptic, and she tolerated the sprinkle formulation. She then had complete resolution of all seizures types after a slow increase of the dose to 875 mg/day.

Past medical history was negative. There was no history of febrile seizures, head trauma or brain infection, and there was no family history of epilepsy.

Examination and investigations

The patient's general and neurological examinations were unremarkable. A brain magnetic resonance imaging scan was normal and an EEG on medication was normal. Her valproate level was 62 mg/l. A muscle biopsy was negative for ragged red fibers.

Diagnosis

Juvenile myoclonic epilepsy.

Treatment and outcome

The patient wanted very much to get pregnant, but had a history of prolonged menstrual cycles of 39–40 days since the onset of menarche at the age of 12. She noted no change in her menses when she began taking valproate regularly, but she was told by her gynecologist that she was likely having anovulatory cycles. She was currently taking folate 4 mg/day. There was no family history of birth defects, including spina bifida.

The patient became pregnant while taking valproate at 875 mg/day and folate. At 16 weeks' gestation, fetal ultrasound showed evidence of spina bifida, cleft palate and hydrocephalus. The pregnancy was terminated. Consultation with a geneticist about the outcome of the pregnancy was obtained, with the opinion that perhaps not all of the fetal malformations could be attributed to valproate. Both parents were Hispanic of Jewish heritage.

The patient wanted to become pregnant again but insisted on not taking any medicine to prevent seizures this time. She continued a high-folate diet and also took a prenatal vitamin preparation plus an additional 3 mg/day of folate (with her prenatal vitamin preparation she would be getting 4 mg), since it was thought that a genetic component was present in the outcome of the first pregnancy. However, she noted that now that she was off valproate, taking the extra folate seemed to produce myoclonic jerks and she gradually tapered off the folate with resolution of the myoclonus. She gradually developed increasing myoclonus as the pregnancy advanced, but she took no antiepileptic drugs. A normal girl was delivered at term.

Postnatally, she was restarted on valproate, but she had continued myoclonus with doses up to 1750 mg/day and she had two generalized convulsions associated with exhaustion. She is currently stable with the addition of topiramate 200 mg/day and clonazepam 0.25 mg/day. Valproate has been reduced to 750 mg/day.

Commentary

This case illustrates many of the difficulties in managing women of reproductive potential with epilepsy. The American Academy of Neurology guidelines for the management of women with epilepsy state that women should be maintained on the antiepileptic drug that best controls seizures,[1] given the low risk of fetal malformations with exposure to antiepileptic drugs and the lack of clear-cut safety or superiority of any single antiepileptic drug in this setting, combined with the risk of seizures to the fetus during pregnancy. The fetus in this case developed abnormally in the presence of valproate, although the patient was

308

taking a low dose, which decreases the risk of fetal malformations.[2,3] The case was further compounded by the question raised of an independent genetic component producing the abnormal fetal outcome.

This patient was taking a higher dose of folate that is generally advocated by epileptologists, yet this did not prevent spina bifida. Paradoxically, when she was not taking valproate, the high-dose folate seemed to exacerbate her myoclonic seizures. There is some evidence in animals and in a few clinical studies that high doses of folate may be epileptogenic. Intracerebral injections of folate have produced myoclonus in chronically implanted, nonepileptic rats.[4] A study of eight patients with epilepsy and low initial folate levels found that injection of very high doses of folate (7–20 mg) produced seizures and EEG activation in six of the patients.[5] In another study of 15 schizophrenic patients with comorbid epilepsy, folate administration improved mood and decreased aggressiveness but was associated with an increase in seizures in three of the patients and increased EEG epileptiform activity in six of the patients.[6] As suggested in one case report, an altered blood–brain barrier may be a factor in increasing the risk of seizures in a patient with epilepsy taking supplemental folate.[7]

Finally, after the pregnancy, the formerly effective treatment regimen was no longer nearly as effective, and this may be at least in part to due situational factors, such as sleep deprivation and increased stress.

What did I learn from this case?

It was reinforced to me that even low doses of valproate can be associated with birth defects. I did not expect it in this case because of the low dose of valproate used together with the high dose of folate.

Furthermore, I realized that resuming medication after a medication-free pregnancy (during which many seizures occurred) may not produce the same stellar results it had before the pregnancy, for reasons that are probably complex but that must include situational factors.

Finally, I learned that my patient's reliable reports of increased seizures with high-dose folate may be supported by existing literature.

How did this case alter my approach to the care and treatment of my epilepsy patients?

I am more careful now to assess seizure frequency when using more than 1 mg/day of folate, and I realize that the 'right' dose for women with epilepsy is unclear at this time. I also feel more cautious about reassuring patients that resuming medications after a prolonged medication-free period, particularly if seizures have occurred during the medication hiatus, can once again produce

309

seizure control. Although situational factors were probably present in this case, I am nagged by the possibility that this patient's seizures during pregnancy may have been epileptogenic in origin.

References

1. Report of the Quality Standards Subcommittee of the American Academy of Neurology. Practice parameter: management issues for women with epilepsy (summary statement). *Neurology* 1998;**51**:944–8.

2. Omtzigt JG, Nau H, Los FJ, Lindhout D. The disposition of valproate and its metabolites in the late first trimester and early second trimester of pregnancy in maternal serum, urine, and amniotic fluid: effect of dose, co-medication, and the presence of spina bifida. *Eur J Clin Pharmacol* 1992;**43**:381–8.

3. Lindhout D, Omtzigt JG. Teratogenic effects of antiepileptic drugs: implications for the management of epilepsy in women of childbearing age. *Epilepsia* 1994;**35(suppl 4)**:S19–S28.

4. Tremblay E, Berger M, Nitecka L, Cavalheiro E, Ben-Ari Y. A multidisciplinary study of folic acid neurotoxicity: interactions with kainate binding sites and relevance to the aetiology of epilepsy. *Neuroscience* 1984;**12**:569–89.

5. Ch'ien LT, Krumdieck CL, Scott CW Jr, Butterworth CE Jr. Harmful effect of megadoses of vitamins: electroencephalogram abnormalities and seizures induced by intravenous folate in drug-treated epileptics. *Am J Clin Nutr* 1975;**28**:51–8.

6. Ueda S, Shirakawa T, Nakazawa Y, Inanaga K. Epilepsy and folic acid. *Folia Psychiatr Neurol Jpn* 1977;**31**:327–37.

7. Eros E, Geher P, Gomor B, Czeizel AE. Epileptogenic activity of folic acid after drug induced SLE. *Eur J Ostet Gynecol Reprod Biol* 1998;**80**:75–8.

Case 79

STATUS EPILEPTICUS IN A HEAVY SNORER

Peter Höllinger, Christian W Hess and Claudio Bassetti

History

A 50-year-old railwayman suffered from idiopathic absence seizures until the age of 16 years and had been seizure-free without antiepileptic treatment since then. Hypothyroidism and arterial hypertension were adequately treated. He was a heavy, habitual snorer. His wife witnessed nocturnal apnoeas and he reported excessive daytime sleepiness (e.g. falling asleep when watching television or when travelling in the train or in the car as a passenger). One day after lunch he was tired and nervous and shortly thereafter had three generalized tonic–clonic seizures in succession, corresponding to tonic–clonic status epilepticus. The patient was treated with intravenous benzodiazepines, phenytoin and muscle relaxation, followed by intubation. He was transferred to our department.

Examination and investigations

On admission the patient was intubated and unconscious as a result of the sedatives and relaxants. His body mass index was 42.5, indicating that he was massively overweight. There were no focal neurological deficits, and a computed tomography scan of the brain was normal.

The patient became seizure-free after intubation and muscle relaxation and he was able to be extubated the next day. An EEG performed 1 day after the status epilepticus showed a mild slowing of the background activity (around 8 Hz) but was otherwise normal. An EEG performed 2 days after the status epilepticus was completely normal. A magnetic resonance imaging scan of the brain and a lumbar puncture also revealed normal results.

The Epworth Sleepiness Score estimated for the 3 months before the status epilepticus was abnormal, with 19 points (a normal score being less than 10); this was consistent with the history of excessive daytime sleepiness.

Polysomnography performed 9 days after admission showed severe obstructive sleep apnoea with an apnoea–hypopnoea index of 74 (a normal index being less

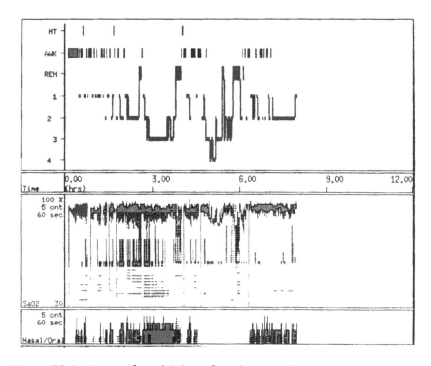

Figure 79.1: Tests performed 9 days after admission. The patient's hypnogram (top) (MT, movement time; AWK, awake). Oxygen saturation (middle). The occurrence of apnoeas and hypopnoeas (bottom).

than 10) and 53 oxygen desaturations per hour (normal being less than 3) (Fig. 79.1). The mean oxygen level during desaturations was 83, and the minimal oxygen desaturation level was 68 %. Sleep latency was 21 minutes, total sleep time was 357 minutes, rapid eye movement (REM) latency was 123 minutes, stage transitions numbered 144 and sleep efficiency was 74 %. Stage 1 sleep accounted for 18 % of the sleep period, stage 2 for 24 %, REM sleep for 8 % and slow wave sleep for 18 %.

Diagnosis

Generalized idiopathic epilepsy with status epilepticus and obstructive sleep apnoea.

312

Treatment and outcome

Treatment with nocturnal continuous positive airway pressure (CPAP) was initiated, with good compliance. Owing to the history of absence seizures in childhood, the antiepileptic drug treatment phenytoin was replaced with valproate, which, however, had to be discontinued because of severe generalized exanthema. Carbamazepine was not tolerated either (again because of generalized exanthema). Finally, phenylbarbital was tried and found to be well tolerated.

In the absence of clinical seizures, EEGs 4 and 9 months later showed frequent generalized epileptiform activity in the form of spike wave bursts without clinical correlates, occurring approximately every 6 minutes.

A control polysomnography performed 1 year after the initiation of CPAP treatment showed normal findings with an apnoea–hypopnoea index of less than 1, and 0.3 oxygen desaturations an hour (Fig. 79.2). Sleep latency was 6 minutes,

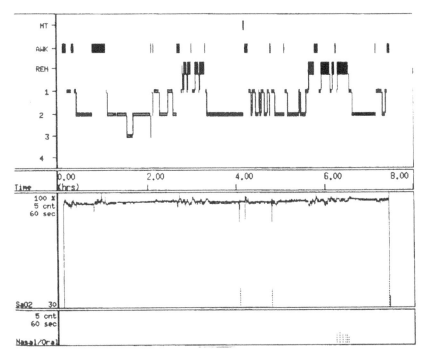

Figure 79.2: *Tests performed 1 year after the initiation of CPAP treatment. The hypnogram (top) is much less fragmented than the earlier test and there is more REM sleep. There are no episodes of oxygen desaturation (middle). There are no episodes of apnoea or hypopnoea.*

313

total sleep time was 384 minutes, REM latency was 155 minutes, stage transitions numbered 78, and sleep efficiency was 85 %. Stage 1 sleep accounted for 20 % of the sleep period, stage 2 for 52 %, REM sleep for 14 % and slow wave sleep for 2 %.

The Epworth Sleepiness Score had normalized to 5 points and the multiple sleep latency test was also normal, with a mean sleep latency of 12.5 minutes (normal being less than 10 minutes).

Two years after the status epilepticus, the patient remains seizure-free on 300 mg phenylbarbital, works to full capacity and is highly satisfied with his CPAP treatment.

Commentary

Why did we choose this case?

This patient's history highlights one possible pathogenic interaction between obstructive sleep apnoea and epilepsy. We hypothesize that this patient's childhood epilepsy remained asymptomatic for many years until the detrimental effect of obstructive sleep apnoea triggered an episode of status epilepticus. Although the exact time of onset of signs and symptoms of obstructive sleep apnoea cannot be determined precisely from the patient's history, he clearly exhibited symptoms of obstructive sleep apnoea (snoring, apnoeas and sleepiness) for a few months before the episode of status epilepticus. In addition he was massively overweight, which is a well known risk factor for obstructive sleep apnoea.

Furthermore, the patient remained clinically seizure-free after treatment with antiepileptic drugs and CPAP, despite the persistence on EEG of generalized spike-wave activity. Control polysomnography demonstrated a complete normalization of the initial sleep disordered breathing, thus excluding persistent obstructive sleep apnoea as a cause of persisting EEG abnormalities. The patient was sleepy before the inititation of CPAP treatment and showed marked lessening of excessive daytime sleepiness with CPAP (with normalization of the Epworth Sleepiness Score from 19 to 5 points), which explained his compliance with the treatment device.

Since additional investigations excluded factors known to cause status epilepticus, including for example fever or inflammatory or structural brain pathology, we postulate that status epilepticus arose from an idiopathic predisposition for generalized epilepsy (as manifested by childhood absence seizures) and severe obstructive sleep apnoea.

What did we learn from this case?

In patients with a hitherto well-controlled seizure disorder and recently increasing seizure frequency, new onset of epileptic seizures, or status epilepticus, it is obviously important to exclude such causes as degenerative, structural or inflammatory brain disease or poor compliance to drug treatment. In the absence of such factors, one should also ask about symptoms of obstructive sleep apnoea such as snoring, observed apnoeas and excessive daytime sleepiness. Fatigue or sleepiness in patients under antiepileptic drug treatment should not automatically be attributed to the drug, since a treatable sleep disorder, including obstructive sleep apnoea, might underlie this specific complaint.[1] In the presence of obstructive sleep apnoea, CPAP treatment should be considered, although at best 80 % of patients in larger series may be compliant with this treatment.[2] Poor compliance is especially likely in patients who do not report excessive subjective daytime sleepiness.

Our group has shown that the frequency of epilepsy and obstructive sleep apnoea is higher than what could be estimated by pure coincidence, suggesting a specific pathogenic link. Obstructive sleep apnoea induces sleep fragmentation caused by recurrent arousals and thus leads to sleep deprivation, which is well known to precipitate epileptic seizures.

Obviously, obstructive sleep apnoea represents only one of several potential pathogenic mechanisms in the aetiology of seizures. Hence, despite optimal treatment with CPAP, seizures may persist. The effect of CPAP treatment on seizure frequency in a single patient may be difficult to estimate considering the fact that most patients already receive antiepileptic drug treatment and that CPAP is prescribed only as an adjunctive treatment. Prospective studies with larger samples of patients with obstructive sleep apnoea and epilepsy are needed.

References

1.   Malow BA, Fromes GA, Aldrich MS. Usefulness of polysomnography in epilepsy patients. *Neurology* 1997;**48**:1389–94.

2.   Strollo PJ, Rogers RM. Obstructive sleep apnea. *N Engl J Med* 1996;**334**:99–104.

Further reading

Höllinger P, Bassetti C, Gugger M, Hess CW. Epilepsy and obstructive sleep apnea. *Neurology* 2000;**54(suppl 3)**:A27.

315

Case 80

A BOY WITH EPILEPSY AND ALLERGIC RHINITIS

Kazuie Iinuma and Hiroyuki Yokoyama

History

A 5-year-old boy with partial epilepsy and allergic rhinitis was hospitalized for optimal seizure control. Eventually, combined antiepileptic treatment with valproate 400 mg/day, zonisamide 80 mg/day and clonazepam 0.8 mg/day resulted in complete seizure control.

About 6 months later, he was given ketotifen 1.0 mg/day for treatment of allergic rhinitis. A few days later, he started having partial seizures, with or without loss of consciousness, two or three times a day. According to his mother, his seizures had previously been aggravated by ketotifen when it has been prescribed by a local doctor during the spring and autumn.

Thereafter, ketotifen was replaced with terfenadine 60 mg/day. After the switch from ketotifen to terfenadine, the patient regained excellent seizure control. There was no obvious change in the serum concentrations of his anticonvulsant medications when the allergy medication was changed.

Examination and investigations

We examined the effect of intravenous D-chlorpheniramine, a centrally acting histamine H_1 antagonist, on the patient's EEG after signed informed consent was obtained from his parents. The occurrence of spikes was calculated before and after administration of D-chlorpheniramine to evaluate its effect on seizure susceptibility.

The administration of D-chlorpheniramine significantly increased the number of spikes compared with those observed before treatment (Fig. 80.1). Figure 80.2 shows an increase of spikes on the EEG after D-chlorpheniramine administration.

316

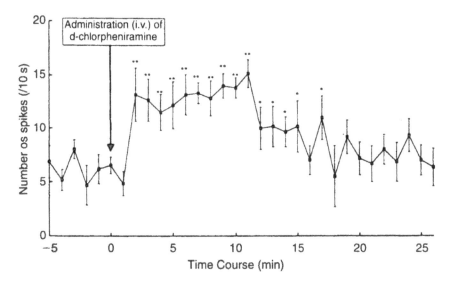

Figure 80.1: *EEG activation by* D-*chlorpheniramine. Spikes were measured over a 10-second period, and averaged during 1 minute before and after the administration of intravenous* D-*chlorpheniramine. Administration of* D-*chlorpheniramine significantly increased the number of spikes, compared to pre-treatment. Significant differences: *p<0.05, **p<0.01 versus the number of spikes before the administration, as determined by ANOVA followed by Duncan's test.*

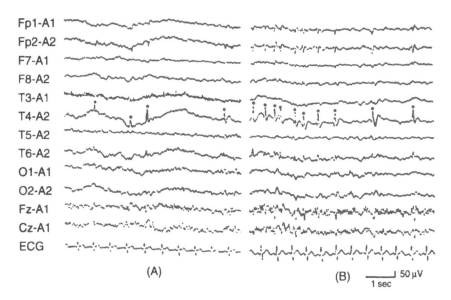

Figure 80.2: *Sample EEG before (A) and after (B) the administration of* D-*chlorpheniramine.*

Diagnosis

Partial epilepsy with seizure exacerbation by ketotifen, an antihistaminic agent.

Treatment and outcome

After switching from ketotifen to terfenadine, the patient was seizure free for 8 years. His antiepileptic drugs were then gradually reduced and discontinued.

Commentary

According to the literature, histamine H_1 antagonists occasionally produce convulsions in healthy children, especially pre-school age children.[1-4] The antihistamines are commonly used in patients with allergic disorders, including patients with epilepsy.

Our patient lost optimal seizure control during treatment with ketotifen; epileptic discharges markedly increased after loading with D-chlorpheniramine, a histamine H_1 antagonist; however, terfenadine, one of the new generation antihistamines with little penetration into brain, did not exacerbate seizures in this patient. These observations strongly support the contention that his seizure exacerbation was due to ketotifen and was probably the result of the blockade of central histamine H_1 receptors. Experiments have shown an inhibitory effect of histamine in a variety of seizure models.[5-7]

What did we learn from this case?

First, we learned that histamine H_1 receptor antagonists might aggravate seizures.

Secondly, we observed that terfenadine did not exacerbate the patient's seizures, possibly because of minimal brain penetration.

Thirdly, we discovered that EEG monitoring during D-chlorpheniramine administration could be used to examine the susceptibility of particular patients with epilepsy to antihistamines. We now believe that this class of drugs should be avoided in patients with epilepsy.

References

1.   Churchill JA, Gammon GD. The effect of antihistaminic drugs on convulsive seizures. *JAMA* 1949;**141**:18–21.

2.   Mueller MD. Phenylpropanolamine, a nonprescription drug with potentially fatal side effects. *N Engl J Med* 1983;**308**:653.

3.   Bernstein E, Diskant BM. Phenylpropanolamine: a potentially hazardous drug. *Ann Emerg Med* 1982;**11**:311–5.

4.   Schwartz JF, Patterson JH. Toxic encephalopathy related to antihistamine–barbiturate antiemetic medication. *Am J Dis Child* 1978;**132**:37–9.

5.   Onodera K, Tuomisto L, Tacke U, Airaksinen M. Strain differences in regional brain histamine levels between genetically epilepsy-prone and resistant rat. *Meth Find Exp Clin Pharmacol* 1992;**14**:13–6.

6.   Freeman P, Sturman G, Wilde P. Elevation of histamine levels but not H2-receptor blockade influences electrically-induced seizure threshold in mice. *J Psychopharmacol* 1990;**4**:313.

7.   Yokoyama H, Onodera K, Maeyama K, *et al.* Histamine levels and clonic convulsions of electrically-induced seizures in mice: the effects of α-fluoromethylhistidine and metoprine. *Naunyn-Schmiedeberg Arch Pharmacol* 1992;**346**:40–5.

319

Case 81

Weight Gain, Acne And Menstrual Disorder In A Woman With Partial Epilepsy

Jouko Isojärvi

History

A 23-year-old woman had several tonic–clonic seizures at the age of 16 and was treated with carbamazepine for some years. Thereafter the medication was tapered off and she remained seizure-free until she started to experience complex partial seizures at the age of 22.

Interictal EEG showed paroxysmal slow waves and some sharp waves in the left temporal region. Magnetic resonance imaging of the brain was normal. The patient was considered to have partial epilepsy originating from the left temporal lobe. Oxcarbazepine was started at 300 mg twice daily. She remained seizure-free, but during the first 10 months of treatment she gained 6 kg in weight, her acne became worse and she started to experience menstrual disorders. Her menstrual cycle changed from 28 days to 35–42 days.

Examination and investigations

On clinical examination the patient had acne on her face and shoulders. Ovarian ultrasonography showed polycystic ovaries. Her serum testosterone level was elevated to 5.0 nmol/l (normal range 0.4–2.7 nmol/l).

Diagnosis

Left temporal lobe epilepsy and polycystic ovarian syndrome.

Treatment and outcome

Oxcarbazepine was switched to carbamazepine 200 mg/day twice daily. The patient remained seizure-free on carbamazepine, and over the next few months the acne on her face and shoulders diminished and her menstrual cycle became shorter and more regular. After 6 months of carbamazepine treatment, she had had three regular cycles (duration 28 days). One year after the switch, ovarian ultrasonography still showed polycystic ovaries. However, the serum testosterone level had decreased and the serum sex hormone-binding globulin levels had increased, resulting in decreased bioactive androgen levels (the free androgen index had diminished from 9.5 to 4.4).

Commentary

I chose this case because it is an interesting example of the association between reproductive endocrine disorders, epilepsy and antiepileptic drugs. It is well known that reproductive endocrine disorders, and especially polycystic ovarian syndrome, are over-represented among women with epilepsy. It has been suggested that temporal lobe epilepsy with left temporal focus, in particular, is associated with the development of polycystic ovarian syndrome.

On the other hand, it appears that some antiepileptic drugs, especially valproate, may be associated with or may even promote the development of polycystic ovarian syndrome. Carbamazepine is known to reduce the bioactivity of androgens; theoretically, it may therefore protect against hyperandrogenism and the development of polycystic ovarian syndrome. Oxcarbazepine is not known to be associated with endocrine abnormalities.

What did I learn from this case?

This case was a practical example of an epilepsy-associated reproductive endocrine problem. It is probable, in this patient, that hyperandrogenism and polycystic ovarian syndrome were associated with left-sided temporal lobe epilepsy, although the possibility that oxcarbazepine promoted hyperandrogenism and related symptoms cannot be excluded.

More importantly, I have learned that the association of epilepsy with reproductive endocrine disorders should be more widely acknowledged and factored into the choice of antiepileptic drugs. This is especially important in young women with epilepsy. Carbamazepine is a good choice for treating women with partial epilepsy, especially those with left-sided temporal lobe epilepsy, who may be at increased risk of developing polycystic ovarian syndrome.

Further reading

Herzog AG, Seibel MM, Schomer DL, Vaitukaitis JL, Geschwind N. Reproductive endocrine disorders in women with partial seizures of temporal lobe origin. *Arch Neurol* 1986;**43**:341–6.

Isojärvi JIT, Laatikainen TJ, Pakarinen AJ, Juntunen KTS, Myllylä VV. Polycystic ovaries and hyperandrogenism in women taking valproate for epilepsy. *N Engl J Med* 1993;**329**:1383–8.

Isojärvi JIT, Laatikainen TJ, Pakarinen AJ, Juntunen KTS, Myllylä VV. Menstrual disorders in women with epilepsy receiving carbamazepine. *Epilepsia* 1995;**36**:676–81.

Vainionpää LK, Rattya J, Knip M, *et al.* Valproate-induced hyperandrogenism during pubertal maturation in girls with epilepsy. *Ann Neurol* 1999;**45**:444–50.

322

Case 82

Seizures And Behavior Disturbance In A Boy

Sookyong Koh

History

The patient is a 12-year-old, right-handed, sixth-grade boy with complex partial seizures, oppositional defiant disorder, attention deficit–hyperactivity disorder, depression, psychosis and a non-enhancing lesion in the left medial temporal lobe.

He initially presented at 4 years of age with 6 hours of unresponsiveness and decreased respiratory effort that required intubation. The head computed tomography (CT) scan was normal. Two years later, he returned because of monthly episodes of forceful swallowing, staring and fidgeting with his hands followed by a period of disorientation. With these spells, which lasted 'a couple of minutes', he would talk rapidly and incoherently with slurred and garbled speech about things that did not apply to the current situation such as 'the cat is in the refrigerator'. At times, he would not recognize his mother and would respond to his mother's placing her hand on his back by saying, 'that's a policeman's hand'. His sister once asked him 'Are you all right?' and he responded, 'I will be if you wake me up'.

He also described visual changes associated with the spells. For example, while looking at a chair it might become a table, a table might become a television and so on. He described apparent auras consisting of a feeling of 'weirdness' or 'fuzziness in my head'. Besides reporting 'sometimes I find myself in a different place than when I started', he had been found lying next to his bicycle, his bed and his school desk, apparently after falls.

In addition to his typical complex partial seizures with rare generalization, he experienced multiple daily episodes of 'floaty feelings', during which he felt 'fuzzy' and 'floaty' as if in a cloud. He also complained of 'dead feelings', when he became limp and unable to move his limbs. He described 'room seizures', when he did not know where he was, thought he was in a room where he had previously been and felt he was going back in time.

He also experienced severe headaches that were 'caused by balls permeating from my head rolling down my face'. During these headaches, he clutched his

323

head, screamed with pain and became completely limp and unresponsive for a brief period. After these headaches he would vomit. Once, after four successive episodes, he described vivid visual hallucinations, such as seeing his dead aunt or seeing evil and good fighting on the wall.

He related a story about his imaginary friends Shelly, who is good, and Philip, who is bad. Philip has been with him almost constantly and interfered with his everyday activities since he was 5 years old. Philip tells him to punch himself at times, and it was Philip who also told him to swallow broken glass (which he had done). It was Philip, too, who caused 'floaty feelings' and 'dead feelings'. Gabapentin made Philip more visible whereas methylphenidate 'fights off Philip and makes Philip calm'. He referred to valproate as a 'shield' against Philip and carbamazepine as a 'sword'.

The patient was maintained on high therapeutic doses of both carbamazepine and valproate. He had been on carbamazepine monotherapy for the first 2 years after diagnosis. Gabapentin was tried for 3 months before being discontinued because of worsening 'dead feelings'. He has had a fluctuating response to his antiepileptic drugs – at best, one or two seizures a month, at worst, three seizures a week with multiple daily episodes of 'floaty feelings'.

Over the years, he has had escalating behavioral dyscontrol, leading to many crises at school and home, fist fights, confrontation with teachers and threats of expulsion. He had tried to hurt himself by swallowing shards of glass and overdosing on his anticonvulsants. He has reported feeling very, very sad and helpless. He has been treated by a psychiatrist with methylphenidate and haloperidol.

Examination and investigations

The patient was admitted to the hospital for presurgical evaluation with video-EEG monitoring. On the admission examination, he presented with 'I am a dickweed' written across his abdomen. He was talkative and inattentive. He had difficulty reciting a short story from memory and wrote, with poor penmanship, 'this season seems like an endless conclusion compared to our winter it seems an illusion'. There was posturing of the right hand on stressed gait and clumsy rapid alternating movements. While his antiepileptic drugs were withheld over the ensuing few days, he became increasingly agitated, ripped his telemetry wires off his head, jumped over the bed and ran out of the room. The outburst escalated and finally necessitated four-point leather restraints, as well as the administration of diazepam, chloral hydrate and lorazepam.

The interictal EEG showed focal sharp waves and continuous slowing over the left mid- to anterior temporal lobe. His 'floaty feelings' were without concomitant EEG correlate.

324

A head magnetic resonance imaging (MRI) scan showed a non-enhancing T2-weighted hyperintense lesion that involved the entire anterior tip and undersurface of the left temporal lobe and extended posteriorly to involve the medial portion. The lesion measured approximately 4 cm by 2.5 cm by 3 cm and had not changed in appearance or size on yearly head MRIs over a 6-year period.

Neuropsychological testing showed a large discrepancy between verbal IQ (120) and performance IQ (79).

Diagnosis, treatment and outcome

The patient underwent left temporal lobe lesionectomy under the guidance of intraoperative electrocorticography at the age of 12 – 6 years after the initial presentation of partial seizures. Pathology revealed a hamartoma.

After the operation, the patient suffered no neurological deficit, but rather could recall remote childhood memories. He is not only free of seizures, but also free of psychosis. The patient continues on valproate, carbamazepine and methylphenidate for continued aggression and 'mood swings', and he attends a residential school for behavioral modification. He remains seizure-free on last follow up, nearly 3 years after the surgery.

Commentary

Neuropsychiatric consequences of poorly controlled temporal lobe epilepsy can be truly devastating. This is particularly evident for seizures that begin in childhood. In one study, nearly one-quarter of the 100 children with temporal lobe seizures followed to adulthood had IQs of less than 70; only 15 of all children were recorded as showing no form of personality difficulty at any time; 26 suffered from the hyperkinetic syndrome; 36 exhibited catastrophic rage, and nine developed schizophreniform psychosis.[1]

This case illustrates the central focus of many patients with epilepsy and of their families – behavioral difficulties. Behavioral problems, once the seizure disorder has become less psychologically dramatic to people in the child's environment, are often considered by the parents and teachers as more difficult to cope with than the epilepsy itself.[2] In addition, a recent study on long-term prognosis of seizures with onset in childhood[3] reports the startling finding of significantly increased risk of death in patients with epilepsy, especially in those whose seizures were not in remission. Patients with epilepsy since childhood were also more likely to remain unmarried, unemployed and childless.

What did I learn from this case?

I often wondered, together with the patient's family, what would have happened if the surgery was performed earlier. Could we have prevented this child's school failure, psychosis, depression, suicidal attempts and behavioral deterioration as well as his seizures if the surgery had been performed at the time of his initial presentation? What if, at age 4, a head MRI had been done instead of a CT scan and the hamartoma had been detected and then removed? Early surgery in my patient may not only have stopped the seizures but may also have prevented further brain injury from the seizures and the side effects of the antiepileptic drugs. Removal of the abnormal tissue might have spared the patient and his family 6 years of ordeal and allowed the remainder of his developing brain to be free of the undesirable influences of the abnormal epileptic tissue.[4]

How did this case alter my approach to the care and treatment of my epilepsy patients?

Surgery for intractable, catastrophic seizures in young children has become more established in recent years. This case impressed me that treatment of seizures, especially for the developing brain, should be 'decisive and prompt'.[5] I now consider early surgery under the appropriate circumstances.

References

1. Lindsay J, Ounsted C, Richards P. Long-term outcome in children with temporal lobe seizures: 3. Psychiatric aspects in childhood and adult life. *Dev Med Child Neurol* 1979;**21**:630–6.

2. Gillberg C. Psychiatric and behavioral problems in epilepsy, hydrocephalus and cerebral palsy. In: Aicardi J, ed. *Diseases of the nervous system in childhood (Clinics in Developmental Medicine No 115–118)*. London: Mac Keith Press; 1992.

3. Sillanpää M, Jalava M, Kaleva O, Shinnar S. Long-term prognosis of seizures with onset in childhood. *N Engl J Med* 1998;**338**:1715–22.

4. Holmes GL. Surgery for intractable seizures in infancy and early childhood. *Neurology* 1993;**43(suppl 5)**:S28–S37.

5. Moshe SL. Intractable seizures in infancy and early childhood. *Neurology* 1993;**43(suppl 5)**:S2.

Case 83

ABULIA IN A SEIZURE-FREE PATIENT WITH FRONTAL LOBE EPILEPSY

Ennapadam S Krishnamoorthy and Michael R Trimble

History

A 32-year-old medically retired civil servant was referred to our clinic by his general practitioner. He had a history of epilepsy from the age of 16 years, and 3 years earlier, on referral to a university hospital, he had been correctly diagnosed with frontal lobe epilepsy. Neuroimaging studies had shown right frontal pathology. Therapy with topiramate had been instituted, which led to complete cessation of seizures. However, over the 18-month period between then and his consultation with us, he had developed a very prominent lack of motivation, though he remained seizure-free. This was diagnosed as depression and treated with fluoxetine for 18 months with little effect. In addition there was a complaint of erectile dysfunction and impaired ejaculation that appeared to predate these complaints.

While waiting to be seen in our clinic his clinical condition worsened significantly. He became profoundly withdrawn, stopped taking care of himself, did not eat for days on end, had not opened his mail and had not washed for a considerable time. While he was somewhat depressed, the most prominent feature was his profound lack of will to engage in goal-directed behaviour (abulia). Unlike people with depression that is severe enough to result in significant self-neglect, he did not have mood-congruent delusions or hallucinations, nor did he entertain nihilistic or suicidal ideas.

His general practitioner replaced fluoxetine with reboxetine, and his family intervened and took care of him. He was also seen by a local psychiatrist, who documented these developments, and by the uroneurologist in our hospital, who recommended sildenafil for the erectile dysfunction.

With the institution of reboxetine, and perhaps the use of sildenafil (on one occasion), his seizure control was destabilized and he developed a flurry of seizures. Nonetheless, his motivation improved, he began to engage in purposeful goal-directed behaviour, his appetite became better and he began to gain weight. Although there was no change in his mood and he remained somewhat miserable, his clinical state improved markedly and his abulia ceased.

327

Examination

When examined in the clinic, the patient was somewhat anxious and he reported long-standing low self-esteem. He attributed his low self-esteem, as well as his sexual dysfunction, to epilepsy. There were no psychotic features or major depressive ideation. He did, however, give a good account of the very prominent syndrome characterized by lack of motivation that he had suffered from, in the absence of seizures, while on treatment with topiramate, and which had remitted when his seizures returned.

Diagnosis

Alternative psychosis in a patient with frontal lobe epilepsy presenting as a frontal lobe syndrome characterized by abulia.

Treatment and outcome

Because the patient's symptoms had remitted with the re-emergence of seizures, it was recommended that the dose of anticonvulsant drugs should be titrated to allow the occasional breakthrough seizure. The patient was referred to a sexual dysfunction clinic. When last reviewed in our clinic, his improvement with regard to abulia was maintained and he continued to have the occasional seizure.

Commentary

This case clearly illustrates the complex relationships between epilepsy and psychiatric disorders, ranging from the more common and better-accepted agonistic relationship, to the less common and often hotly debated antagonistic relationship – the forced normalization of Landolt[1] and the alternative psychoses of Tellenbach.[2]

This case also shows that distinct, possibly localization-related, neuropsychiatric syndromes do exist in epilepsy and are often mistaken for common psychiatric disorders such as depression.

Furthermore, this case aptly demonstrates the significance of the disability that sometimes results from anticonvulsant-induced neuropsychiatric disorders, which may arise, paradoxically, as a consequence of seizure control.

What did we learn from this case?

This case taught us several important lessons.

First, it is automatically assumed that good seizure control is the panacea for all the patient's ills. While this is certainly true for the vast majority of patients, there is a distinct subset of patients in whom we see an antagonistic relationship between seizure control and mental health. We learn from this case that it may be better for some patients to have the occasional seizure, rather than aggressively pursuing the ideal of complete seizure control. As Landolt somewhat crudely put it: 'It appears that there are some patients with epilepsy who need to have seizures in order to be mentally sane'.[3]

Secondly, a number of people fail to recognize the distinct behavioural syndromes that accompany neurological and neuropsychiatric disorders. Abulia, the inability to engage in goal-directed behaviour, is one such syndrome, commonly seen with lesions of the basal ganglia and frontal lobes.[4] According to experts that we have surveyed, the syndrome does have some very distinct characteristics, such as difficulty in initiating and sustaining purposeful actions, reduced social interactions and reduced interest in usual pastimes, reduced emotional responsiveness and spontaneity, and reduced spontaneous speech and movement.[5] Abulia is often mistaken for depression and treated as such. In this case, treatment with antidepressant drugs was beneficial in that it destabilized the patient's seizure control, leading to remission of the abulia.

Thirdly, even those clinicians who acknowledge the existence of the antagonistic relationship between epilepsy and psychiatric disorders often believe that the only presentation of the psychiatric disorders is with psychotic symptoms. This could not be further from the truth. The alternative psychoses, often accompanied by forced normalization of the EEG, are a spectrum of disorders that range from traditional psychosis to affective disorder, anxiety disorder and even non-organic complaints.[6] In our experience, alternative psychoses can also present as discrete neuropsychiatric syndromes such as abulia and even the syndrome of episodic dyscontrol. Putative mechanisms include kindling in subcortical structures, secondary epileptogenesis and alternating states of GABAergic and glutaminergic preponderance, influenced by complex interactions with dopamine.[7] Anticonvulsant drugs, particularly those such as topiramate that increase γ-aminobutyric acid levels, are well known to lead to alternative psychosis with or without forced normalization of the EEG.[8]

Furthermore, although the alternative psychoses are usually acute, they often develop insidiously. Recently we have proposed criteria for the diagnosis of this condition that we hope will encourage epileptologists to establish prospective studies.[9]

Fourthly, most anticonvulsant drugs (both new and old) do produce neuropsychiatric symptoms or syndromes in some patients that are often ignored

329

or remain undiagnosed. These syndromes can cause a significant level of disability, as this case highlights, and need to be identified and managed properly.

Finally, this case serves to remind us that psychotropic drugs, especially antidepressants, are proconvulsant and may precipitate seizures. On this occasion the offending agent was reboxetine, a newer antidepressant. The seizure, however, proved helpful in the patient's diagnosis and remission.

References

1. Landolt H. Serial EEG investigations during psychotic episodes in epileptic patients and during schizophrenic attacks. In: Lorentz De Haas AM, ed. *Lectures on epilepsy*. Amsterdam: Elsevier; 1958:91–133.

2. Tellenbach H. Epilepsie als Anfallsleiden und als Psychose. *Nervenar* 1965;36:190–202.

3. Schmitz B. Forced normalization: history of a concept. In Trimble MR, Schmitz B, eds. *Forced normalization and alternative psychoses of epilepsy*. Petersfield: Wrightson; 1998:7–24.

4. Bhatia KP, Marsden CD. The behavioural and motor consequences of focal lesions of the basal ganglia in man. *Brain* 1994;117:859–76.

5. Vijayaraghavan L, Krishnamoorthy ES, Brown RB, Trimble MR. Abulia: a survey of British neurologists and psychiatrists. *Movement Disorders* (in press).

6. Wolf P. Acute behavioural symptomatology at disappearance of epileptiform EEG abnormality: paradoxical or forced normalisation. In: Smith D, Treiman D, Trimble MR, eds. *Neurobehavioural problems in epilepsy*. New York: Raven; 1991:127–42.

7. Krishnamoorthy ES, Trimble MR. Mechanisms of forced normalization. In: Trimble MR, Schmitz B, eds. *Forced normalization and alternative psychoses of epilepsy*. Petersfield: Wrightson; 1998:193–207.

8. Trimble MR. Forced normalization and the role of anticonvulsants. In: Trimble MR, Schmitz B, eds. *Forced normalization and alternative psychoses of epilepsy*. Petersfield: Wrightson; 1998:169–78.

9. Krishnamoorthy ES, Trimble MR. Forced normalization: clinical and therapeutic relevance in mood disturbances, psychoses and epilepsy. *Epilepsia* 1999;40(suppl 10):S57–S64.

Case 84

THE CONTINUING PLACE OF PHENOBARBITAL

Fumisuke Matsuo

History

This male patient experienced his first seizure in 1978 at the age of 15. It was a generalized convulsion that occurred early in the morning during sleep and lasted approximately 5 minutes, as have all of his subsequent seizures. EEG was abnormal and his family doctor initiated phenobarbital 120 mg/day. The phenobarbital dose was raised to 180 mg/day after his second seizure 9 months later.

A subsequent EEG in 1981 was normal. The phenobarbital was reduced by 60 mg every other day. Soon after this, the patient suffered another seizure, and phenobarbital was increased back to 180 mg/day. In October 1982, he left for an 18-month church mission, which radically altered his eating and sleeping habits. Two seizures occurred over the next 6 months and his phenobarbital was increased to 240 mg/day. The dose was further increased to 360 mg/day in January 1984 after another seizure that was unrelated to non-compliance. After being seizure-free for 2 years, the patient decreased phenobarbital to 300 mg/day.

Over the next 12 years, in consultation with a neurologist, he attempted further phenobarbital dosage reductions down to 200 mg daily, but breakthrough seizures occurred and the dose was continued at 300 mg/day.

Investigations

The patient's sister, 7 years younger, suffered refractory generalized epilepsy from the age of 2 years, with a frequency of four or five seizures a month. She died a sudden and unexplained death at the age of 24. The family doctor arranged for all six siblings to undergo EEGs when our patient experienced his first seizure. Two of the siblings had abnormal EEGs, but neuroimaging was normal in both of these siblings.

331

Treatment and outcome

At his wife's urging, the patient saw another neurologist when he was aged 36. The neurologist felt that the patient's quality of life would be better with a different medication, and initiated carbamazepine. When the carbamazepine dose reached 800 mg/day, the phenobarbital dose was reduced by 50 mg every 3 weeks. During the transition, the patient had two seizures; by October 1999 the phenobarbital dose was 50 mg/day and the carbamazepine dose was 1200 mg/day. The next month, he had a mild seizure, noted involuntary muscle jerking and began experiencing severe double vision.

Phenobarbital was discontinued and he had several additional seizures over the next few months. Lamotrigine was added and titrated over 2 months to 400 mg/day in two divided doses, and carbamazepine was reduced to 800 mg/day in two divided doses.

The patient continued to have seizures and therefore restarted phenobarbital. On a regimen of phenobarbital 100 mg/day, carbamazepine 200 mg/day and lamotrigine 400 mg/day in two divided doses, he suffered from tiredness but his seizures were completely controlled.

Diagnosis

Syndrome of familial epilepsy with nocturnal recurrences.[1]

Commentary

Phenobarbital was able to control this patient's seizures, although the patient and his wife were concerned about adverse neurobehavioral symptoms at high doses. Carbamazepine not only failed to control the seizures at maximally tolerated doses, but it may also have precipitated non-convulsive generalized seizures.[2] Lamotrigine may prove satisfactory in this patient, but ultimate control may require the use of valproate as monotherapy or in combination.[3]

What did I learn from this case?

I learned that it might take decades in some patients with very infrequent seizures to assess the results of different treatment regimens. This patient suffered an average of one seizure a year, including some precipitated by minor changes in antiepileptic drug regimens. This patient's history also highlights the difficulty involved in evaluating possible discontinuation of prophylaxis with antiepileptic drugs even after prolonged periods of freedom from seizures.[4] This case illustrated to me that the efficacy of antiepileptic drugs is notoriously difficult to assess in certain provoked epilepsy syndromes, and that such assessments may result in negative notions about the role of antiepileptic drugs in such patients.[5]

How did this case alter my approach to the care and treatment of my epilepsy patients?

I am more sensitive now to the fact that the lives of patients with very infrequent seizures could be disrupted by the occurrence of a seizure, even when they are exclusively nocturnal as in this patient. I am also more cautious about discontinuing phenobarbital.[6]

References

1.   Berkovic SF, Scheller IE. Genetics of the epilepsies. *Curr Opin Neurol* 1999;12:177–82.

2.   Snead OC, Hosey LC. Exacerbation of seizures in children by carbamazepine. *N Eng J Med* 1985;313:916–21.

3.   Brodie MJ, Yuen AW. Lamotrigine substitution study: evidence for synergism with sodium valproate. *Epilepsy Res* 1997;26:423–32.

4.   American Academy of Neurology. Practice parameter: a guideline for discontinuing antiepileptic drugs in seizure-free patients: summary statement. *Neurology* 1996;47:600–2.

5.   Friis ML, Lund M. Stress convulsions. *Arch Neurol* 1974;31:155–9.

6.   Buchthal F, Svenmark O, Simonsen H. Relation of EEG and seizures to phenobarbital in serum. *Arch Neurol* 1968;19:567–72.

Case 85

TREAT THE PATIENT, NOT THE BLOOD LEVELS

A James Rowan

History

The patient is a 70-year-old woman who was seen in January 1999 for evaluation of her seizures and difficulty walking. She was accompanied by one of her three daughters, who had never seen an event. Seizure onset was in December 1996, coincident with an episode of encephalitis. She apparently was quite ill – at the time she was intubated and cared for in the intensive care unit, where she was treated with phenytoin.

She made a good recovery, but in April 1997 she suffered her second seizure. Therapeutic changes at the time are unknown, but by the summer of 1998 she was having seizures every month.

The patient recalls nothing of her seizures save that they are preceded by a smell of ammonia and by tingling in her fingers and toes. Her daughter said that on most occasions the patient would be taken to a local emergency department where the dosages of her medications would be altered. When asked what antiepileptic drugs she was taking, the patient was uncertain but the daughter said she was taking a combination of carbamazepine and valproate of uncertain dosage. Examination of various containers and pharmacy records failed to elucidate the matter. The daughter thought she might be taking carbamazepine 100 mg/day and valproate 2500 mg/day.

When asked about her mother's gait, the daughter said her mother became progressively unsteady some months ago. A doctor prescribed a walker, explaining that the patient was getting older and some gait difficulty was to be expected. The daughter also noted that her mother had slowed down and was having trouble functioning on her own.

Examination and investigations

On examination, the patient presented as an alert older woman. She weighed 109 kg. She had marked gait difficulty and used her walker with slow steps and a

334

broad base. Without the walker she was markedly ataxic, falling to either side. At station she was unsteady with both her eyes open or closed. There was mild sustention tremor that increased during finger–nose maneuvers. Rapid alternating movements were clumsy. There were a few beats of nystagmus to both right and left lateral gaze. The neurological examination was otherwise unremarkable.

A rapid work-up was ordered, including records of her hospitalizations and emergency department visits. A magnetic resonance imaging (MRI) scan of the brain revealed evidence of cortical atrophy along with small vessel ischemic changes in the white matter. An EEG showed right hemispheric slowing with rare right temporal sharp waves. Her serum valproate level was 51.2 μg/ml; carbamazepine level was 7.8 μg/ml.

Diagnosis

Neurotoxicity secondary to antiepileptic medication.

Treatment and outcome

The patient was seen again in February 1999. At that time she said she was stressed and depressed. She had recurrent feelings 'like a rush', and was taking alprazolam 0.25 mg from time to time. During this visit the actual dosage of her medications was ascertained as being carbamazepine 1100 mg/day and valproate 4200 mg/day.

It was decided to effect a radical change in the patient's antiepileptic drug regimen by changing to lamotrigine monotherapy. Accordingly, lamotrigine 25 mg every other day was added to her current antiepileptic drugs. After 2 weeks, gradual reduction of valproate was begun (25 % of the total daily dose every 2 weeks) while lamotrigine was increased every 2 weeks. When valproate was discontinued, the patient was still receiving her usual dose of carbamazepine plus lamotrigine 100 mg/day. By the end of March 1999 she was somewhat less ataxic and had been seizure-free for about 5 weeks. By mid-April, at which time her valproate dose was 1000 mg/day she had improved and could walk alone with good stride, although she was still ataxic. Her tremor remained. One week later she had a seizure.

By mid-May she was on carbamazepine 900 mg/day and lamotrigine 200 mg/day. Her gait was much improved, there was no tremor and she was in better spirits. She no longer required a walker. Three weeks later lamotrigine was at 400 mg/day and carbamazepine was at 300 mg/day. There was only mild unsteadiness of gait. No further seizures were reported. In mid-July she reported a seizure 2 weeks previously. At that time she was taking lamotrigine 500 mg/day. She felt well but thought she was still unsteady. The examiner, however, who was standing outside his office, saw her running down the street because she was late. Formal gait testing showed her to be able to perform tandem walking with some support. In September she reported one or two small seizures. Her gait was quite good, and she required minimal support at tandem. Three was no tremor or appendicular ataxia, and there was no nystagmus. The patient was in reasonably good spirits, and her interaction with her daughters was feisty.

Commentary

A 70-year-old woman with seizures resulting from encephalitis was seen because of poor seizure control and severe gait difficulty. She was taking a combination of carbamazepine and valproate, but despite increasing doses of both drugs, experienced increased seizure frequency accompanied by progressive ataxia.

Serum levels of both drugs were within the therapeutic range. The MRI scan revealed cerebral atrophy and white matter changes; the EEG showed right hemispheric slowing and some sharp waves. The patient was crossed over to lamotrigine monotherapy with resolution of her ataxia and a decline in seizure frequency.

The patient presented with a classic problem of chasing seizures with increasing dosage of multiple (in this case two) antiepileptic drugs. The yardstick used for dosing strategy was the therapeutic range of the administered drugs. The result was increasing drug toxicity with concomitant failure to control seizures.

What did I learn from this case?

The main lesson from this case relates to the interpretation of the so-called therapeutic range and its application to the elderly population. The therapeutic range is a statistical statement based on a large cohort of patients. The concept is that maximum seizure control will be realized in most patients when serum levels are within the stated limits. Subtherapeutic levels are said to be associated with increased seizures, whereas supratherapeutic levels are associated with toxic manifestations. There are, however, many exceptions to these observations, based on individual metabolic characteristics and tolerance.[1]

The problem is compounded in the elderly. They often take multiple medications, have reduced cerebral reserve and generally have decreased tolerance to drug side effects. Moreover, it is known that it is difficult to obtain high levels of valproate when it is administered with an enzyme inducer such as carbamazepine.[2] In addition, valproate increases the level both of free

336

carbamazepine and of carbamazepine 10,11 epoxide, which is thought to be responsible for many of the toxic effects of carbamazepine.[3,4] These interactions can lead to drug toxicity despite apparently 'therapeutic' serum levels of the two drugs. Thus, the finding of therapeutic levels in this case despite the large doses was rendered meaningless.

Some of the antiepileptic drugs that have been introduced since 1992 offer potential benefits to elderly patients with seizures. In particular, several of these drugs have favorable side effect profiles while offering equivalent seizure control. In general, drug interactions with the newer agents are fewer, a particular advantage in the elderly, who each take an average of between five and six medications for various medical conditions, and sometimes many more.[5,6] The older agents such as phenytoin and carbamazepine have many interactions with other compounds.[7] In general, the newer antiepileptic drugs have fewer drug interactions and more favorable side effect profiles. It may well be that one or more will prove effective and tolerable in the elderly. Additional studies of the new antiepileptic drugs in the elderly are needed. At this time a multicenter, double-blind study (Veterans' Affairs Co-operative Study number 428) comparing carbamazepine, lamotrigine and gabapentin in older patients with newly diagnosed seizures is in progress.[8]

It was clear that this patient's current drugs had to be replaced with another agent. Based on its efficacy and tolerability profile, lamotrigine appeared to be a reasonable choice.[9] In a patient receiving valproate, lamotrigine must be introduced very slowly, a maneuver that appears to reduce the potential of rash, one of the known complications of lamotrigine therapy. Valproate is lowered after lamotrigine is introduced, and then after valproate has been stopped the inducing agent is tapered. The reason for this order is the differential effects of valproate and carbamazepine on the half-life of lamotrigine – valproate doubles the half-life of lamotrigine while carbamazepine halves it.[10] Thus, the potential of early lamotrigine toxicity is reduced. Subsequent reduction of carbamazepine then increases the effectiveness of lamotrigine.

How did this case alter my approach to the care and treatment of my epilepsy patients?

This case illustrated to me the importance of considering the side effects of antiepileptic drugs as a major factor in selecting drug therapy for the elderly. Close attention to the patient's neurological condition and quality of life, rather than laboratory values and seizure counts, should prevent untoward consequences.

References

1. Bourgeois BFD. Pharmacokinetics and pharmacodynamics in clinical practice. In: Wyllie E, ed. *The treatment of epilepsy: principles and practice*. Baltimore: Williams and Wilkins; 1996:728–36.

2. Mattson RH, Cramer JA. Valproate: interactions with other drugs. In: Levy RH, Dreifuss FE, Meldrum BS, Mattson RH, Penry JK, eds. *Antiepileptic drugs*, 3rd ed. New York: Raven; 1989:621–33.

3. Haidukewych D, Zielinski JJ, Rodin EA. Derivation and evaluation of an equation for prediction of free carbamazepine concentration in patients with valproic acid. *Ther Drug Monit* 1989;11:528–32.

4. Bertilsson L, Tomson L. Clinical pharmacokinetics and pharmacological effects of carbamazepine and carbamazepine 10,11 epoxide: an update. *Clin Pharmacokinet* 1986;11:177–98.

5. Cloyd JC. Clinical pharmacology of antiepileptic drugs in the elderly: practical applications. *Consultant Pharmacist* 1995;10:9–15.

6. United States General Accounting Office. Prescription drugs and the elderly. GAO/HEHS-95–152, July 1995.

7. Leppik LE, Wolf D. Drug interactions in the elderly with epilepsy. In: Rowan AJ, Ramsay RE, eds. *Seizures and epilepsy in the elderly*. Boston: Butterworth–Heinemann; 1997:291–302.

8. Rowan AJ. Reflections on the treatment of seizures in the elderly population. *Neurology* 1999;51(suppl 4):S28–S33.

9. Ramsay RE, Pellock JM, Garnett WR, Sanchez RM, *et al*. Pharmacokinetics and safety of lamotrigine (Lamictal) in patients with epilepsy. *Epilepsy Res* 1991;10:191–200.

10. Messenheimer JA. Lamotrigine. *Epilepsia* 1995;36(suppl 2):S87–S94.

Case 86

A Patient With Epilepsy Slips Down Some Attic Stairs

Rajesh C Sachdeo

History

The patient is a 63-year-old white man who was admitted to a community hospital with status epilepticus and then transferred to my facility the next day for further evaluation and management.

The patient had a history of seizures since the age of 16 years (etiology and type unknown) and had been well controlled on phenobarbital and phenytoin since then. His seizures consisted of arm and leg shaking with loss of consciousness and occasional incontinence. Six months before admission, he slipped down some stairs and sustained head trauma with loss of consciousness for 10 minutes. At that time, he did not seek medical attention because he felt well. Over the ensuing 6 weeks, the patient developed increasing lethargy, memory impairment, decreased sensation on the right side of his body, headache and visual impairment.

A subdural hematoma was diagnosed and evacuated. He initially did well, but after several weeks he developed increasing lethargy progressing to loss of consciousness. He had a second burr hole (3 months before the present admission) and again he did well but required a third evacuation about 3 weeks before admission.

Beginning about that time, his seizures increased to a frequency of about five a day. They were typically nocturnal and characterized by focal shaking of the right arm or leg with secondary generalization. He had recently been prescribed sustained-release oral theophylline for asthma control in addition to prednisone, and his seizure exacerbation was attributed to the theophylline.

At the time of admission, the patient was on:

- carbamazepine 800 mg/day in four divided doses;
- phenobarbital 180 mg/day in three divided doses;
- phenytoin 400 mg/day in four divided doses;
- sustained-release theophylline 800 mg/day in two divided doses; and
- prednisone 15 mg/day.

Examination and investigations

On examination, the patient had a decreased attention span, poor performance of serial sevens, dysdiadochokinesia and mild tremor. An EEG done on admission revealed bilateral mild slowing. A computed tomography (CT) scan of the brain showed postsurgical changes of the left calvarium and a left parietal subdural fluid collection. The carbamazepine level was low.

Diagnoses

Seizures since childhood, assumed to be partial onset, and recent head trauma.

Treatment and outcome

Based on the absence of seizures on EEG, phenobarbital and phenytoin were discontinued. The carbamazepine dose was increased over 3 days to 1600 mg/day. The patient was seizure-free for 2 days and then had a generalized tonic–clonic seizure, which was initially thought to be secondary to phenobarbital withdrawal. However, when the EEG showed epileptiform discharges in the right frontotemporal area and generalized spike–wave activity, valproate 750 mg/day in three divided doses was started.

The next day, the patient developed complex partial status epilepticus, terminated with intravenous diazepam. The carbamazepine dose was then increased to 1800 mg/day. In addition, theophylline was discontinued and replaced by albuterol with consultation of the pulmonary service. After 1 week on valproate, the patient developed intolerable vertigo and nystagmus, which necessitated discontinuation of the drug. He was then discharged from the hospital 2 days later.

Three days after discharge, the patient was readmitted because of two generalized seizures, and he had two more seizures on the day after admission. He had sustained a laceration of his left eyebrow. A CT scan showed no new changes, but an EEG showed focal epileptiform discharges as well as generalized spike–wave discharges. He was successfully treated with phenytoin 200 mg intravenously and then with oral phenytoin; he was started again on valproate 1000 mg/day and carbamazepine reduced to 1400 mg/day.

An EEG 18 months later showed mild generalized slow wave activity together with sharp and slow wave complexes in the right anterior temporal region. Four years after the initial presentation, the patient had a normal EEG and was eventually weaned off the carbamazepine.

340

Commentary

This patient had an antecedent history of seizures since the age of 16, which were not well characterized but were assumed to be partial onset. At the age of 63 he sustained a fall, which required three surgical evacuations of a subdural hematoma. The head trauma clearly was a risk factor for partial seizures. An EEG demonstrated right frontotemporal epileptiform discharges that generalized, thereby confirming partial epilepsy.

On the assumption that the patient had partial seizures and that polytherapy may not have been necessary, his drug regimen was simplified to carbamazepine monotherapy. At that point, generalized tonic–clonic seizures emerged, suggesting the possibility that the patient's lifelong seizure disorder was due to a generalized epilepsy syndrome. Valproate was therefore added.

It is well known that carbamazepine can exacerbate generalized epilepsies such as childhood absence epilepsy, juvenile myoclonic epilepsy, generalized tonic–clonic seizures and atonic or myoclonic seizures. A subsequent EEG in this patient confirmed two types of epileptiform abnormalities – focal discharges with secondary generalization and generalized epileptiform patterns consistent with primary generalized epilepsy.

What did I learn from this case?

Ockham's razor does not always prevail! William of Ockham was a Franciscan logician who lived in England in the 13th century. Ockham is credited with the saying 'entities should not be multiplied unnecessarily'. Thus, the principle of parsimony has been called Ockham's razor. The practice of clinical neurology is predicated upon this rule of parsimony – we strive to localize a single lesion that explains all the symptoms under one diagnosis. In this case, Ockham's razor failed us, since the patient had two different types of seizure disorders at once – complex partial seizures with secondary generalization and primary generalized tonic–clonic seizures.

Furthermore, this case points out the importance of obtaining a complete history of any antecedent seizures. This patient's seizure at the age of 16 was considered to be of uncertain etiology. Perhaps, if the patient's chart or an earlier EEG had been available, his epilepsy would have been more accurately characterized. At times, a family history of epilepsy can also be helpful.

How did this case alter my approach to the care and treatment of my epilepsy patients?

This case taught me that different seizure types, as identified by the international classification system, are not mutually exclusive. Now I do not rule out the

341

possibility of the co-occurrence of a primary generalized epilepsy and an acquired symptomatic complex partial seizure disorder in appropriate patients. I am mindful of choosing antiepileptic drug regimens for such patients that are likely to be beneficial and not potentially detrimental.

Further reading

Snead OC, Hosey LC. Exacerbation of seizures in children by carbamazepine. *N Engl J Med* 1985;313:916–21.

Case 87

BILATERAL HIP FRACTURES IN A 43-YEAR-OLD WOMAN WITH EPILEPSY

Dieter Schmidt

History

The patient is a 43-year-old heavy smoker with a history of idiopathic generalized epilepsy with absences since childhood and generalized tonic–clonic seizures, often on awakening.

She stopped taking primidone on the recommendation of her neurologist in July 1998 after being completely seizure free for several years. In October of the same year she was hospitalized for an ischemic middle cerebral artery stroke with transient left sided hemiplegia and received low dose heparin while she was bed-ridden. At 7:30 in the morning of October 10 she had a generalized tonic–clonic seizure that lasted 1 to 2 minutes according to the nurse's report. Afterwards the patient complained about moderate pain in both upper legs and difficulty moving her legs in bed. She received an intravenous infusion of 4 mg clonazepam over several hours and oral carbamazepine treatment was started. At 14:00 she had her second tonic–clonic seizure.

Diagnosis

Bilateral hip fracture in a patient with idiopathic generalized epilepsy following a relapse of tonic–clonic seizures.

Investigations

Two hours later, an X-ray revealed bilateral hip fractures (Fig. 87.1), which were successfully operated on the next day. The surgeon told the neurologist who had cared for her in the hospital that he was surprised how brittle her bones had been.

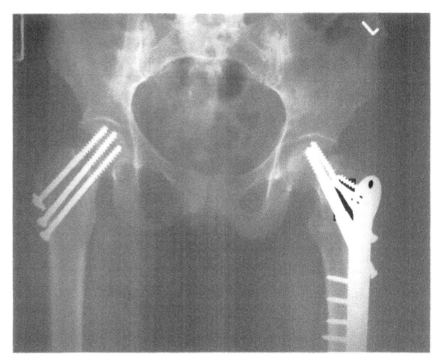

Figure 87.1: *Bilateral hip fracture in a 43-year old woman with epilepsy following a single tonic clonic seizure. A second one occurred several hours later. The X-ray shown here was taken following surgery the next day. A medial femoral neck fracture is seen on the right side and a pertrochanteric fracture on the left side.*

Outcome

A lawyer acting on behalf of the woman later charged that better treatment after the first seizure would have prevented the second one and the fractures, and for good measure suggested that bodily violence against the patient by hospital staff might have caused the fractures. I learnt about the case when I was asked to give an expert opinion in the ensuing legal controversy.

Commentary

Why did I choose this case?

I chose this case for two reasons. First, I was interested in why a middle-aged patient would suffer from bilateral hip-fractures while having a tonic–clonic seizure in bed, and second, I had never heard about bilateral leg pain following a seizure which is different from the well-known post-ictal back pain or general muscle ache.

344

What did I learn from this case?

When I first heard about this case, I had known from experience that
tonic–clonic seizures in bed without falls may cause compression fractures of
the lower thoracic or upper lumbar spine, resulting in back pain for a few weeks.
Enzyme-inducing antiepileptic drugs may uncommonly cause osteomalacia in
otherwise healthy people, putting them at risk for fractures. Patients with poor
nutrition or gastrointestinal disease may be at even higher risk. The relative risk for
fractures is increased twofold in patients with epilepsy (CI 1.5 2.5).[1] Bilateral
fractures have been reported in individual patients[2] and one report singled out
bilateral hip fractures in institutionalized patients with epilepsy.[3,4] In a further
report, muscular contractions were identified as the cause of bilateral hip fractures
during a tonic -clonic seizure, as occurred in our patient.[5] In total, about 0.3 % of
patients with epilepsy suffer fractures after seizures, not including those after falls.
In summary then, the patient suffered from seizure-related bilateral hip fractures, a
rare but nevertheless well-described complication of a tonic -clonic seizure.

How did this case alter my approach to the care and treatment of my epilepsy patients?

If a patient complains about pain immediately following a seizure, I look for
bone fractures even when the patient did not fall as a consequence of the seizure.
I am particularly aware of this possible complication in patients on long-term
therapy with enzyme-inducing antiepileptic drugs, because of their increased risk
for latent or overt osteomalacia and seizure-associated bone fractures. Further, I
try to use non-enzyme inducing antiepileptic drugs, if possible, to minimize the
risk of anticonvulsant-induced osteomalacia.

Finally, I am more cautious when withdrawing antiepileptic drugs in adult
patients who have had a remission of their seizures for at least two years because
of the morbidity associated with recurrent seizures.

References

1. Vestergaard P, Tigaran S, Rejnmark L, Tigaran C, Dam M. Fracture risk is
    increased in epilepsy. *Acta Neurol Scand* 1999;**99(5)**:269 75.

2. Lohiya GS, Tan-Figueroa L. Eighteen fractures in a man with profound mental
    retardation. *Ment Retard* 1999;**37(1)**:47 -51.

3. Ribacoba-Montero R, Salas Puig J. Simultaneous bilateral fractures of the hip
    following a grand mal seizure. An unusual complication. *Seizure* 1997;**6(5)**:403–4.

4. Desai KB, Ribbans WJ, Taylor GJ. Incidence of five common fracture types in an
    institutional epileptic population. *Injury* 1996;**27(2)**:97–100.

5. Van Heest A, Vorlicky L, Thompson RC. Bilateral central acetabular fracture
    dislocations secondary to sustained myoclonus. *Clin Orthop* 1996;**324**:210–3.

Case 88

PICKING A WRONG ANTIEPILEPTIC DRUG FOR A 9-YEAR-OLD GIRL

Peter Uldall

History

This patient was diagnosed with childhood absence epilepsy at the age of 4 years by the local paediatric department. She was treated with valproate with a good result. She developed normally and was seizure-free for 3 years. When she was 7 years old, her mother tapered off the medicine by herself. The next year passed apparently without seizures – at least nobody noticed any. By the time she was 9 years of age, however, it became obvious that she was having frequent absences, and valproate treatment was re-instituted by the local paediatric department. Now, however, she complained of adverse effects, including vomiting, abdominal discomfort and weight gain. She was re-admitted three times and a new EEG was performed. At this time, some focal traits were seen in the EEG (Figs. 88.1 and 88.2).

On suspicion of complex partial seizures, a trial of vigabatrin was undertaken. The seizures increased; she was re-admitted and treatment was changed to valproate syrup. The adverse events continued, however, and she refused to take any medicine orally. Then she was put on valproate suppositories. This resulted in unstable plasma levels, diarrhoea and continuing absences. Furthermore, she was wetting the bed and she had learning disabilities, no friends and no self-confidence. She had never had generalized tonic–clonic seizures.

Examination and investigations

The patient, together with her mother, was admitted to a tertiary epilepsy hospital for 4 weeks. Her mother was a single, insecure woman, who had two other children and was only just able to manage to keep her job. Video-EEG showed typical absences. During admission she was observed in the school at the hospital. The girl and her mother were intensively informed and educated about epilepsy. A neuropsychological examination showed that the patient had normal intelligence and only subtle cognitive problems. The neurological examination was normal.

346

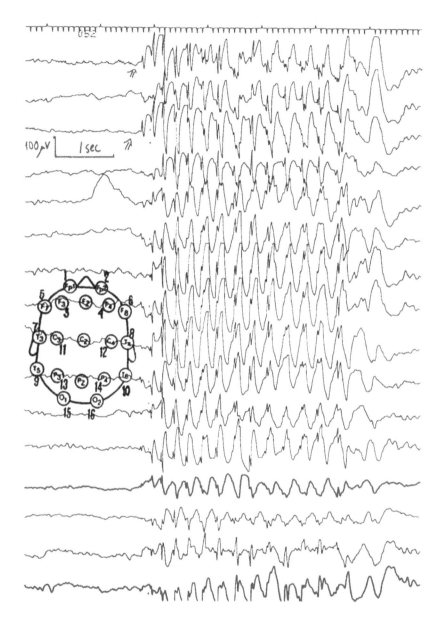

Figure 88.1: EEG from the patient with idiopathic generalized epilepsy (absences). The focal onset (L. prefrontal & L. frontal region) of the generalized spike-wave discharge can be seen (arrows).

347

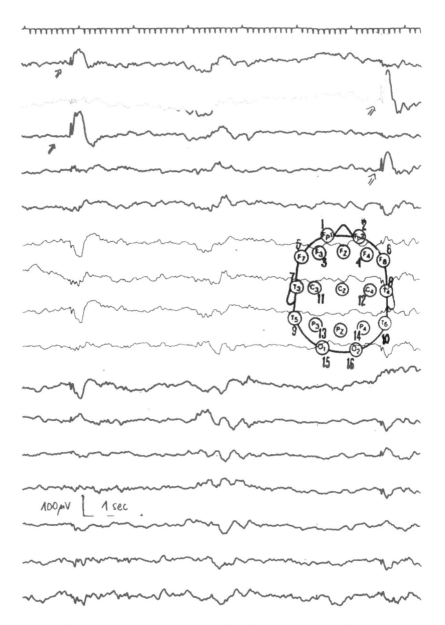

Figure 88.2: *(Light sleep), two independent frontal spike wave discharges are seen (arrows).*

Diagnosis

Childhood absence epilepsy.

Treatment and outcome

When the mother and the girl were shown the video-EEG, they realized what the problem was and finally became motivated to try a new drug. The girl was started on ethosuximide syrup without any adverse events. The absences disappeared and the child slowly regained her self-confidence. It was possible to get leave for the mother from her job for 2 months so that she could support the child. The daughter was able to regain her confidence about her school performance. The bed wetting disappeared after the valproate was tapered off (it had previously been unsuccessfully treated with a reward of 5 Danish kroner for each dry night and a penalty of 2 Danish kroner for each wet night). At discharge the patient could return to her school without problems, and the EEG was normal.

Commentary

Why did I choose this case?

This case highlights issues that are important for the paediatric neurologist. First, it shows that apparently focal paroxysms on the EEG can be seen in otherwise typical absence epilepsy. This must not lead to the conclusion of a localization-related epilepsy with complex partial seizures.

Second, the case underlines the fact that the management of epilepsy extends far beyond the classification of the epilepsy syndrome and the prescription of an antiepileptic drug. In many cases the psychological, educational and social problems are at least as important as the seizures and their treatment. Information on epilepsy and acceptance by the patient and the patient's family of the epilepsy is mandatory in order to obtain good compliance.

What did I learn from this case?

The diagnosis of absence epilepsy is not always easy. Some absences can last up to 20–30 seconds with elements of automatisms. If a non-experienced neurologist describes some focal traits at the EEG and the patient does not respond to valproate, the clinician may erroneously believe that it is a case of complex partial seizures.

349

Because of the failure of treatment resulting from the use of a wrong antiepileptic drug (vigabatrin in this case) and an unsuitable route of administration, as well as the adverse events that resulted, the confidence of the patient and her mother in treatment and in the doctors was lost. The mother could not persuade the child to take her medicine and because of ongoing seizures and adverse events (such as bed wetting) the child lost her self-confidence at school. In this way, a vicious cycle began.

In such a case, comprehensive re-evaluation is necessary, and this may be difficult to handle in an out-patient clinic. During admission, several supportive talks with other girls with epilepsy, the nurses, school teachers and psychologists made it possible to change the situation. A video-EEG is a very powerful tool, not only for diagnostic purposes, but also for education of patients and relatives. In this case the girl and her mother could see for themselves what was going on, and they both realized the importance of treatment. Even a video without EEG could be used in this situation. The neuropsychological examination was necessary to convince the girl herself and her teachers that she had sufficient abilities to continue in her mainstream school. Adverse events must always be taken seriously, even minor ones. Bed wetting is often overlooked. In this case, the treatment may actually have been worse than the disease.

In conclusion, this case illustrates that information and correct syndrome diagnosis is crucial not only in the severe intractable cases of childhood epilepsy, but also in the benign syndromes, when we should be able to give our patients a normal life.

An important message from this case and from several audit studies, not least in teenagers, is that the treatment process should include management of global health and daily function of the child from the social, educational and psychological points of view – then it will be possible to change the life of children with epilepsy.

Case 89

WITH EPILEPSY YOU NEVER KNOW

Walter van Emde Boas

History

While living in the tropics, Mrs F had her first generalized convulsion at the age of 3½ years in association with a fever, which was possibly malarial. She was born after a normal pregnancy of healthy Caucasian parents and had normal psychomotor development.

Seven years later she had a second generalized convulsion, which was provoked by sleep deprivation. At the time a neurologist examined her. Physical examination was normal. The EEG showed right posterior focal slowing but no epileptiform discharges. A computed tomography (CT) scan showed a small, contrast-enhancing lesion in the right frontal lobe. After a negative angiography study, the tentative diagnosis of angioma was changed to cerebral cysticercosis, although cerebrospinal fluid titers remained negative.

Anticonvulsant treatment with phenytoin and carbamazepine was started but did not prevent occasional generalized seizures, which were consistently provoked by sleep deprivation and jet lag after long flights. Brief absence-like episodes, sometimes with mild automatisms, started at the age of 14 years and continued despite treatment up to maximum tolerated doses with carbamazepine and phenytoin. When she was 16 years of age, phenytoin was replaced by valproate because of progressive gingival hyperplasia but this had no effect on the seizures. The possible option of epilepsy surgery was suggested but rejected by the patient and her parents until they could return permanently to the Netherlands.

Examination and investigations

The first time I saw Mrs F she had just turned 18. Generalized seizures had not occurred for more than 20 months but she reported between one and three brief 'absence' spells a day and complained about drowsiness and impaired concentration caused by her medication (valproate 1000 mg/day in two divided doses and carbamazepine 800 mg/day in two divided doses).

Physical examination was normal, as before, but the interictal EEG now showed irregular slow waves and occasional spike-and-wave discharges over the right anterior region without consistent focal characteristics. A magnetic resonance imaging scan of the brain showed a small (approximately 2.5 cm), well-demarcated round lesion in the anteriomedian part of the right frontal lobe, probably a cavernoma, without signs of progression in comparison to the previous CT scans.

During EEG with video monitoring, the 'absences' turned out to be brief complex partial seizures with arrest reaction, loss of contact and partial amnesia but without additional clinical signs. An ictal EEG showed some attenuation of ongoing activity, followed by an increase of irregular theta and delta activity over both anterior regions, with slight preponderance to the right but otherwise without convincing lateralizing or localizing features.

Diagnosis

Symptomatic frontal lobe epilepsy characterized by complex partial seizures with anterior frontal or frontopolar clinical characteristics.[1]

Treatment and outcome

Epilepsy surgery was discussed again. At that time (1989) it was believed that intracranial EEG and video monitoring were mandatory in all cases without unequivocal scalp EEG localization, even in the presence of a lesion. Mrs F and her parents did not consider her sufficiently socially or medically impaired to warrant such studies. Furthermore she wanted to finish high school during that summer and it was decided to postpone further procedures.

She switched to controlled-release carbamazepine, which improved her diurnal alertness, and she successfully took her final examinations. She immediately applied for and obtained a scholarship for a 3-year college education in the USA, starting within 3 months. Presurgical evaluation was thus further postponed.

Over the next 3 years her complex partial seizures gradually became more severe, and secondary generalized seizures recurred occasionally. The dose of controlled-release carbamazepine was increased to 1200 mg/day in two divided doses, and phenytoin was added but then withdrawn again when disfiguring hirsutism developed. Repeat EEG with video monitoring during a brief holiday in the Netherlands (in 1991) showed more elaborate complex partial seizures, including vocalizations, oro–alimentary automatisms and some hypermotor automatisms of the arms.[2] The ictal EEG remained poorly localizing.

After graduation, Mrs F returned to the Netherlands for further consultation.

352

At this time her seizure pattern had become more disabling and included frequent urinary incontinence during complex partial seizures. A third video–EEG suggested clinical involvement of the anteriofrontal area as well as the anterior cingulate, insular–opercular and mesial frontobasal areas,[1] suggesting a progressive type of frontal lobe epilepsy.[3] Ictal scalp EEG still remained equivocal but late ictal and postictal slowing predominated over the right frontal lobe. Our surgical approach of lesional epilepsy had changed, following the second Palm Desert Meeting on Epilepsy Surgery,[4] and surgery was offered without further invasive procedures.

A partial right frontal lobe resection was performed, including complete lesionectomy, and Mrs F became seizure-free as of December 1992. She successfully completed health-care-related studies and started a private practice in yet another faraway country. Treatment was gradually reduced to monotherapy with controlled-release carbamazepine 200 mg/day, and follow-up consultations became rare.

In 1998 she wrote to me saying that she was experiencing a problem with insurance because of her epilepsy, despite having been seizure-free for more than 5 years. I advised her to consider herself healed, and to stop her controlled-release carbamazepine gradually over the next 4 months and then to try again with the insurance company. I included a letter to the company, stating that in her case the epilepsy had been surgically cured and that seizure recurrence was extremely unlikely. Four months later I learned that she had relapsed. Since then she has been on controlled-release carbamazepine 800 mg/day in two divided doses, without significant side effects and thus far without further seizures.

Commentary

What did I learn from this case?

First of all I learnt from her that epilepsy is a disorder that people can cope with. Despite significantly disabling seizures, this brave and motivated young woman, assisted by an understanding and supportive family, managed to pursue and achieve the goals of her own choosing, most often on her own terms.

Secondly I learnt that epilepsy surgery is indeed an elective type of surgery – medical urgencies can be offset by social urgencies and the process of evaluation and surgery must be optimized accordingly.

From the case of Mrs F I also learnt that epilepsy can be a progressive disorder, even in lesional epilepsy that is associated with a static, non-malignant structural lesion.[3]

From her, more than from others, I learnt that epilepsy surgery rarely relieves patients from their seizure disorder. In most patients who undergo surgery, we are able to change an intractable epilepsy into a treatable condition, yet with the need for lifelong drug treatment of a perennial lingering and threatening disorder.

Finally I learnt to realize my own limitations better. I had advised this young woman that she was cured of her epilepsy because I wanted to believe her to be cured, *not* because I knew that she was.

With epilepsy you never know.

References

1. van Emde Boas W, Velis DN. Frontal lobe epilepsies. In: Meinardi H, volume ed. *The epilepsies, part II*. In Vinken PJ, Bruyn GW, eds. *Handbook of clinical neurology (revised series)* vol 73(29). Amsterdam: Elsevier;2000:37–52.

2. Lüders H, Acharaya J, Baumgartner C, *et al*. Semiological seizure classification. *Epilepsia* 1998;39:1006–13.

3. van Emde Boas W. Longitudinal evolution of frontal lobe complex partial seizures: a progressive seizure syndrome? In: Wolf P, ed. *Epileptic seizures and syndromes*. London: John Libbey; 1994:408–15.

4. Engel J, ed. *Surgical treatment of the epilepsies*. 2nd ed. New York: Raven; 1993.

V

Unexpected Solutions

Case 90

WHEN ANTIEPILEPTIC DRUGS FAIL IN AN INFANT WITH SEIZURES, CONSIDER VITAMIN B6

Mary R Andriola

History

The patient is a 3½-year-old girl with a normal perinatal history, normal growth and development, and a negative family history.

She first presented at 8 months of age with partial seizures involving the left hand and arm. A routine EEG and a video-EEG, without an event, were normal, as was a magnetic resonance imaging (MRI) scan of the brain. She was treated with carbamazepine and was seizure-free for 2 months.

She then presented with partial motor seizures, which again began in the left hand but then generalized. Her carbamazepine regimen was adjusted. Two weeks later, at 11 months of age, she was hospitalized with recurrent multiple seizures. These still had a focal component with twitching of the left face but frequent generalization. In the pediatric intensive care unit she received intravenous fosphenytoin, phenobarbital and lorazepam. There was only a partial clinical response at first and then the seizures became intractable with decreased interictal responsivity. When she was given intravenous pyridoxine (vitamin B$_6$), the seizures stopped.

Examination and investigations

When the patient presented at 11 months of age with left facial twitching, she was noted to have spike–polyspike–wave activity from the right hemisphere. Video-EEG monitoring revealed seizures developing independently and multifocally from either the right or left hemisphere. Following treatment with intravenous antiepileptic drugs in the pediatric intensive care unit, the EEG was diffusely slow. When the seizures became intractable, the EEG was markedly abnormal with polymorphic slow wave activity and frequent rhythmic 1-Hz slow-and-sharp wave activity. With the administration of intravenous pyridoxine

100 mg, the sharp activity was rapidly replaced by diffuse slowing, which persisted for a number of days.

Diagnosis

Pyridoxine-dependent seizures.

Treatment and outcome

Carbamazepine and phenobarbital were quickly tapered and the patient was maintained on pyridoxine 100 mg/day. Her mental status gradually improved, as did her developmental skills. At 1 year of age, approximately 1 month after beginning pyridoxine therapy, she had a normal neurological examination, a normal EEG and a normal MRI scan.

She has continued to grow and develop normally, and is maintained on pyridoxine 100 mg/day. She experienced a single seizure at about 2 years of age when she had a febrile illness and had missed a dose of pyridoxine. This was a brief and self-limited seizure. Her parents were instructed to give her pyridoxine 200 mg whenever she has a febrile illness.

Commentary

This girl first presented when she was 8 months old with partial seizures that initially responded to carbamazepine. When her seizures recurred, with partial onset but secondary generalization, they became intractable and EEGs suggested multifocal onset, eventually showing diffuse slowing and 1-Hz spike-and-slow wave activity.

The intravenous administration of pyridoxine was both diagnostically and therapeutically specific for pyridoxine-dependent seizures. This was an unusual presentation, out of the neonatal period, with partial seizures that initially appeared to respond to carbamazepine. Such unusual or atypical cases have been reported but there are less than 100 total cases of pyridoxine-dependent seizures in the literature. Cases have been reported with onset up to 3 years of age.

What did I learn from this case?

Pyridoxine-dependent seizures require a high index of suspicion. From this case, I learned that intractable seizures in an infant may be related to pyridoxine dependency even if the seizures do not have their onset in the neonatal period.

The most important aspects of this infant's gradual clinical evolution were progressively abnormal EEGs and decreased responsivity of the patient in spite of multiple antiepileptic drugs that were being appropriately administered. This had to be distinguished from the sedating effects of medications.

How did this case alter my approach to the care and treatment of my epilepsy patients?

I consider administering intravenous pyridoxine to a child whose seizures become intractable and refractory to antiepileptic drugs when there is no known etiology. A markedly abnormal interictal EEG also suggests that a metabolic etiology should be pursued. Pyridoxine-dependent seizures is a rare disorder, and a high index of suspicion must be present if it is to be diagnosed properly; treatment of affected children can be almost miraculously effective.

Further reading

Bankier A, Turner M, Hopkins IJ. Pyridoxine-dependent seizures: a wider clinical spectrum. *Arch Dis Child* 1983;**58**:415–8.

Goutieres F, Alcardi J. Atypical presentations of pyridoxine-dependent seizures: a treatable cause of intractable epilepsy in infants. *Ann Neurol* 1985;**17**:117–20.

Krishnamoorthy KS. Pyridoxine-dependency seizure: report of a rare presentation. *Ann Neurol* 1983;**13**:103–4.

Mikati MA, Trevathan E, Krishnamoorthy KS, Lombroso CT. Pyridoxine-dependent epilepsy: EEG investigations and long-term follow-up. *Electroencephalogr Clin Neurophysiol* 1991;**78**:215–21.

Case 91

A 12-YEAR-OLD BOY WITH DAILY CLONIC SEIZURES

Eloy Elices and Santiago Arroyo

History

A 12-year-old right-handed boy started to have seizures at the age of 5 years. At first the seizures consisted of clonic jerking of the left lower extremity, most prominent in the foot.

Within a few weeks, the seizures evolved into epilepsia partialis continua, which was eventually controlled, several months later, on a combination of carbamazepine and clobazam.

Soon after this, the patient started to have:

- daily clonic seizures of his left lower extremity (again most prominent in the foot);
- left-sided motor seizures occurring between six and eight times a month and beginning either in the foot or hand, followed by Todd's paralysis for several minutes; and
- several myoclonic jerks of the left leg each day.

At the age of 11, the patient reported three new types of episodes:

- left hand paresthesias lasting up to 1 minute;
- episodes of bilateral auditory or visual illusions; and
- right versive seizures with drooling, abnormal pharyngeal sensation and preserved consciousness.

These events occurred on a weekly to monthly basis despite multiple trials of antiepileptic drugs (phenytoin, valproate, carbamazepine, primidone, phenobarbital, clonzepam, piracetam, clobazam and prednisone) used at different doses and in different combinations. He also received three 5-day courses of inmunoglobulins without significant success.

The patient's motor development was normal. After the age of 6, he became progressively slower when performing his usual tasks, which his parents and teachers attributed to difficulties with attention and concentration. Moreover, he was increasingly more hyperactive and impulsive. These behaviours did not improve with several changes in his antiepileptic drugs.

Beginning at the age of 12, the patient developed a slowly worsening left hemiparesis, more pronounced in the leg, which progressed in a step-wise fashion.

The patient's parents were not related to each other and there had been no problems with his delivery. His past medical history was unremarkable and he had normal developmental milestones. A maternal uncle, who had a few convulsive seizures during infancy that were easily controlled with medication, had been seizure-free for many years without medication.

Examination and investigations

Neurological examination when the patient was 9 had shown a left hemiparesis with hyper-reflexia (before this his strength and reflexes had been normal). The hemiparesis was symmetrical, mild (4/5) and stable for several years, when it rapidly progressed over 2 3 months to complete functional loss of the hand, left motor neglect and mild hypoesthesia of the left hand. No neurological deficits were found on the right side.

A brain magnetic resonance imaging (MRI) scan performed at age 7 was reported as normal but subsequent MRI scans showed radiological deterioration (Fig. 91.1).

Video-EEG monitoring at age 11 showed independent multifocal right hemisphere seizures simple partial motor seizures (left leg clonic activity), secondarily generalized seizures (with motor component prominent over the left extremities), and simple partial auditory seizures.

Serial neuropsychological tests showed a continuous decline in his neuropsychological performance, including cognitive slowing.

A right temporal pole biopsy was performed in 1998 when he was age 12. This confirmed the diagnosis of Rasmussen's encephalitis. No viral inclusions were found in the tissue and cerebrospinal fluid studies for viral serologies, and GluR3 antibodies were negative.

Diagnosis

Rasmussen's encephalitis.

Treatment and outcome

When the patient lost function in his left hand at the age of 12, a functional hemispherotomy was carried out. Following the operation, his seizures greatly improved – he only had occasional right frontal onset EEG-confirmed simple partial seizures (bilateral blinking), and these were easily controlled with

360

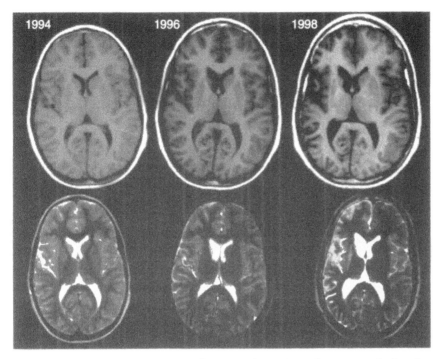

Figure 91.1: *Progressive atrophy of the right hemisphere, first seen in the basal ganglia, leading eventually to the near-disappearance of the caudate and lenticular nuclei. In addition, hyperintensity of these nuclei was seen in the early stages. No radiographic abnormalities were seen in the left hemisphere.*

adjustments to his drug dosages. His intellectual performance improved significantly, as did his behaviour. The left hemiparesis did not prevent him from walking within 2 weeks after surgery and he is undergoing intense rehabilitation for his left arm.

Commentary

Although Rasmussen's encephalitis has been a fairly well known disease for over 40 years, its incidence is very low. Our patient presented with several interesting and characteristic features:

- he had several types of seizures, which included motor signs, somatosensory symptoms, and auditory and visual semiology. The presence of multiple unilateral seizure types and epilepsia partialis continua is very suggestive of Rasmussen's encephalitis;

- the hemiparesis appeared 4 years after the onset of the seizures and was very mild until 3 years later, when it became rapidly progressive (in 2 months he was hemiplegic);
- brain MRI scans showed striking and progressive hemispheric changes – hemiatrophy, hyperintense signals and basal ganglia involvement.

What did we learn from this case?

Although there are no prospective studies of serial MRI scans in patients with Rasmussen's encephalitis, our patient's studies provide a good example of the radiological progression typical of this disease. We have looked with particular interest at these MRI abnormalities, because we are not aware of any other disease that shares similar characteristics. Since a certain diagnosis can only be achieved by brain biopsy, we have become aware of the need for diagnostic studies that would point to the diagnosis before brain atrophy occurs.

How did this case alter our approach to the care and treatment of our patients with epilepsy?

We waited until the child lost the functional use of his hand to do the biopsy and then perform the hemispherotomy, even though the diagnosis of chronic encephalitis had already been assumed. The optimal time to perform surgery is a controversial subject. Some clinicians propose waiting until the patient has hemiparesis and others advocate performing the hemispherectomy before the hemiparesis is complete in order to avoid the neuropsychological impairment, years of seizures and social handicap that are associated with this otherwise relentless disease. The debate is still ongoing.

Further reading

So NK, Andermann F. Rasmussen's encephalitis. In: Engel J, Pedley T, eds. *Epilepsy. A comprehensive textbook*. Philadelphia: Lippincott–Raven;1997:2379–88.

Tien RD, Ashdown BC, Lewis DV, *et al*. Rasmussen's encephalitis: neuroimaging findings in four patients. *AJR Am J Roentgenol* 1992;158:1329–32.

Vining EP, Freeman JM, Brandt J, *et al*. Progressive unilateral encephalopathy of childhood (Rasmussen's syndrome): a reappraisal. *Epilepsia* 1993;34:639–50.

Case 92

Vigabatrin Treatment In A Patient With Visual Field Defects: What To Do?

Roy G Beran

History

The patient was first seen when he was aged 35 years, when he moved from interstate. He developed epilepsy at the age of 18 months in the setting of pneumonia. His birth was difficult and complicated by perinatal cyanosis.

His typical seizures were complex partial, although he also had simple partial seizures that occasionally progressed to secondarily generalised tonic–clonic seizures. The most frequent episodes were described as losing contact with his environment and having automatisms, especially of his left upper limb. When first seen he had tried phenobarbital, primidone, phenytoin, carbamazepine, valproate, vigabatrin and lamotrigine.

A significant reason for his move interstate was psychosocial disintegration. He had a failed marriage and had moved back to live with his elderly mother. He was unemployed and had virtually lost contact with his daughter and former wife. Two years after the initial consultation, he would still experience seizures provoked by correspondence received from his daughter, and he coped with this by taking short-acting benzodiazepine medication half an hour before reading the letters. This approach prevented further such seizures.

In 1997, he had been seizure-free for almost 2 years on a combination of valproate (1 g twice daily), vigabatrin (1 g twice daily) and lamotrigine (100 mg twice daily). As a consequence, he was given permission to resume driving. This revitalized his self-confidence and he was able to return to full employment. Through the greater social contact that employment provided, he met, courted and married his second wife, moved into separate accommodation and now lives a full and independent life.

Examination and investigation

When reports of visual field defects associated with the use of vigabatrin emerged, he underwent formal visual field testing with Goldmann and

363

Humphries perimetry, which confirmed bilateral upper quadrant nasal field defects.

Diagnosis

Vigabatrin-associated visual field defect, symptomatic partial epilepsy.

Treatment and outcome

The visual field findings were discussed with the patient and he was given the option of stopping the vigabatrin and considering an alternative antiepileptic medication. After discussion with his wife, the patient opted for continuing vigabatrin and ongoing monitoring of the field defect to determine its progression. He based this decision on the fact that he was symptom-free and enjoying a full and active life. He was extremely afraid that cessation of vigabatrin might cause recurrence of seizures.

As of June 2000, he was taking valproate 1 g twice daily, lamotrigine 100 mg twice daily and vigabatrin 1 g twice daily. His field defect remained stable.

Commentary

This is the case of a mature man whose life had been devastated as a result of the consequences of epilepsy, with loss of marriage, job, independence and self-esteem. This has been successfully modified and reversed by combination therapy, including vigabatrin, but he was found to have visual field defects, presumed to be associated with vigabatrin.

What did I learn from this case?

The first lesson to be learnt from this case is the beneficial use of short-acting benzodiazepines to treat situationally related reflex epilepsy. This man experienced seizures in response to the emotions provoked by contact from his estranged daughter. Taking the benzodiazepines half an hour before such provocation, at a time that was appropriate (he would be unable to drive if the benzodiazepine caused sedation), gave him protection from these seizures and allowed him to maintain his seizure-free status.

The second lesson to be absorbed from this case is the devastating social burden of epilepsy. Conversely, the message that this case provides is how the maintenance of seizure-freedom can allow a patient who was rendered totally

364

isolated and dependent from uncontrolled seizures to resume a full and active life.

The final message from this case is the need to respect the patient as an autonomous agent who has the right to determine what they do or do not accept as treatment options. The patient had visual restriction to 40°, which is really quite substantial, and had the opportunity to see his own fields as mapped out by a neuro-ophthalmologist.

In discussing this issue with the patient, we could not guarantee that he would remain seizure-free if we stopped vigabatrin or that an alternative treatment regimen would be as effective. Furthermore, we could not provide confirmation that stopping vigabatrin would reverse the deficit, nor could we advise that maintenance of vigabatrin would result in further deterioration.

In the face of all these negatives and in the absence of any symptoms or clinical signs with examination, such as visual confrontation, this patient made the informed decision to remain on his medications, including vigabatrin. He has been followed for more than 3 years and has maintained the identical constriction of visual fields that we have learned to associate with vigabatrin, without progression.

It could thus be argued that he has exercised his right of autonomy and informed consent, despite our fears for his potential loss of vision. His decision would appear to have been correct because his lifestyle has remained intact and his vision has not deteriorated.

Case 93

A Child With Attention Deficit Disorder, Autistic Features And Frequent Epileptiform EEG Discharges

Frank MC Besag

History

This male patient first presented to our service at 6.5 years of age. Although there was no history suggestive of birth trauma, seizures commenced at 6 days of age with a prolonged period of unconsciousness that lasted 2 or 3 days, during which he had several convulsions. After this illness he was initially lethargic.

His milestones were delayed. He crawled at 12 months of age, walked at 20 months and was not able to utter more than three words until 20 months of age. At 23 months he fell off the bed when playing and struck his head. Although he was not knocked unconscious, he fell deeply asleep the following day and had a series of seizures in which he appeared blank for a few seconds and his pupils were dilated. Two months later he had a prolonged convulsion that had to be terminated with emergency treatment in hospital.

He continued having prolonged convulsions at 2-week to 3-month intervals, usually stopped with 15 mg rectal diazepam. From about 5 years of age he also developed blank spells during which he stared and was unresponsive. These occurred three to six times a day on 4–7 days a week. From age 5 years he also developed episodes in which his eyeballs flicked up and to the left side while his mouth was pulled down and to the left; his left hand came up and adopted a claw-like posture. These episodes lasted between 40 seconds and 1 minute. They occurred three or four times weekly when he was first seen.

Examination and investigation

When the patient first presented to our service, at 6.5 years of age, he was very overactive. It was difficult to obtain EEGs because of the overactivity, but they showed copious spike–wave activity. At that time he was being treated with carbamazepine and phenytoin. In addition to very poor concentration span and a high degree of motor overactivity, he also had some striking autistic features. He appeared to be in a world of his own, could not carry out a conversation and gave poor, fleeting eye contact. However, he had developed a special skill of reciting nursery rhymes. If someone uttered the first few words of a nursery rhyme he would continue with the rhyme. At around 6 years of age his ability to recite nursery rhymes was far superior to that of any other child at his school or indeed any of the adults.

Dilated ventricles were noted on a computed tomography (CT) scan at 2.5 years of age. A repeat CT scan at 10 years of age showed marked atrophy of the right hemisphere. He had a very mild left hemiparesis, tending to drag his left leg when walking. However, he could run quite fast and play football.

Diagnosis

Attention deficit disorder, frequent epileptiform discharges and autistic features.

Treatment and outcome

Following a review of the antiepileptic medication, the phenytoin was tailed off and valproate was added. He was also treated with acetazolamide for a period. The epileptiform discharges on the EEG resolved. He became calm, lost his motor overactivity and was able to engage in rewarding two-way conversations. He began to enjoy social interaction greatly.

It was subsequently possible to discontinue both the acetazolamide and the valproate, leaving him on carbamazepine monotherapy. By the age of 19 years, he typically had no more than one seizure a year and the EEG showed only a non-specific excess of slow wave activity with occasional right-sided sharp waves of dubious significance. Although he enjoyed social interaction and derived great pleasure from interacting with his parents and carers, he was markedly eccentric. The intonation and content of his speech was typical of an individual with Asperger syndrome. He had developed many skills of daily living but continued to require a moderate degree of supervision to enable him to live within society.

Commentary

This case illustrates that epilepsy may present in ways that lead to evaluation and management by psychiatrists or paediatricians rather than paediatric neurologists.

This patient's initial presentation at 6.5 years was striking both because of gross attention-deficit disorder and overactivity and because of the autistic features. It appears that both of these clinical disorders were the result of frequent epileptiform discharges that were fragmenting his concentration and affecting his ability to interact with the world around him. When these frequent epileptiform discharges responded successfully to treatment he was able to develop rewarding interactions with other people, and the gross overactivity and attention deficit resolved. However, he then presented with a different clinical picture, reminiscent of Asperger syndrome.

I have now seen several young people who have presented with a similar clinical picture in the mid-to-late teenage years, having gone through a period in earlier childhood when frequent epileptiform discharges occurred. It would appear that children who have frequent epileptiform discharges that largely prevent them from having the easy two-way interaction with the world that most children experience may subsequently have difficulties with social interaction even after the epileptiform discharges have resolved. It appears that this is the reason why this patient presented with strong features of Asperger syndrome in his late teenage years even though the epileptiform discharges were well controlled at that time.

What did I learn from this case?

First, I learnt that children who present with attention-deficit disorder and overactivity may be having frequent epileptiform discharges that are breaking up their ability to concentrate and to interact with others. Treatment of these discharges can result in the resolution of the attention-deficit disorder and overactivity and can enable them to have a meaningful, rewarding interaction with the world around them.

Second, if a child is prevented from having the usual two-way social interaction with the world around him or her during a critical phase of development because of frequent epileptiform discharges, he or she may continue to have social interaction problems, presenting with an Asperger-like picture, long after the discharges have been treated or have resolved.

Third, the implication of these cases is that early energetic treatment of epileptiform discharges might both resolve the autistic features at the time and even prevent the development of permanent Asperger-like characteristics with the accompanying social interaction difficulties.

Further Reading

Asperger H. Die 'Autistischen Psychopathien' im Kindesalter. *Archiv für Psychiatrie und Nervenkrankheiten* 1944;117:362–8.

Wing L. Asperger's syndrome: a clinical account. *Psychol Med* 1981;11:115–29.

Harris JC. *Developmental neuropsychiatry. Assessment, diagnosis, and treatment of developmental disorders.* Vol II. Oxford, Oxford University Press; 1995:221–8.

Case 94

COMPLETE SEIZURE CONTROL IN A 14-YEAR-OLD BOY AFTER TEMPORAL LOBECTOMY FAILED

Martin J Brodie

History

A 14-year-old autistic, learning-disabled boy had been experiencing fortnightly clusters of 10–20 partial and secondary generalized seizures before his referral in July 1992.

He had been born by emergency caesarian section in response to fetal distress and had an Apgar score of 4 on delivery. Seizure activity developed following three prolonged febrile convulsions early in his first year of life and continued throughout childhood, despite removal of a damaged left temporal lobe at the age of 3 years. He was aggressive before the clusters of seizures, which were always followed by complex automatisms. His parents found his constant wandering particularly difficult to cope with. Treatment on referral was with phenytoin monotherapy. He had received carbamazepine, valproate, phenobarbital and bromide in the past.

Adding vigabatrin to the phenytoin did not improve his seizure control and worsened his behaviour. Lamotrigine produced a modest reduction in the number of seizures. The patient's family then moved from the area. When he was referred again in November 1996, his treatment consisted of phenytoin 300 mg/day (concentration 80 μmol/l) and lamotrigine 500 mg/day (concentration 21 μmol/l). Seizure frequency had worsened. The numbers of bi-monthly clusters had not increased, but each cluster now consisted of 20 or more complex partial seizures with frequent secondary generalization over a period of 2–3 days.

Examination and investigations

Neurological examination was essentially normal. The patient had stereotypic behaviour and marked gum hypertrophy. A surface EEG showed excess slow wave activity but no epileptiform discharges. Brain imaging was not undertaken.

370

Diagnosis

Partial-onset seizures secondary to perinatal hypoxic brain damage in an autistic, learning-disabled young man.

Treatment and outcome

Phenytoin was withdrawn and the lamotrigine dose was increased to 800 mg/day in two divided doses. This regimen produced a modest reduction in the frequency and severity of seizures. The cautious addition of low-dose topiramate led to a marked improvement in alertness and behaviour.

This young man has remained seizure-free since September 1998 on lamotrigine 800 mg/day in two divided doses (concentration 66 μmol/l) and topiramate 75 mg/day (25 mg in the morning and 50 mg at bedtime; concentration 6 μmol/l).

Commentary

The combination of high-dose lamotrigine and low-dose topiramate resulted in complete seizure control with improvement in the patient's quality of life and that of his family. Temporal lobectomy and previous treatment with carbamazepine, valproate, phenobarbital, bromide, phenytoin, phenytoin–vigabatrin and phenytoin–lamotrigine had been unsuccessful.

My recent studies suggest that in nearly 40 % of patients, seizures will not come under control with a single antiepileptic drug. It is therefore essential to develop therapeutic strategies for combining antiepileptic drugs in patients with difficult-to-control epilepsy. Without a detailed knowledge of the pathophysiology underlying seizure generation and propagation, it seems reasonable to choose drugs with different and potentially complementary modes of action. Attention also needs to be paid to the range of efficacy, side-effect profile and propensity for adverse interaction. This strategy is particularly relevant for patients with learning disabilities, who often present with multiple seizure types and always represent a major management challenge. The best evidence in support of this approach has been provided by results with lamotrigine and valproate, which is universally regarded as a 'synergistic' combination.

When taking the history from a patient with refractory epilepsy, the clinician must review not just previous attempts at single-drug therapy but also what combinations of antiepileptic drugs (and in what dosages) have been tried. A

371

range of different strategies should be used until the best outcome is obtained. Some patients respond best to three-drug combinations, particularly valproate, lamotrigine and topiramate. The older agents clobazam and acetazolamide should not be forgotten. The aim should be seizure freedom unless there is a good reason to be less ambitious. Sometimes the patient and doctor need to take a 'time out' from manipulations of antiepileptic drugs. Nevertheless, if at first you don't succeed, try, try and try again!

What did I learn from this case?

There is now an increasingly wide range of new antiepileptic drugs to try in addition to the traditional agents. Using these drugs in rational combinations results in substantial improvement in seizure control in many more patients than ever before. I believe that both lamotrigine and topiramate contributed to the excellent outcome in this patient in a way that we do not yet fully understand. This sort of observation sets up a hypothesis that can be tested scientifically (Fig. 94.1).

This patient represents one in a small series that has changed my clinical practice. We now have an ongoing research programme exploring the use of adjunctive topiramate in patients with learning disability that involves a

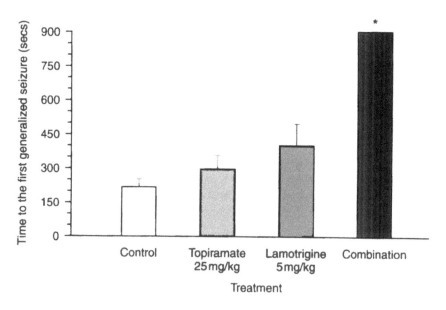

Figure 94.1: *Effect of lamotrigine and topiramate singly and in combination in preventing pentylenetetrazol-induced seizures in adult Imperial Cancer Research mice.*

prospective baseline and predetermined end-points. So far, 64 patients have been recruited to the study. The preliminary results look encouraging with 25 % seizure-free.

Further reading

Brodie MJ, French JA. Management of epilepsy in adolescents and adults. *Lancet*; 2000;**356**:323–9.

Brodie M J, Yuen AWC and the 105 Study Group. Lamotrigine substitution study: evidence for synergism with sodium valproate? *Epilepsy Res* 1997;**26**:423–32.

Dichter MA, Brodie MJ. New antiepileptic drugs. *N Engl J Med* 1996;**334**:1583–90.

Hannah JA, Brodie MJ. Epilepsy and learning disabilities: a challenge for the next millennium. *Seizure* 1998;**7**:3–13.

Kwan P, Brodie MJ. Early identification of refractory epilepsy. *N Engl J Med* 2000;**342**:314–19.

Stephen LJ, Sills GJ, Brodie MJ. Lamotrigine and topiramate may be a useful combination. *Lancet* 1998;**351**:958–9.

Stephen LJ, Sills GJ, Brodie MJ. Topiramate in refractory epilepsy: a prospective observational study. *Epilepsia*; 2000;**41**:977 -80.

Case 95

ICTAL CRYING IN A 32-YEAR-OLD WOMAN

Edward B Bromfield

History

A 32-year-old woman, who had had a single febrile seizure at the age of 1 year, was well until a head-on motor vehicle collision at the age of 24, caused by another driver. She had 2-day retrograde amnesia and 5-day anterograde amnesia, subdural and subarachnoid hemorrhages, and bifrontal and left inferior temporal contusions.

She was treated prophylactically with antiepileptic drugs. She developed a rash from phenytoin and phenobarbital but not from carbamazepine. She later began having episodes of palpitations and a strange bodily sensation, followed by right upper and lower extremity paresthesias with nausea and inability to speak. These episodes lasted 1–2 minutes each. There was a sense of confusion, with variable preservation of comprehension and memory. Months later, when she had a prolonged confusional state that culminated in three convulsions, these episodes were recognized as seizures. Her dosage of carbamazepine was increased, but seizures persisted at a frequency of one or two a week. Lamotrigine was added but was then stopped when she had a second episode of status epilepticus. Gabapentin was added, possibly with some benefit, but later she was weaned off gabapentin in favor of valproate. Increasing doses of carbamazepine and valproate resulted in gastrointestinal distress, sedation and dizziness without improvement in seizure control.

Despite residual naming and memory problems after rehabilitation, she was able to complete law school and pass the bar exam. She tried working for a law firm but had to resign, more because of seizures than cognitive limitations. She and her husband were highly motivated to have a child, although they were concerned about the potential risks of seizures and the patient's antiepileptic drug on the baby. The patient decided to attempt conversion to gabapentin monotherapy. This was accomplished over several months, with no change in seizure frequency or severity.

374

Examination and investigations

Examination was notable for mild dysnomia, right-sided clumsiness and right hyper-reflexia. Neuropsychological testing demonstrated average global functioning, decreased naming, and memory deficits greater for verbal memory than for visuospatial memory.

A magnetic resonance imaging scan showed prominent central and cortical atrophy and two areas of encephalomalacia in the inferior left temporal lobe.

Inpatient video-EEG monitoring showed bilateral anterior–mid-temporal sharp waves and spikes occurring twenty times more frequently on the left than the right. After gabapentin was reduced, she had two complex partial seizures arising from the left anterior temporal lobe, the second of which generalized after 10 minutes. During the seizures, she held her left hand over her mouth, extended her right arm, and opened and closed the right hand; she appeared in profound distress and cried intermittently. Ictal single photon emision computed tomography showed marked hyperperfusion in the inferolateral left temporal region.

Subsequently, left temporal and frontoparietal subdural electrodes were implanted. Numerous interictal discharges and electrographic seizures were recorded from the left inferior temporal lobe. Because of the patient's reluctance to taper gabapentin aggressively, only one clinical seizure was recorded, showing a regional left inferior temporal onset. Language mapping showed interference with naming and reading when posterior temporal contacts were stimulated.

An intracarotid amobarbital test initially showed poor memory bilaterally. She recognized only two stimuli out of eight on left-sided injection and three out of eight on right-sided injection; however, she had profound shivering and anxiety during the left-sided injection. When this test was repeated during invasive monitoring, she recognized seven stimuli out of eight.

Diagnosis

Post-traumatic neocortical temporal lobe epilepsy.

Treatment and outcome

A tailored left temporal lobectomy was performed, using intraoperative language mapping and confirmatory electrocorticography. Pathological examination revealed neuronal loss and gliosis in the neocortex and hippocampus, together with focal neocortical hemosiderosis.

Three months after surgery, the patient's gabapentin was tapered and she had a secondarily generalized seizure. Gabapentin was increased, birth control was stopped, and she conceived within 1 month. She has since remained seizure-free except for a single aura during the second trimester of her pregnancy. One year after temporal lobectomy, she gave birth to a healthy baby boy. Repeat neuropsychological testing showed stable naming deficits and some memory improvement. She now works part-time for an advocacy organization.

Commentary

This patient had post-traumatic left temporal lobe, neocortical epilepsy. Her seizures included prominent contralateral somatosensory manifestations, which probably reflected spread to the second sensory area in the frontal operculum. This area mediates sensation either contralaterally or bilaterally, often in the distal extremities.[1] She also had the unusual phenomenon of ictal crying.[2]

In the setting of phenytoin and possible phenobarbital allergies, partial response to gabapentin, and poor response to carbamazepine and valproate, the patient tolerated gradual conversion to gabapentin monotherapy without any increase in the frequency or severity of her seizures. Although gabapentin has shown efficacy as a sole agent,[3] it has not been systematically compared to other antiepileptic drugs, and meta-analyses have shown a lower response rate.[4]

Tailored left temporal lobectomy resulted in freedom from seizures, excluding an unsuccessful early postoperative attempt at medication reduction[5] that was done because of the patient's desire to minimize medications before conception.[6] Despite the multifocal nature of the insult, post-traumatic temporal lobe epilepsy can have a high surgical success rate.[7]

What did I learn from this case?

I learned that gabapentin monotherapy can be as effective as other drugs that are generally viewed as more potent. The case also reinforced the possibility of contralateral somatosensory symptoms and ictal crying as manifestations of temporal lobe (neocortical) epilepsy, and also the possibility of a good surgical outcome despite a known multifocal injury.

This patient also taught me how strongly a patient's desire to minimize risk during pregnancy can guide decision making, even with limited information. Finally, I realized how social supports and a realistic view of one's limitations and capacities can lead to excellent recovery from a potentially devastating injury.

How did this case alter my approach to the care and treatment of my epilepsy patients?

I am more likely now to view gabapentin monotherapy as a viable option in

376

selected patients. I am also more positive about surgical and psychosocial prognosis after major head injury that leads to intractable epilepsy.

References

1. Penfield W, Jasper H. *Epilepsy and the functional anatomy of the human brain*. Boston: Little, Brown, 1954.

2. Offen ML, Davidoff RA, Troost BT, Richley ET. Dacrystic epilepsy. *J Neurol Neurosurg Psychiatry* 1976;**39**:824–34.

3. Chadwick DW, Anhut H, Greiner MJ, *et al*. A double-blind trial of gabapentin monotherapy for newly diagnosed partial seizures. *Neurology* 1998;**51**:1282 8.

4. Chadwick DW, Marson T, Kadir Z. Clinical administration of new antiepileptic drugs: an overview of safety and efficacy. *Epilepsia* 1996;**37(suppl 6)**:S17 S22.

5. Schiller Y, Cascino GD, So EL, March WR. Discontinuation of antiepileptic drugs after successful epilepsy surgery. *Neurology* 2000;**54**:346–9.

6. Quality Standards Subcommittee, AAN. Practice parameter: Management issues for women with epilepsy (summary statement). *Neurology* 1998;**51**:944–8.

7. Mathern GW, Babb TL, Vickrey B, Melendez M, Pretorius JK. Traumatic compared to non-traumatic clinical–pathologic associations in temporal lobe epilepsy. *Epilepsy Res* 1994;**4**:129–39.

Case 96

HEALING BEGINS WITH COMMUNICATING THE DIAGNOSIS

Orrin Devinsky

History

The patient is a 48-year-old right-handed man with a history of atypical nocturnal behaviors. There was a vague history that as a child he had episodes during sleep that were similar to the recent episodes witnessed by his wife. The frequency and the intensity of these events had increased over the past 5 years. He had been evaluated by six neurologists, including two epileptologists, and had undergone two video-EEG monitoring studies and three admissions to sleep disorder centers for polysomnography. Various diagnoses were made, the most common of which was conversion disorder with non-epileptic seizures.

During a 3-day inpatient video-EEG monitoring study that was conducted 6 weeks before our initial evaluation, he had multiple nocturnal episodes. During a typical episode he awakened with return of posterior alpha-wave activity and then suddenly grabbed his left knee screaming in pain and calling for assistance as soon as possible. Previous medical, rheumatological and orthopedic evaluations of his left knee were unremarkable. During some episodes, there was mild clonic activity in the left upper extremity. The episodes were associated with intense emotional expression, tachycardia, diaphoresis, facial flushing and increased respiratory rate. The episodes would occur over a period of 20–45 minutes. After the recent video-EEG monitoring study he was sent home after a supportive discussion of non-epileptic conversion episodes and a recommendation for psychiatric counseling and possible psychopharmacology if an underlying mood disorder was identified. An anxiety disorder was also considered.

The patient was seen in outpatient follow-up 2 weeks later, and both he and his wife were very resistant to the diagnosis of conversion disorder. During a prolonged discussion he expressed his frustration with the medical system and what he perceived as the lack of a clear answer despite very extensive testing. This reflected his failure to accept the diagnosis of conversion non-epileptic events. He was admitted for another video-EEG monitoring study to review his episodes and to look more carefully at his sleep activity to make certain that there was no

378

evidence of an atypical parasomnia. However, before the admission he suffered from an anterior wall myocardial infarction and underwent emergency angioplasty. He continued to have the nocturnal episodes, which were witnessed in the coronary care unit. A different group of neurologists were called in for consultation and thought that these episodes were psychiatric in origin. An additional neurologist suggested the diagnosis of an atypical Tourette's syndrome.

The patient was sent home. One week later he had another myocardial infarction in a different cardiac distribution and ruptured a papillary muscle, requiring emergent open-heart surgery for mitral valve repair and three-vessel bypass. He continued to have the nocturnal episodes in the postoperative period, causing significant concerns that they would contribute to additional cardiac injury.

He was readmitted for video-EEG monitoring and again his atypical episodes were recorded. His alpha rhythm would return out of sleep and he would grab his left knee. He would then curse and scream. He would be belligerent towards the nursing staff who attended him, and was in a state of heightened sympathetic nervous system activity for a period of 20–45 minutes.

On discussion with the patient that there were no EEG correlates, he and his wife again became very upset and said, 'We knew that already. What is the diagnosis? Don't tell us it is a conversion disorder'.

A review of the literature revealed that some patients with panic disorder had their episodes exclusively limited to night-time, possibly accounting for up to 2.5 % of all patients with panic disorder. This diagnosis was made and the biological nature of panic disorder was emphasized.

Diagnosis

Panic disorder.

Treatment and outcome

The patient was started on clonazepam 0.5 mg at bedtime, which was increased to 1.0 mg at bedtime. He has been free of episodes since that time (12 weeks), with stable cardiovascular function.

Commentary

This patient has episodes for which the ultimate diagnosis is still uncertain and controversial. This man, like many others, was very hesitant to accept the

379

diagnosis of a conversion disorder, although it is likely that part of his disorder was attributable to that entity. However, the repeated presentation of this diagnosis to him and appropriate counseling did not lead to any improvement in his symptoms and unfortunately may have contributed to some of the stress that ultimately precipitated two myocardial infarctions and the need for angioplasty and open heart surgery.

What did I learn from this case?

I learned that the borderline between neurology and psychiatry is a shifting one. In this case, finding a biological explanation (panic disorder) that may not have been the best scientific answer (or even a justifiable clinical explanation) was nonetheless clearly beneficial for the patient's clinical condition and psychological well-being.

How did this case alter my approach to the care and treatment of my epilepsy patients?

I now understand the therapeutic importance of being willing to change my shift of attention and style of presentation to patients and their families in a very individualized manner.

Case 97

AN UNUSUAL CASE OF SEIZURES AND VIOLENCE

Robert S Fisher

History

The patient was a 24-year-old right-handed man with convulsions, postictal psychosis and seizure-associated aggressive behavior. He had been well until the age of 11, when he developed viral encephalitis, which resulted in coma and acute seizures. No causative organism was isolated. He recovered, suffering only some residual short-term memory and attentional problems. Seizures recurred several months after the encephalitis. These were of a complex partial type, often with secondary generalization. The first warning of seizure onset was a sense of fear, followed by confusion, growling like a 'caged bear' and hyperalertness. The patient would be unaware of conversation, and would not recall episodes that transpired during the seizures.

Seizure frequency increased over the next few years until he was having many seizures a week. By the age of 18, the patient was beginning to experience elements of postictal psychosis, with religious rumination and a sense that he was somehow 'special' in the scheme of the world. Intrusive paranoid thoughts about people trying to harm him also were expressed during the postictal state. As time progressed, postictal psychosis became more frequent and more prolonged, and the patient did not return to a baseline normal psychiatric state between seizures.

By the age of 20, the patient would jump up during a seizure from a reclining or seated position and run across the room, sometimes slamming into objects and injuring himself. If he encountered people during his seizure, he might strike them or push them away. On one occasion, he physically lifted his father and hurled him into a wall. The most disturbing incident occurred when he had a seizure onset while sitting next to his mother, who was going through the day's mail. During the seizure, he picked a letter opener off the table, and stabbed his mother in the side. Fortunately, her physical injury was slight.

The patient was committed involuntarily to a hospital for the criminally insane, when no other facility would accept him. While in this hospital he attacked several of the other patients during seizures. During one seizure, he put his fist through a glass window and pulled back against a glass shard, cutting his hand severely. He then ran around the room brandishing the shard. Following this behavior he was locked in a padded room in isolation.

Examination and investigations

The neurological examination fluctuated with proximity to a seizure. Within days of most seizures the patient showed an organic psychosis with religious preoccupation and failure to recognize place and time. At a time more than one week from a seizure, he was fully oriented, conversant and without focal neurological signs, but depressed about his life circumstances. One seizure was observed in the clinic – he roared and then leapt up and out of the room. He ran straight down the clinic corridor towards an open door connecting with the clinical laboratory, screaming all the way. Laboratory phlebotomists heard and saw him coming and slammed the door shut. The patient ran forcibly into the closed door, slumped to the ground and had a tonic–clonic convulsion.

Routine EEGs, video-EEG monitoring and invasive recordings from eight electrodes (eight contacts on each) disclosed multifocal bilateral seizure onset in the temporal amygdalar and superior frontal regions, as well as diffuse interictal spiking. A magnetic resonance imaging scan showed no focal lesion and no specific mesial temporal sclerosis.

Diagnosis

Multifocal partial epilepsy with postictal violence.

Treatment and outcome

Most of the usual seizure medications that were available at the time (before 1994) were tried, either without benefit or with intolerable side effects. Given the desperate and unusual nature of this case, a meeting was convened of the hospital ethics committee together with the parents (his legal guardians) to review all possible therapeutic options.

A decision was made to perform bilateral stereotaxic amygdalotomies, since both amygdalas appeared to be heavily involved in the origin of his seizures. The hippocampi were spared. This procedure was technically successful but completely ineffective against his epilepsy and provided no benefit for his postictal violence.

A decision then was made to perform stereotaxic radiofrequency lesions of the cingulate bundles bilaterally in the anterior superior medial frontal regions. The rationale for this procedure was two-fold:

- interruption of the spread of seizures via the circuit of Papez and the cingulum bundle; and
- possible benefit of cingulotomy for intractable violence.

After the cingulotomies, the patient was lethargic and nearly mute for approximately 5 days. He then began to talk and became normally animated, appearing less depressed than before surgery. Memory and cognitive functions showed no decline from the preoperative (somewhat impaired) baseline.

After the cingulotomy, the patient's seizures and intermittent psychotic ruminations continued as before, but over 3 years of follow-up, none of the seizures led to running or violent actions. He was released from hospital to home on conventional antiepileptic and neuroleptic medications. One day, when sitting on the couch next to his mother, he suddenly stood up, roared like a bear, then turned to her and said, 'Just kidding'. She was not amused!

Commentary

People with epilepsy very rarely harm anyone but themselves during seizures.[1] A review of videotapes from 5400 people with epilepsy, including 19 with reported aggressive behavior during seizures, showed violence during or after a seizure to be uncommon.[2] The so-called epilepsy defense – claiming that a crime was due to epilepsy – is rarely justified or effective,[3] although exceptions do occur.[4]

This was one of my most memorable cases as an exception to the rule of non-aggression during seizures. Even in this extreme instance, however, the aggression was unfocused, non-directed, unplanned, and along the line of a striking out at anything in the field of attention.

The association of aggression with postictal psychosis may not be coincidence, since at least one study[5] has found the risk for violent postictal behavior to be much higher in those with postictal psychosis. Details of the seizures and EEG patterns may be less important for assessing the risk of epilepsy-associated aggression than several variables related to baseline psychopathology and cognitive ability.[6] These factors may also be of key importance as well for interictal violence.[7]

The use of stereotaxic lesions to treat epilepsy in this context raises several controversial practical and ethical questions. Were we treating the patient's epilepsy, his behavior or both? Was this a type of psychosurgery, a set of techniques with dubious background?[8] Stereotaxic cingulotomy has been claimed to be effective for uncontrolled aggression, obsessive–compulsive disorder and several other psychiatric conditions.[9] The ethics of such surgery were considered in this case, and the relevant ethical issues have also been discussed in the medical literature.[10]

What did I learn from this case?

Epilepsy is such a broad and varied family of disorders that blanket statements rarely hold true without exception. Most seizures do not precipitate violence, but some do. Any violence is likely to be unplanned, undirected and inadvertent. Unusual cases call for 'out-of-the-box' thinking about therapies. In such circumstance, help from objective ethical review and human consent committees can help to make sure that the actions that are taken are likely to be in the best interests of the patient.

How did this case alter my approach to the care and treatment of my epilepsy patients?

I advise families, friends and health-care workers to be cautious in their delivery of first aid to all delirious patients, including those in the midst of or in the wake of a seizure. The best approach is usually one of gentle guidance, reorientation and reassurance, rather than physical restraint.

References

1. Fenwick P. The nature and management of aggression in epilepsy. *J Neuropsychiatry Clin Neurosci* 1989;1:418–25.

2. Delgado-Escueta AV, Mattson RH, King L, *et al*. Special report. The nature of aggression during epileptic seizures. *N Engl J Med* 1981;**305**:711–6.

3. Treiman DM. Violence and the epilepsy defense. *Neurol Clin* 1999;**17**:245–55.

4. Ramani V, Gumnit RJ. Intensive monitoring of epileptic patients with a history of episodic aggression. *Arch Neurol* 1981;**38**:570–1.

5. Kanemoto K, Kawasaki J, Mori E. Violence and epilepsy: a close relation between violence and postictal psychosis. *Epilepsia* 1999;**40**:107–9.

6. Mendez MF, Doss RC, Taylor JL. Interictal violence in epilepsy. Relationship to behavior and seizure variables. *J Nerv Ment Dis* 1993;**181**:566–9.

7. Devinsky O, Bear D. Varieties of aggressive behavior in temporal lobe epilepsy. *Am J Psychiatry* 1984;**141**:651–6.

8. Diering SL, Bell WO. Functional neurosurgery for psychiatric disorders: a historical perspective. *Stereotact Funct Neurosurg* 1991;**57**:175–94.

9. Ballantine HT Jr, Bouckoms AJ, Thomas EK, Giriunas IE. Treatment of psychiatric illness by stereotactic cingulotomy. *Biol Psychiatry* 1987;**22**:807–19.

10. Bouckoms AJ. Ethics of psychosurgery. *Acta Neurochir Suppl (Wien)* 1988;**44**:173–8.

Case 98

SEIZURE RELAPSE 13 YEARS AFTER SUCCESSFUL SURGERY

John R Gates

History

The patient was a 15-year-old, right-handed, white male with no previous head injury or CNS infection who began having seizures in September 1978. They were characterized by a 'dizzy feeling' and an inability to respond or speak during an event, although afterwards he could remember and reply to what had been said. He also felt a tingling in his left foot spreading up into the thigh and often had left arm stiffening. These episodes were occurring every 2–3 days. He also had a history of medication-controlled tonic–clonic seizures.

Examination and investigations

At the time of the evaluation, he was on valproate and mesantoin. He had failed phenytoin, phenobarbital, and primidone. The neurological examination was remarkable for mild upper motor neuron weakness of the left upper extremity with decreased, rapid, alternating movements of the left hand and decreased tapping of the left foot. Somatosensory testing was within normal limits. Deep tendon reflexes were symmetrical. Gait was normal. His CT scan revealed an avascular cystic mass in the right parietal area. Surface video-EEG recording confirmed partial seizure onset in the right parietal area. A subdural electrode array was placed.

Diagnosis

Parietal lobe epilepsy.

Treatment and outcome

Functional cortical mapping and epileptogenic localization were performed resulting in a resection, as demonstrated in Figs 98.1 and 98.2. Pathology revealed a grade I–II astrocytoma. He had no deficit from the intervention. Subsequently he completed a course of radiation therapy. After this intervention and while being maintained on both phenytoin 500 mg and carbamazepine 1200 mg per day, he obtained complete seizure control with yearly imaging showing no change in the tumor.

Thirteen years later he began to have simple partial somatosensory seizures behind his left knee. An imaging study showed increased size of the tumor in the

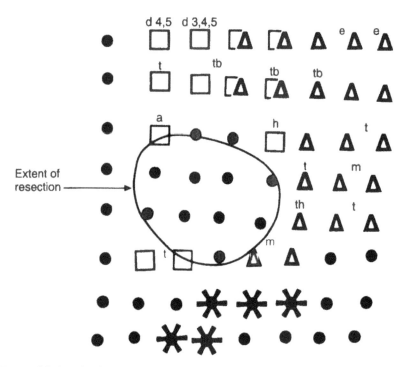

Figure 98.1: *The diagram shows the superimposition of the data gathered from stimulation studies from the patient who was implanted with a 64-contact subdural grid. The grid is over the right hemisphere (anterior is to the right, posterior to the left, the temporal region is inferior, and the frontal and parietal regions represented in the superior portion of the photograph). The squares identify somatosensory function; the triangles refer to motor function; 'd' identifies hand digits as numbered; 't' refers to tongue; 'tb' to thumb; 'e' to eyes; 'a' to arm; 'm' to mouth; and ** refers to a sensation of hearing.*

386

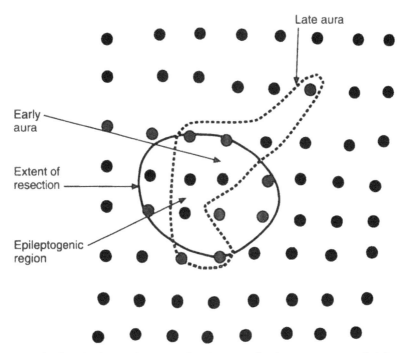

Figure 98.2: *The broken line identifies the area of epileptogenesis recorded from the grid. The early and late aura regions are identified. The extent of resection is identified by the solid line.*

right posterior frontal lobe with enlargement of both the cystic component and the adjacent T2 signal. He subsequently returned to surgery for a more localized resection performed stereotactically. No deficits were noted post operatively. This time, the pathology revealed a grade II oligodendroglioma. The old surgical slides were pulled and re-read as consistent with a grade II oligodendroglioma. After the stereotactic resection, he was maintained on gabapentin monotherapy 600 mg bid. He has continued to be seizure-free.

Commentary

Why did I choose this case?

This patient had a tumor in a location that two other institutions had been uncomfortable pursuing because of the belief that it was in the anatomical primary motor strip.

Since he did not have a significant sensory or motor deficit in the left upper extremity, though he had some mild tone changes, we elected to perform the subdural electrode array placement. The absence of a deficit indicated to us that the tumor was not in the motor strip. The variability and the location of the primary motor strip and its incredible plasticity has been repeatedly observed.[1,2] Consequently, in the absence of a deficit the function must be subserved elsewhere than the classical anatomical zones.

What did I learn from this case ?

The remarkable course of this neoplastic process now spans 20 years from the patient's first seizure. The 15-year-old boy is now a man in his early 30s who had recurrence of the tumor, yet we were able to resect it without further deficit because of the remarkable consistency of the functional cortical map over time. This is one of the longest maps to second resection that we have made and underscores the durability of cortical functional mapping with subdural electrode array.

Another aspect of this case is the remarkable variability of primary CNS neoplasia. When I first received the pathology report on this young man, I dreaded that in five or at most 10 years he would be dead. Instead, I followed him every year for a period of 15 years until the tumor recurrence and subsequent resection.

We have an arrangement. Every year he 'visits' the tumor and confidently 'leaves' it in my office until his return the next year. Of all the parameters followed, including neuropsychological testing, MRI scanning, neurological exam, and seizure frequency and type, it was the seizure frequency and type that was the most sensitive indicator of recurrence that prompted us to re-image at an earlier date than our regularly scheduled annual appointment.

References

1. Gates JR. Presurgical evaluation for epileptic surgery in the era of long-term monitoring for epilepsy. In: Puzzo MLJ (ed). *Neurosurgical aspects of epilepsy*. American Association of Neurological Surgeons: Park Ridge, IL, 1992:59–72.

2. Gates JR, Dunn ME. Presurgical assessment and surgical treatment for epilepsy. *Acta Neurologica Belgica* 1999;**99**:291 -4.

Case 99

ATTACKS OF GENERALIZED SHAKING WITHOUT POSTICTAL CONFUSION

James S Grisolia

History

A 36-year-old woman was admitted for dilatation and curettage following a spontaneous abortion. This was one of multiple miscarriages in her attempt to have a child with her husband. After the procedure, she began to have multiple attacks of generalized shaking that lasted about 30 seconds each. Although the patient appeared unconscious during each attack, she often reported the sense of being able to hear health personnel talking during the attacks, and she suffered no postictal change whatsoever.

The patient had already received diazepam 10 mg intravenously followed by phenytoin 1 gram intravenously before neurological consultation. There was a previous history of rare apparent faints with a few tonic movements, generally occurring perimenstrually, and a history of multiple sclerosis, with minor residual co-ordination loss in the right leg.

Examination and investigations

The patient was somnolent owing to the effect of the intravenous medications, but she was easy to rouse. There was nystagmus in all directions of movement, which had not been present during the examination on admission. The remainder of the neurological examination was remarkable only for reduced rapid alternating movements in the right foot, which from the history was a residual effect of her multiple sclerosis.

The patient's EEG, blood pressure and cardiac rhythm were monitored during the episodes. No changes were seen in any studies.

Diagnosis

Psychogenic pseudoseizures.

389

Treatment and outcome

The patient was gently confronted with the fact that these attacks were 'stress-induced' attacks rather than 'epileptic' attacks. She offered the observation that as she went into each attack, she had a feeling that she was 'going away', just as she would 'go away' when her mother beat her when she was a little girl.

Further inquiry established that she had a very difficult and stressful relationship with her mother, who subjected her to emotional and physical abuse. Sexual abuse by the mother or anyone else was denied. When offered the suggestion that her miscarriage undoubtedly was a significant acute stressor, she agreed, saying that she and her husband very much wanted children. I suggested that her maternal desire might include a desire to repair the relationship with her own mother by a healthy relationship with her own daughter, and that the frustration of this desire by the miscarriage might have triggered the 'going away' response from her youth. The patient looked astonished for an instant, then readily agreed. I offered the hope that now that she understood the process and its origins, she was unlikely to have further pseudoseizures.

Under the vicissitudes of managed care, she was lost to follow-up until 6 years later, when she was referred back to me for follow-up of her stable multiple sclerosis. In the interim, she and her husband had weathered five miscarriages to have a lovely daughter. On occasion, she has had rare attacks conforming to a clinical diagnosis of convulsive syncope, but has never had sustained shaking or repetitive attacks.

Commentary

The association of psychogenic pseudoseizures with early life trauma is now well recognized. However, pseudoseizure cases that are commonly encountered in clinical practice demonstrate significant psychiatric morbidity, conforming to diagnoses of borderline personality organization, somatization disorder or other character pathology. Overall, the pathologies associated with early life trauma form a complex spectrum, with well-established neuroendocrine and cognitive pathologies still under study.

The profound character pathology associated with many pseudoseizure patients frustrates all clinicians. While much of this pathology arises from the original trauma and the reaction to it, prolonged ineffective treatment of pseudoseizures could contribute significantly to learned dependency, somatic preoccupations, depression and distrust of health-care providers.

What did I learn from this case?

This patient was unique in presenting as a high-functioning person who responded to an acute psychodynamic intervention, with apparent cure over a very long follow-up. Her case follows a less complicated psychodynamic conversion paradigm, responding to a traditional 'talking cure'.

How did this case alter my approach in the care and treatment of my patients with epilepsy?

My experience with this patient has encouraged me to attempt to diagnose pseudoseizures early, rather than at the end of a long, failed course of multiple medications. While direct intervention is usually unlikely to be as successful as it was in this case, I try to clarify the difference between 'epileptic' and 'stress-induced' seizures for the patient and the family, attempting to impart this opinion in a manner that is congenial with their medical beliefs and understanding. I avoid distinguishing between 'real' and 'fake' seizures. The revelation that anticonvulsants and emergency trips to hospital are unavailing comes as good news to some and as a threat to others. When there is significant character pathology, maintaining supportive contact with the patient appears valuable, both to avoid a fresh round of misdiagnosis and to provide reassurance to psychotherapists and others involved in the patient's care.

Further reading

Arnold LM, Privitera MD. Psychopathology and trauma in epileptic and psychogenic seizure patients. *Psychosomatics* 1996;37:438–43.

Krumholz A. Nonepileptic seizures: diagnosis and management. *Neurology* 1999;**53** (suppl 2):576–83.

Lesser RP. Psychogenic seizures. *Neurology* 1996;46:1499–507.

Van der Kolk BA, Pelcovitz D, Roth S, *et al*. Dissociation, somatization and affect dysregulation: The complexity of adaptation to trauma. *Am J Psychiatry* 1996;153:83–93.

Case 100

LENNOX–GASTAUT SYNDROME WITH GOOD OUTCOME ASSOCIATED WITH PERISYLVIAN POLYMICROGYRIA

Marilisa M Guerreiro

History

The patient is a 10-year-old right-handed boy with a history of dysarthria and seizures. He started having seizures at 3 years of age. They began with generalized tonic–clonic seizures. After a couple of weeks he started having drop-attacks and absence spells, which progressively increased in frequency, occurring up to 50–60 a day.

He was diagnosed with Lennox–Gastaut syndrome and underwent several unsuccessful trials of valproate, clobazam, phenobarbital, clonazepam, phenytoin, carbamazepine and lamotrigine. Excellent control was finally achieved with topiramate 200 mg/day; for the past 4 years, he has averaged one generalized tonic–clonic seizure a year.

He was born after an uneventful pregnancy. Delivery was normal. Psychomotor development was borderline (walking at 18 months) but speech development was delayed. He has marked dysarthria and has a history of choking and feeding difficulties during infancy. He also has a history of learning disabilities but made progress in his studies and now attends a regular class, two grades behind the expected level for his age.

His younger brother is followed by a speech therapist and his mother has articulation problems under stress.

Examination and investigations

On examination, he presented with striking dysarthria, drooling, moderate restriction of tongue movements (he is unable to protrude his tongue completely), difficulty in whistling and blowing, and an abnormally brisk jaw jerk. Deep tendon reflexes were hyperactive. The remainder of the neurological examination was normal.

Brain magnetic resonance imaging (MRI) revealed bilateral perisylvian

392

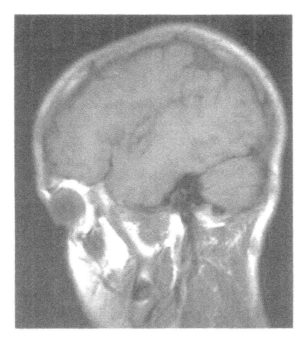

Figure 100.1 *Sagittal T1-weighted image showing diffuse polymicrogyria around the Sylvian fissure.*

polymicrogyria (Fig. 100.1). His brother had asymmetrical perisylvian polymicrogyria on MRI and his mother had similar, unilateral findings.

Diagnosis

Lennox–Gastaut syndrome due to perisylvian polymicrogyria.

Commentary

The main features of perisylvian syndrome are pseudobulbar palsy, cognitive deficits and epilepsy. The variability of the clinical picture is remarkable. Not all patients present with all the main features. On the contrary, they may present with soft signs, as was the case in this patient's mother. She had no complaints and had never been examined. Dysarthric speech seems to be the main feature of this syndrome, and it occurs in approximately 75 % of patients. Variable cognitive deficits and epilepsy occur in 50–75 % of patients.

Imaging findings show a broad spectrum of abnormalities. Unilateral polymicrogyria correlates with milder or absent pseudobulbar signs, and

393

bilateral, extensive anatomic involvement correlates with worse pseudobulbar symptoms and signs. Bilateral asymmetric lesions may be present in affected people even though malformations may not be detectable with current MRI techniques.

A genetic basis in some patients with cortical dysplasia is becoming increasingly apparent. Band heterotopia or the double cortex syndrome and bilateral periventricular nodular heterotopia have been associated with X-linked transmission. Perisylvian syndrome may be familial. In this case it appears to be genetically heterogeneous. There are some families in which autosomal dominance is the most likely mode of inheritance; patterns in other families suggest X-linked transmission.

What did I learn from this case?

I learnt that Lennox–Gastaut syndrome may be medically treated and sometimes responds well to treatment with antiepileptic drugs. It is an age-dependent epilepsy syndrome with many different possible etiologies. I believe its prognosis depends on the underlying cause more than on the treatment itself.

In addition, we are learning that cortical dysgenesis comprise a spectrum of developmental malformations with different intrinsic epileptogenicity according to the specific pathology. Polymicrogyria probably stands on the benign side of this spectrum.

Further reading

Guerreiro MM, Andermann E, Guerrini R, *et al*. Familial perisylvian polymicrogyria: a new familial syndrome of cortical maldevelopment. *Ann Neurol* 2000;**48**:39–48.

Kuzniecky R, Andermann F, Guerrini R, *et al*. Congenital bilateral perisylvian syndrome: study of 31 patients. *Lancet* 1993;**341**:608–12.

Palmini A, Gambardella A, Andermann F, *et al*. Intrinsic epileptogenicity of human dysplastic cortex as suggested by corticography and surgical results. *Ann Neurol* 1995;**37**:476–87.

Case 101

TEMPORAL LOBE RESECTION IN A PATIENT WITH SEVERE PSYCHIATRIC PROBLEMS

Reetta Kälviäinen

History

A 40-year-old right-handed woman had suffered from asphyxia at birth and began to have frequent epileptic seizures from the first day of her life.

At first the seizures were generalized tonic–clonic seizures, but later the dominant seizure type was complex partial seizures with *dejá vu* and amnesia lasting for 1–2 minutes. While amnestic, the patient usually had orofacial automatisms and sometimes rhythmic movements with her right lower extremity.

During childhood the patient had suffered from difficult-to-control seizures and was overprotected by her parents. However, she became independent when her generalized seizures were controlled with dual therapy with carbamazepine and valproate. Because she still had one or two complex partial seizures a month, she was offered surgical evaluation, but she refused.

She married and had two children, and eventually she owned her own small firm. Suddenly, at the age of 30, she suffered a series of six generalized seizures, became psychotic and was hospitalized. The psychotic episode relapsed after 1 year and the patient became severely depressed, requiring treatment with high-dose neuroleptics, antidepressants and benzodiazepines.

The patient had to give up working. Her husband left her, taking their children. She had to move back in with her father, who had not coped well with her epilepsy when she was a child. Moreover, he abused alcohol.

When she was 37, she was put on olanzapine and the dosages of her other psychoactive drugs were reduced.

Examination and investigations

The patient underwent a surgical evaluation at the age of 38. Magnetic resonance imaging (MRI) clearly revealed left-sided hippocampal sclerosis. Additionally, the

395

posterior part of the left hemisphere was smaller than the right and there was white matter hyperintensity behind the trigonum consistent with the history of asphyxia at birth.

Multiple interictal scalp EEGs had been performed over the years, demonstrating left temporal abnormalities. During video–EEG monitoring, only one complex partial seizure was recorded. Although she stared motionlessly, there were no EEG changes. Subsequently left temporal sharp theta activity was recorded. Interictally, sharp theta activity was also recorded maximally from the region of the left sphenoidal electrode. Difficulties in memory tasks were predominantly verbal; no frontal deficits were seen.

Diagnosis

Mesial temporal lobe epilepsy.

Treatment and outcome

The patient's psychiatrist felt that she needed full psychiatric support but was capable of going through epilepsy surgery. Her antiepileptic drug regimen was optimized before surgery with carbamazepine, topiramate and clobazam. She remained on olanzapine and had frequent discussions with psychiatrists.

A left hippocampectomy and amygdalectomy were performed at the age of 39. Pathologic analysis of the resected tissue demonstrated severe focal neuronal loss in the hippocampus. In the first year after surgery, she had no seizures, moved to her own apartment and started to work again.

Commentary

This case shows that MRI is helpful in selecting optimal candidates for surgical treatment of temporal lobe epilepsy. Before high-resolution MRI was available, surgical candidates frequently required invasive EEG monitoring with depth or strip electrodes in the temporal lobe.

More recently, preoperative investigations have been limited to scalp EEG monitoring, MRI, neuropsychologic testing, and – at some centers – positron emission tomography or single photon emission computed tomography. This is a significant advance, particularly for patients like this woman who have MRI evidence of hippocampal pathology and who do not have to undergo invasive monitoring, which might have predisposed her to the possible psychiatric complications of long-term subdural or depth EEG monitoring.

What did I learn from this case?

The relative contraindications to epilepsy surgery include interictal psychosis, persistent interictal thought disturbance or depression, and severely dysfunctional family dynamics. My patient did suffer from all of these conditions, yet I still believed that many of these problems were related to her intractable mesial temporal lobe epilepsy. Fortunately, her temporal lobe epilepsy could be clearly and effectively localized, and she did in fact benefit from surgery. Consistent with my impression, her seizure control and also her behavioral situation and overall quality of life improved.

Further reading

Engel J, Shewmon DA. Who should be considered a surgical candidate? In: Engel J, ed. *Surgical treatment of the epilepsies*. New York: Raven Press; 1993:23–34.

Flor-Henry P. Ictal and interictal psychiatric manifestations in epilepsy: specific or non-specific? A critical review of some of the evidence. *Epilepsia* 1972;**13**:767–72.

Thadani VM, Williamson PD, Berger R, *et al*. Successful epilepsy surgery without intracranial EEG recording: criteria for patient selection. *Epilepsia* 1995;**36**:7–15.

Trimble M. *The psychoses of epilepsy*. New York: Raven Press; 1991.

397

Case 102

AN OPEN MIND CAN BENEFIT THE PATIENT

Kaarkuzhali Babu Krishnamurthy

History

The patient was a 35-year-old right-handed woman with a history of recurrent seizures since the age of 2 years. She was the product of a full-term, uneventful pregnancy and delivery, and she achieved her developmental milestones at the appropriate ages. At first, her seizures were associated with high fever, but they later began occurring without fever. A typical seizure for her began with an aura of a bad taste, followed by nausea and a rising abdominal sensation. This would progress to loss of awareness, during which she would run or wander. She could converse relatively normally during the postictal period, but was quite aggressive and amnesic. Bystanders often mistook her postictal behavior for drunkenness and assumed she was mentally ill.

She completed high school, but could not begin college or hold down any type of employment. She was married briefly, and was the sole parent of a 6-year-old child. She had tried eight antiepileptic drugs in monotherapy and combinations without improvement in her seizure frequency. A magnetic resonance imaging (MRI) scan revealed a left frontal lobe heterotopia.

She was referred to me for a presurgical evaluation. At the time of my initial evaluation, she was experiencing between 6 and 12 seizures a month.

Examination and investigations

Surface video-EEG monitoring demonstrated independent, bitemporal interictal discharges. Clinical seizures were poorly localized. Neuropsychological testing suggested subtle left frontal dysfunction.

Since there was lack of concordance between her clinical and EEG data, the patient underwent depth electrode monitoring. The onset of her clinical seizures localized to the right amygdala, but the ictal activity then spread rapidly to the left hippocampus. Electrical stimulation through the implanted depth electrode in the right amygdala reproduced her clinical symptoms without affecting her EEG, while stimulation through the left hippocampal electrode produced some EEG changes without reproducing her clinical symptoms.

Diagnoses

Right temporal lobe epilepsy and left frontal heterotopia.

Treatment and outcome

The patient underwent a right temporal lobectomy. Pathological examination of the resected tissue was consistent with hippocampal sclerosis. During the year that elapsed after our initial meeting, her father was diagnosed with Alzheimer's disease, her mother developed breast cancer, and a close male friend was diagnosed with testicular cancer.

Since the lobectomy, she has been maintained on carbamazepine monotherapy. Approximately twice a year, she attempts to decrease her dose by 100–200 mg/day, which inevitably leads to breakthrough seizures. Otherwise, she has been seizure-free. Neuropsychological testing 18 months after surgery revealed only a mild decline in her nonverbal memory compared to presurgery performance, which was not an unexpected finding. After completing a vocational rehabilitation program, she went to work as an office manager and executive secretary. Most recently, she began a romantic relationship with a man whom she met at a self-help program and is contemplating marriage and, perhaps, pregnancy.

Commentary

This patient's life was complicated by seizures as well as difficult social and family situations, which became exacerbated during the period leading up to her surgery. She did not have the support system in place to help her through the presurgical evaluation and recovery period. However, with the input of the epilepsy treatment team, we concluded that her social situation was likely to get significantly worse in the near future because of the nature of the illnesses of her parents and friend, and that her loved ones would be happier knowing that she was helping herself.

What did I learn from this case?

This case serves as a nice reminder that dual pathology can occur in epilepsy. Her clinical semiology was strongly suggestive of a temporal focus, but the presence of the left frontal heterotopia was what prompted her referral for a surgical evaluation. Fortunately, we pursued invasive monitoring to clarify the picture, because resection of the appropriate region resulted in a significant improvement in seizure control and overall quality of life. This is contrary to suggestions in the literature that resection of the lesion as well as the epileptic focus are important. In this woman's situation, however, resection of the visible lesion would probably have resulted in some loss of motor function. Thus, we must treat the patient as an individual, distinct from group statistics in the literature.

The second significant point for me is that, while psychosocial support is very important for patients considering epilepsy surgery, there is no absolute level of support quality or quantity that should determine whether to proceed to surgery. I initially considered this patient's unfortunate home situation to be a contraindication for surgery. I was convinced, however, by her epilepsy nurse specialist that the time of anticipated surgery was likely to be a 'calmer' period in this patient's life than the next few months.

How did this case alter my approach to the care and treatment of my epilepsy patients?

I now keep a very open mind when working with patients who are considering epilepsy surgery. Before resorting to neuroimaging or EEG monitoring, I find it most helpful to localize seizure onset based on a description of the seizures by the patient or witnesses. Then, if the MRI data does not match the localization as predicated by the clinical features of the patient's seizures, I am reminded by this case that the presence of a single visible lesion does not preclude a second lesion, perhaps not apparent on the MRI, that may be responsible for the patient's epilepsy.

I value the multidisciplinary approach to epilepsy surgery that I am able to provide patients. Having epilepsy nurse specialists and social workers advise me about the pros and cons of the timing of epilepsy surgery was the key to this patient's successful outcome. If my original view had prevailed, her surgery would have been delayed and she might not have been able to rise above her grief.

Further reading

Li LM, Cendes F, Andermann F, *et al*. Surgical outcome in patients with epilepsy and dual pathology. *Brain* 1999;**122**:799–805.

Clarke DB, Olivier A, Andermann F, Fish D. Surgical treatment of epilepsy: the problem of lesion/focus incongruence. *Surg Neurol* 1996;**46**:579–85.

Case 103

AN UNEXPECTED LESSON

Paul M Levisohn

History

I first met G, an almost 3-year-old boy from southern Colorado, on 5 July 1995. He and his family were referred to me for treatment of his poorly controlled epilepsy. G had experienced his first seizure 2 years earlier, just short of his first birthday. Like most families, his parents sought an explanation for his seizures that had meaning to them;[1] they believed at the time that his seizure had occurred because of a fall and bump to the head.

Five months later, G experienced two further seizures, both with generalized motor activity. He was started on phenobarbital, which proved ineffective, as would many other antiepileptic drugs. He experienced frequent seizures as well as several episodes of status epilepticus despite serial treatment with carbamazepine, valproate and clonazepam. Associated symptoms included insomnia, irritability and severe language delay. He was treated with melatonin and chloral hydrate for sleep and carnitine for potential valproate toxicity. Episodes of status epilepticus were treated with rectally administered diazepam.

Seizures became more complex. He experienced events that began with behavioral arrest, followed by lateralized automatisms and tonic eye deviation to either side, perhaps more frequently to the left. Other less well-defined spells also occurred. Trials of other antiepileptic drugs, including investigational medications, proved ineffective.

Developmental testing at the age of 2 years demonstrated severe language delays but otherwise normal developmental functioning. However, his language had deteriorated as his seizures became more frequent; over time, there were concerns regarding more extensive developmental delays.

Examination and investigations

Multiple EEGs were all normal. Imaging studies revealed a benign congenital arachnoid cyst in the right temporal fossa. In October 1996, an evaluation for

401

possible resective epilepsy surgery was initiated. Video-EEG monitoring suggested lateralization to the right hemisphere both in seizure semiology and EEG, although localization was unclear. Ictal SPECT study demonstrated multifocal areas of abnormal activity. A positron emission tomography (PET) scan revealed hypometabolism on the right, including the frontal cortex, the temporal cortex and the parietal cortex.

Diagnosis

Medically refractory seizures (right hemisphere onset) with developmental delay.

Treatment and outcome

Before initiating further work-up for surgery, the family wanted to try the ketogenic diet. The diet resulted in a 3-week seizure-free interval. However, daily seizures then resumed; the seizures were now predominantly asymmetric tonic seizures, along with occasional seizures with a jacksonian march. He also began to experience episodes of left Todd's paresis and dysphasia.

At about this time, his parents divorced, an event which surprised my staff and me since both parents had always attended clinic together with him on a regular (and frequent) basis and seemed to work extremely well together as they sought what was best for their son.

In June 1998 (4 years after he had experienced his first seizure) G underwent a craniotomy for placement of subdural grid electrodes. The study confirmed that many of his seizures were of right frontal origin although the site of onset of others was undefined. Recognizing that a 'cure' was unlikely, his parents nevertheless agreed to proceed with a right frontal lobectomy. They reasoned that perhaps his most troublesome seizures, those leaving him with an increasing amount of left hemiparesis, would resolve.

Unfortunately, the surgery had little impact on G's epilepsy. His subsequent course was punctuated by status epilepticus with associated liver failure from which he gradually recovered; a fractured left arm from a fall related to ataxia (a residual effect of his almost fatal bout of status epilepticus and hepatic failure); poor weight gain and significant neurobehavioral dysfunction that was suggestive of pervasive developmental disorder. A vagus nerve stimulator was placed in July 1998 but appeared to have little impact. His parents requested that the stimulator be removed. However, shortly after turning the stimulator off, his parents noted that his seizures and behavior worsened and stimulation was reinstituted at low current settings. Clobazam was introduced in May 1999 after all commercially available antiepileptic drugs had been tried without success.

402

Whether because of this unusual combination of vagus nerve stimulation and clobazam or because of the 'natural history' of his disorder, G's epilepsy has recently improved. Most of his seizures now occur in sleep and there are no significant postictal residua. His behavior and learning, although still significantly impaired, have improved and he has developed limited language abilities. His mother has completed her bachelor's degree despite developing and apparently surviving ovarian cancer.

Both parents attend clinic together with G despite their divorce. They clearly have agreed to work together to do whatever is necessary for their son. I have suggested treatment with some of the newest antiepileptic drugs but they are not anxious to make any changes at this time. G is doing reasonable well and they have no desire to 'upset the apple cart'.

Commentary

Most of us, I believe, see G's story as a tragedy. A previously normal child develops epilepsy just before his first birthday and despite aggressive treatment with the new tools available for patients with intractable epilepsy, he experiences the full brunt of this disorder – progressive cognitive dysfunction, medication toxicity, injury, nearly fatal status epilepticus and hepatic failure. His parents, too, have born the impact of his disorder, in addition to their divorce and the mother's illness.

Even so, I always look forward to visits from G and his family. His parents are intelligent and warm people who are active participants in their son's care. They welcome my advice and heed my recommendations, but only when it appears appropriate within the context of their lives. They bear no obvious malice or anger for the troubles that their son has experienced. They do not see their son's life or their own lives as tragic.

G has been my teacher. He has tested my skills and learning as I have struggled to deal with his seizures and their impact. In his few years, he has become a textbook of epilepsy treatment at the end of the 20th century – from phenobarbital, the oldest of the antiepileptic drugs, to clobazam, an unapproved drug in the US, from the ketogenic diet to vagus nerve stimulation, from magnetic resonance imaging to functional imaging, he has run the gauntlet. Because of G, I have been forced to rethink what I thought I knew. PET and single photon emission computed tomography studies suggested that resective surgery might indeed result in seizure control, despite the lack of an identifiable lesion.[2-4] However, when intracranial monitoring failed to define a single zone of ictal onset, my goal for resective epilepsy surgery for G was modified from full control of seizures to improved control, a goal accepted by his parents. (Taylor *et al.*[5] provide a discussion about adjusting one's hoped-for outcomes from epilepsy surgery.)

Although I am unconvinced about the role of the ketogenic diet in children with localization-related epilepsy, I was willing to try the diet and have done so subsequently with greater success. At the time of his vagus nerve stimulator implant, G was the youngest child who had been implanted at my hospital and he was the only one from whom I have removed the stimulator.[6] As we have tried to help G, his parents have actively participated in his care, asking appropriate questions and carefully responding to my recommendations.

What did I learn from this case?

G's journey has been mine also, and I am a better physician because of him. The most important lesson I have learned from G and his family has nothing to do with pharmacology or neurophysiology. Rather it is that, as a physician, I have a limited ability to truly alter some patients' lives. If all goes well, I can significantly help children and families with the new tools that are available to me. But for too many children, this is not possible.

And I wonder at the responses of so many families. The families who do best despite apparently tragic circumstances seem to grow in strength under their burden. They bring to life the words of Emily Pearl Kingsley, the mother of a child with Down syndrome, who wrote a brief essay entitled 'Welcome to Holland' in 1987 (reprinted with permission).

Welcome to Holland

I am often asked to describe the experience of raising a child with disability – to try to help people who have not shared that unique experience to understand it, to imagine how it would feel. It's like this ...

When you're going to have a baby, it's like planning a fabulous vacation trip – to Italy. You buy a bunch of guidebooks and make your wonderful plans. The Coliseum. The Michelangelo. David. The gondolas in Venice. You may learn some handy phrases in Italian. It's all very exciting.

After months of eager anticipation, the day finally arrives. You pack your bags and off you go. Several hours later, the plane lands. The stewardess comes in and says, 'Welcome to Holland.'

'Holland?!?' you say. 'What do you mean Holland?? I signed up for Italy. I'm supposed to be in Italy. All my life I've dreamed of going to Italy.'

But there's been a change in the flight plan. They've landed in Holland and there you must stay.

404

The important thing is that they haven't taken you to a horrible, disgusting, filthy place, full of pestilence, famine and disease. It's just a different place.

So you must go out and buy new guidebooks. And you must learn a whole new language. And you will meet a whole new group of people you would never have met.

It's just a different place. It's slower pace than Italy, less flashy than Italy. But after you've been there a while and you catch your breath, you look around ... and you begin to notice that Holland has windmills ... and Holland has tulips. Holland even has Rembrandts.

But everyone you know is busy coming and going from Italy ... and they are all bragging about what a wonderful time they had there. And for the rest of your life, you will say, 'Yes, that's where I was supposed to go. That's what I had planned'.

And the pain of that will never, ever, ever go away ... because the loss of that dream is a very, very significant loss.

But ... if you spend your life mourning the fact that you didn't get to Italy, you may never be free to enjoy the very special, the very lovely things ... about Holland.

How did this case alter my approach to the care and treatment of my epilepsy patients?

Because of G, I too have arrived in a different place. I now know that while in my head I am a neurologist, in my heart I am a pediatrician. I recognize that too often treating epilepsy in children like G will not result in a cure and so for them my goals have to change.

Treating chronic illness is not something I was taught by my professors during my training and I suspect it is rarely taught even today, except by children like G. To treat chronic illness effectively, we must listen to our patients' stories, their narratives.[1] We must not only treat diseases of the nervous system but also illnesses of the whole person.[7] Outcomes cannot be measured only by percentage of seizure reduction or even by quantitative measures of 'health-related quality of life'.[8] Rather, it is by listening to our patients, to their hopes and goals, that we can most help them live in 'Holland'.

I only hope that in my role as teacher and mentor, I can transmit to students and residents everything that G has taught me.

References

1. Good BJ, Del Vecchio Good MJ. In the subjunctive mode: epilepsy narratives in Turkey. *Soc Sci Med* 1994;**38**:835–42.

2. Resnick T, Duchowny M, Jayakar P. Early surgery for epilepsy: redefining candidacy. *J Child Neurol* 1994;**9(suppl 2)**:S36–S41.

3. Juhasz C, Chugani DC, Muzik O, *et al.* Is epileptogenic cortex truly hypometabolic on interictal positron emission tomography? *Ann Neurol* 2000;**48**:88–96.

4. Chugani HT. Imaging: anatomic and functional. In: Wallace S, ed. *Epilepsy in children.* Cambridge: Chapman Hall; 1995:483–506.

5. Taylor DC, Neville BGR, Cross JH. New measure of outcome needed for the surgical treatment of epilepsy. *Epilepsia* 1997;**38**:625–30.

6. Crumrine PK. Vagal nerve stimulation in children. *Semin Pediatr Neurol* 2000;**7**:216–23.

7. Cassell E. Illness and disease. Hastings Center Report 1976;**6**:27–37.

8. Vickery BG, Hays R, Engel J. Outcome assessment for epilepsy surgery: the impact of measuring health-related quality of life. *Ann Neurol* 1995;**37**:158–66.

Case 104

WHEN SURGERY IS NOT POSSIBLE, ALL HOPE IS NOT LOST

Cassandra I Mateo and Brian Litt

History

The patient is a 31-year-old left-handed single white man who was well until 1991, when he fell off a bunk and landed on a concrete floor. He experienced loss of consciousness and amnesia after the fall and had a generalized convulsive seizure 2 days later.

The patient began to have generalized convulsive seizures every other week, with occasional seizure-free periods of 2–3 weeks. There were also brief periods when he had flurries of seizures every other day. He denied auras. Soon after this time he began to experience complex partial seizures. During these events he was noticed to stare, look around with a blank stare on his face; sometimes he would get up and say the words 'hike, hike' at the beginning of these events. Family members noted that he would tap on his legs and body with his hands at times. Complex partial seizures routinely lasted from between 15 seconds and 1 minute. The patient was usually confused postictally and felt weak after the seizures. On average, complex partial seizures occurred approximately every other week. Of note, the patient was often able to speak, though unintelligibly, throughout his seizures.

Past medical history was not significant, other than his history of epilepsy. He was the normal product of a full-term gestation and was actually delivered 1 week post-date. The patient was delivered by Caesarean section because of failure to progress. No hospital stay was required. The patient reached his motor and verbal milestones at appropriate ages and was a good student in school. There was no history of febrile convulsions, meningitis or encephalitis during infancy.

He left school after the tenth grade and then pursued his graduate equivalency degree. He works as a cashier and lives alone. He has relatively few social contacts and has been primarily concerned with getting rid of his seizures so that he could improve his life situation and pursue more rewarding employment. There is no history of drug or alcohol use.

Prior medication trials included maximally tolerated doses of phenytoin, carbamazepine, valproate, lamotrigine, topiramate and gabapentin. Medications at the time of the patient's initial visit were phenytoin and valproate.

Examination and investigations

The patient's general, cardiological and neurological examinations were unremarkable. Previous routine EEGs demonstrated left temporal spikes. Magnetic resonance imaging showed no evidence of hippocampal sclerosis or focal lesion. The patient had been previously recorded in the epilepsy monitoring unit at an outside hospital, where he experienced 13 seizures that were poorly localized, although it was suggested that seizures arose from the left hemisphere. Anterior to mid-temporal epileptiform discharges (at electrodes F7 and T3) were noted interictally. The patient then underwent epilepsy monitoring with intracranial electrodes, which did not define an operable ictal onset zone, owing to technical limitations of the procedure.

The patient was subsequently referred to our center for evaluation. He was admitted for scalp–sphenoidal monitoring, now 1 year after his phase II monitoring. This demonstrated frequent left anterior temporal spike discharges, maximum in amplitude at the left sphenoidal electrode. An ictal EEG showed poorly localized seizures, sometimes with bitemporal onset although usually with greater field seen over the left temporal region.

A positron emission tomography scan showed mild left temporal hypometabolism. Neuropsychological evaluation showed a full-scale IQ of 90, perceptual organization index 99 and verbal comprehension 86, demonstrating subtle language and verbal memory impairment that could be localized to the left temporal region. An amytal test demonstrated his speech to be in the left hemisphere and that the right hemisphere was capable of supporting memory.

The case was discussed in surgical conference and it was felt that the patient was an appropriate candidate for phase II evaluation with bilateral intrahippocampal depth electrodes and a large frontotemporal grid including subtemporal and subfrontal strips on the left side (Fig. 104.1).

Depth electrodes were implanted without event. Seizures were recorded after medication taper. These demonstrated widespread onset in the left anterior frontal, lateral temporal and posterior frontal regions (Fig. 104.2).

Diagnosis

Medically refractory partial seizures, poorly localized to left frontal and temporal lobes.

Treatment and outcome

Options for treatment were considered at epilepsy conference. After careful review of the patient's comprehensive evaluation, it was concluded that the

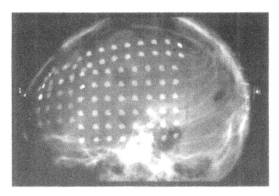

Figure 104.1 *Plain postoperative X-ray of the subdural electrode grids placed over the frontal and temporal regions in this patient. Disc electrodes are embedded in a plastic sheet, with only the active side exposed to brain. Wires are embedded in silastic coverings, which are passed through the skull and scalp to make contact with digital EEG machines used for continuous monitoring.*

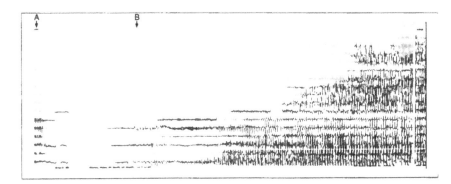

Figure 104.2 *16 Channel intracranial EEG tracing demonstrating seizure onset from the patient's subdural grid placed over the frontal and temporal regions. The first burst of seizure activity is seen at the very beginning of the figure (arrow A). This is followed by another burst and then sustained seizure activity (arrow B). The top 9 channels are recording from the frontal lobe. The bottom 5 channels are recording from the temporal lobe. Note that seizure onset is not sufficiently localized for resective surgery to be a viable option.*

patient would not be a good surgical candidate. It was reasoned that any attempt at resection or subpial transection would have to be widespread, would have little chance of controlling the patient's seizures and might result in severe functional consequences, since both language and verbal memory were found to reside in the region most appropriate for resection. Other options included

409

newer antiepileptic drugs, an investigational antiepileptic drug or vagus nerve stimulation.

After a long discussion, the patient chose a trial of levetiracetam as add-on therapy to his phenytoin. He reported less intoxication and tremor than with his previous combination therapy of phenytoin and valproate. Fortunately, the patient has remained seizure-free for the past 12 months on this new drug combination.

Commentary

As epileptologists, we frequently encounter patients with medically refractory seizures. In such cases, epilepsy surgery is looked upon as the ultimate, most definitive therapeutic approach. Evaluation for epilepsy surgery includes a time consuming, comprehensive battery of tests, often culminating in surgical implantation of invasive electrodes, when scalp monitoring fails to identify the site of seizure onset. These evaluations are expensive, painful and involve risks to the patient.

There is great pressure to perform a definitive therapeutic procedure when this stage is reached. We are frequently put in the position of feeling as if we must do *something* after the patient has been implanted with depth electrodes, subdural strips and grids, even in the face of findings that suggest that this is not wise.

What did we learn from this case?

This case teaches that, despite these pressures, it is better to do nothing than to jeopardize the patient's well being in pursuit of overly aggressive or ill-advised treatment. This case had a 'happy ending', although we have all seen many similar cases that end in disappointment and no improvement in the patient's condition despite enormous cost, effort and personal sacrifice.

How did this case alter our approach to the care and treatment of our epilepsy patients?

We do not lose hope when surgery does not appear possible. We know now that failure to find a surgical solution, even in the face of extensive invasive monitoring, can still be followed by a good outcome. It may be that this outcome may be delayed while new therapeutic approaches catch up with the desperate need of our patients.

This case also reminds us of the limitations of currently available techniques for localizing seizure onset and the inadequacy of our understanding of how cellular networks in the brain generate seizures. Our hope is that, as this understanding grows, there will be fewer and fewer cases like ours.

410

Case 105

INTRACTABLE IDIOPATHIC GENERALIZED EPILEPSY IN A TEENAGE MOTHER

Lina Nashef and David Berry

History

The patient is a 19-year-old woman. After a premature birth, her early development was normal. Simple febrile convulsions occurred at around 6 months of age. At the age of 12 years she developed intractable absences and generalized tonic–clonic seizures. Physical examination and cognition were within normal limits.

The patient's schooling and family life were significantly disrupted by the epilepsy. Her family history was positive: a brother, a paternal half-sister, a cousin and a great-uncle all had young-onset epilepsy.

Details of her initial therapy were unavailable but probably included ineffective treatment with phenytoin and carbamazepine. During her early teens, treatment with valproate and ethosuximide was largely unsuccessful because of non-compliance and side effects, including nausea and vomiting with high-dose ethosuximide and weight gain and irritability with valproate. The patient was started on lamotrigine at the age of 13 and valproate was withdrawn. At the age of 16, ethosuximide was withdrawn and a combination of valproate and lamotrigine was tried again for a few months before returning to monotherapy with lamotrigine. The initial response was limited but, with a gradual increase in the dose and with better compliance, control of the epilepsy improved significantly. Seizure frequency dropped from up to fortnightly generalized tonic–clonic seizures to two generalized tonic–clonic seizures over a 6-month period at the age of 17. At that time she was taking lamotrigine 900 mg/day in two divided doses, with lamotrigine serum levels ranging from 15.6 to 23.4 mg/l. (The timing of the samples in relation to the timing of the last dose was not available.)

The patient was referred to the adult epilepsy service at the age of 17, during her first pregnancy.

411

Investigations

The EEG at presentation supported the diagnosis of generalized epilepsy – it demonstrated generalized high-amplitude, frontally dominant, spike-and-slow-wave paroxysms soon after hyperventilation. In addition, frequent paroxysmal bilateral theta activity was noted, sometimes with small spikes without a consistent focus. Further, 3–3.5 Hz generalized spike–wave discharges were observed in later recordings, as well as occasional right frontoparietal discharges. A photoparoxysmal response was not elicited.

Magnetic resonance imaging, including fluid attenuated inversion recovery (FLAIR) and temporal lobe sequences, was normal. There was no apparent epileptogenic structural abnormality.

Diagnosis

Idiopathic generalized epilepsy; juvenile absence epilepsy subtype.

Treatment and outcome

Seizures occurred more frequently during the patient's pregnancy – by the end of the first trimester she was experiencing weekly generalized tonic–clonic seizures. Lamotrigine level at that time was 6.2 mg/l, dropping 1 month later on the same dose to a nadir of 1.8 mg/l.

Medication compliance (reportedly good) was questioned. She was admitted to the hospital, and although higher lamotrigine concentrations were obtained when the medication was administered under observation, levels nevertheless remained well below those concentrations previously associated with good seizure control on the same dose.

The lamotrigine dose was increased to 1000 mg/day in two divided doses. The maximum level recorded during her pregnancy was 10.7 mg/l. During the second trimester, topiramate 25 mg/day was briefly tried but was not tolerated because of drowsiness. Despite some improvement, seizure control during pregnancy remained suboptimal.

The patient delivered a normal infant and chose not to breast-feed. At the time of delivery, the lamotrigine concentration was 9.9 mg/l, with a cord level of 9.0 mg/l. Fearing the recurrence of seizures, she was reluctant to reduce her lamotrigine back to the previous dose. She gradually developed headaches, dizziness and double vision that worsened 2–3 weeks after delivery. The dose was temporarily reduced and later increased again to 1000 mg/day in two divided doses. Topiramate was reintroduced at a dose 12.5 mg at night; the dose was gradually increased to a total of 200 mg/day.

The patient was still troubled by dizziness about 2 hours after her morning lamotrigine dose and had occasional breakthrough generalized seizures, often late in the afternoon. The regimen was changed to 1000 mg/day in three divided doses (400 mg, 300 mg, 300 mg). This resulted in improved control, with only one brief generalized tonic–clonic seizures over a 6-month period and infrequent absences. She has had no side effects on this regimen.

The patient's serum concentrations of lamotrigine before and during pregnancy and after delivery are shown in Fig. 105.1.

Commentary

We chose this case both to emphasize the wide variations between patients in the therapeutic dose range of lamotrigine and to discuss the use of lamotrigine in pregnancy and the postpartum period, given that lamotrigine is being increasingly used in young women.

Pharmacokinetic interactions between lamotrigine and other antiepileptic drugs are well described. These interactions result in different dose recommendations depending on the concomitant medication regimen.[1] Variability between patients is a prominent feature of lamotrigine pharmacokinetics, which are also influenced by age, pregnancy and disease state.[2-6] Patients who are prescribed lamotrigine may exhibit large differences in dose-to-serum concentration responses.[7] These differences are presumably due to large inter-individual differences in clearance. Serum concentration monitoring can identify patients who have unusual pharmacokinetics and can also reassure clinicians while doses are titrated higher. The recommended dosing schedule for lamotrigine is two doses a day; however, as this case demonstrates, peak concentration toxicity with high doses may be avoided by using three doses a day.

Kirkpatrick et al.[8] reported no clear relationship between lamotrigine levels, side effects and therapeutic response over a wide range of doses and levels. We quote a reference range of 1–15 mg/l, recently confirmed by Morris et al.[9] Although some patients are able to tolerate serum levels in excess of 20 mg/l,[7] the frequency of neurological toxicity rises considerably with levels above 15 mg/l.[7,9,11]

What did we learn from this case?

Although monitoring of lamotrigine concentrations cannot be used to predict seizure control, monitoring can still be useful in an individual case, particularly under changing situations, such as pregnancy and the postpartum period, as in this case. Although reduced compliance probably accounted for some of the initial decrease in lamotrigine concentrations and deterioration in seizure control

413

414

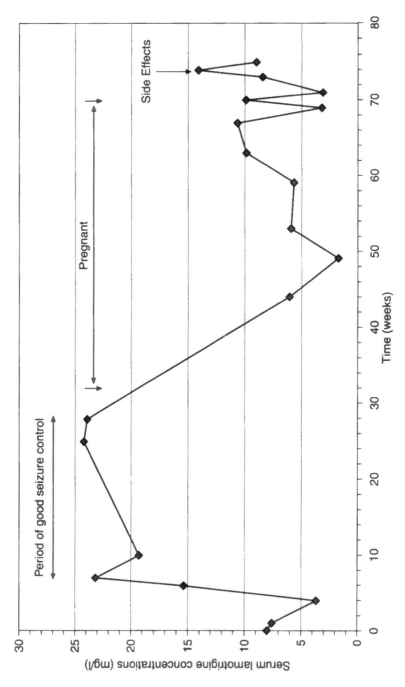

Figure 105.1 Serum lamotrigine concentrations versus time before and during pregnancy and after delivery.

at the end of the first trimester, it is likely that physiological changes also played a part. Tomson et al.,[12] in a very well-documented case report, observed:

- a clinically significant decrease in lamotrigine concentrations during pregnancy with breakthrough seizures;
- a post-partum rise in lamotrigine concentrations; and
- significant concentrations of lamotrigine in breast milk.

One of us (DB) has also reported breast milk concentrations after 34 pregnancies at 40–80 % of serum concentrations.[13] Rambeck et al.[14] recommended breast-feeding but advised that the transfer of lamotrigine during pregnancy and lactation should not be neglected and that the child should be observed for any potential side effects. In this situation advice may need to be individually tailored and, where necessary, guided by blood and breast milk concentrations and clinical monitoring.

In this patient's case, better seizure control has been achieved with high-dose lamotrigine (with side effects minimized using three times a day dosing) in combination with topiramate, which was not tolerated during pregnancy but was reintroduced successfully at low dosage with slow titration.

References

1. Perrucca E. The new generation of antiepileptic drugs: advantages and disadvantages. *Br J Clin Pharmacol* 1996;**42**:531–43.

2. Hussein Z, Posner J. Population pharmacokinetics of lamotrigine monotherapy in patients with epilepsy: Retrospective analysis of routine monitoring data. *Br J Clin Pharmacol* 1997;**43**:457–65.

3. Perrucca E. The clinical pharmacokinetics of new antiepileptic drugs. *Epilepsia* 1999;**40(suppl 4)**:S7–S13.

4. Rambeck B, Wolf P. Lamotrigine clinical pharmacokinetics. *Clin Pharmacokinet* 1993;**25**:433–43.

5. Bartoli A, Guerrini R, Belmonte A, et al. The influence of dosage, age and comedication on steady state plasma lamotrigine concentrations in epileptic children: a prospective study with preliminary assessment of correlation with clinical response. *Ther Drug Monit* 1997;**19**:252–60.

6. Tomson T, Johannessen SI. Therapeutic monitoring of the new antiepileptic drugs. *Eur J Clin Pharmacol* 2000;**55**:697–705.

7. Werz MA, Reed RC. Tolerability and efficacy of very high dose lamotrigine: clinical experience. *Epilepsia* 1999;**40(suppl 7)**:77–8.

8. Kilpatrick ES, Forrest G, Brodie MJ. Concentration-effect and

415

concentration–toxicity relations with lamotrigine: A prospective study. *Epilepsia* 1996;**37**:534–8.

9. Morris FM, Black AB, Harris AL, *et al.* Lamotrigine and therapeutic drug monitoring: retrospective survey following the introduction of a routine service. *Br J Clin Pharmacol* 1998;**46**:547–51.

10. Besag FM, Craven P, Berry DJ, *et al.* The role of blood-level monitoring in assessing lamotrigine toxicity. *Epilepsia* 1998;**39(suppl 6)**:131.

11. Fröscher W, Keller F, Kramer G, *et al.* Serum level monitoring in assessing lamotrigine efficacy and toxicity. *Epilepsia* 1999;**40(suppl 2)**:253.

12. Tomson T, Ohman I, Vitols S. Lamotrigine in pregnancy and lactation: a case report. *Epilepsia* 1997;**38**:1039–41.

13. Berry DJ. The disposition of lamotrigine throughout pregnancy. *Ther Drug Monit* 1999;**21**:450.

14. Rambeck B, Kurlemann G, Stodiek SRG, *et al.* Concentrations of lamotrigine in a mother on lamotrigine treatment and her newborn child. *Eur J Clin Pharmacol* 1997;**51**:481–4.

Case 106

SOMETIMES LESS IS MORE

R Eugene Ramsay and Flavia Pryor

History

The patient is a 32-year-old white woman with a history of 'seizures' starting at the age of 8. These were diagnosed as 'petit mal'. At the age of 16 she began having 'night seizures'. These episodes were very dramatic – the patient would fall out of bed and scream, kick and move her arms as if fighting something. Frequency was between two and 20 episodes a night, and she would awake with injuries secondary to the events. She was seen by several neurologists and psychiatrists and was given a variety of diagnoses, including psychogenic seizures, parasomnia, anxiety and substance abuse. Despite being treated with numerous medications the events continued unchanged.

The patient also has a significant history of physical and psychological abuse that she believes may have some influence on her seizures. She describes herself as 'rather unstable' and has taken diazepam and alprazolam to obtain relief. In the past, the patient acknowledges occasional recreational use of cocaine and marijuana and, on some evenings, using alcohol in order to reduce her anxiety about having seizures.

In 1996 she was diagnosed as having 'sleep terrors' and was treated with clonazepam. Later that year the diagnosis of myoclonic and absence epilepsy was made on the basis of the clinical description by the patient and her mother. She was switched from carbamazepine to divalproex without improvement.

Examination and investigation

In April 1997, EEG video-telemetry was carried out and multiple bizarre events were recorded. These events consisted of posturing of the upper extremity, gesturing and, on one occasion, a backwards roll over the edge of the bed rail, which resulted in the patient falling out of bed. The EEG was normal during the events. Placebo induction was negative. After the induction, however, the patient became drowsy and fell asleep. The next day the patient reported having had an event.

Diagnosis

On the basis of these clinical manifestations, the epilepsy service concluded that the patient had frontal lobe seizures with an interhemispheric focus that precluded epileptiform activity from being seen on the EEG.

Treatment and outcome

On 26 May 1998, the patient continued to have frequent nocturnal seizures. Six days earlier she had a long series at night. Home video of a long nocturnal cluster revealed frequent myoclonic jerks that involved mainly the legs but occasionally would spread into the trunk and arms. These lasted only 1–2 seconds and occurred every 15–60 seconds. This pattern is quite different from what has been recorded in the past. Medications at the time included gabapentin 2400 mg/day and tiagabine 48 mg/day. It was decided that these seizures were different and most prominently appear to be myoclonic in nature. They were probably frontal lobe status with frequent myoclonic jerks. It was agreed to taper tiagabine while starting topiramate 25 mg/day and titrating the dose.

On 30 September 1998, the patient was noted to have had approximately 10 seizure clusters over the previous 2 months. These clusters consisted of microseizures occurring repeatedly over 1–2 hours. The patient had not increased her topiramate as instructed last month because she was concerned that topiramate had increased her seizures. She has continued tiagabine 32 mg/day. The patient was reassured that topiramate was not likely to be worsening her seizures. In fact her seizures had improved and the topiramate was increased to 200 mg/day.

On 17 December 1998, the patient was reported to have done remarkably well. In the previous month she had had only four of her typical frontal lobe seizures. Medications at this time were topiramate 300 mg/day and tiagabine 32 mg/day. Her menstrual periods had returned to normal, she was beginning to exercise and she reported feeling great. She also reported having a mild word-finding difficulty and a short temper. The other more important concern was that she found occasionally her knees buckle and she would fall to the ground. These were not seizure-related falls. She had a very significant abrasion above her left knee as a result of one of these falls. The word-finding difficulty was felt to be secondary to topiramate and the knee buckling to be secondary to tiagabine. This meant that an increase in the dose of either drug could result in more problems. It was agreed to maintain the present regimen and to see if symptoms clear.

On 28 October 1999, the patient was noted to have had a number of

418

medical problems in the past 10 months that resulted in increased seizure frequency. She had 12 seizures in the past month and the knee buckling had continued. It was agreed to taper and discontinue tiagabine since the maximum tolerated dose has been reached, and to increase topiramate to 400 mg/day.

On 12 January 2000 she was noted to have done very badly as the dose of tiagabine was reduced. Review of dosage changes and seizure occurrences revealed that side effects had resolved and seizures were controlled for the short time that she was on tiagabine 20 mg/day. This regimen was reinstated (topiramate 400 mg/day and tiagabine 20 mg/day).

On 25 September 2000, the patient was noted to have been seizure-free for 8 months on topiramate 400 mg/day and tiagabine 20 mg/day. This is really very remarkable since she has in the past experienced 25–30 seizures in a day. She has no side effects from the medication and is doing very well.

Commentary

This patient initially presented with a very confusing clinical picture. Her spells were described as screaming, kicking and moving her arms. Because of a strong family psychiatric history, the unusual character of her seizures, normal EEGs and coexisting anxiety disorder, she was thought by many to have non-epileptic seizures and sleep parasomnia syndrome. The epileptic etiology for her spells became apparent after video-EEG monitoring. Even though the ictal EEG was normal the clinical manifestations were those of frontal lobe motor association seizures. Subsequently, we felt more comfortable employing a more vigorous therapeutic approach, maximizing drug doses until side effects were encountered.

Frontal lobe seizures are notoriously difficult to control. At worst, this patient would experience 15–30 seizures a night. The seizures failed to improve with the older antiepileptic drugs. Although some improvement in seizure control was realized with the use of the newer antiepileptic drugs, complete control eluded us. High doses of tiagabine produced weakness (knee buckling), and increasing doses of topiramate caused some word-finding difficulty, which cleared as the tiagabine was decreased. Seizure control improved as the dose of topiramate was increased and monotherapy was achieved. Unfortunately, her seizures returned. Review of her seizure occurrences and medication changes revealed that she had been seizure-free for the 6 weeks when she had been on a combination of topiramate 400 mg/day and tiagabine 20 mg/day. Therefore this regimen was reinstated and seizure control was again attained. The patient has now been seizure-free for 11 months on this combination.

419

What did we learn from this case?

This case illustrates two important clinical lessons. First, the definite diagnosis of epilepsy and particularly frontal lobe seizures was not clear until video-EEG monitoring was carried out. The second and perhaps more significant lesson is the importance of a careful review of a patient's response to medications. This patient had a partial response to several antiepileptic drugs in combination and in monotherapy; however, total control was achieved only by combined therapy with doses that were lower than those used in monotherapy.

How did this case alter our approach to the care and treatment of our epilepsy patients?

The careful tracking of seizures and medication changes in this case allowed us to realize that seizures came under control only when particular doses of tiagabine and topiramate were used together. We are now more carefully looking for other combinations with a similar synergistic efficacy.

Further reading

Bourgeois BF. New antiepileptic drugs. *Arch Neurol* 1998;**55**:1181–3.

Brodie MJ. Drug interactions in epilepsy. *Epilepsia* 1992;**33(suppl 1)**:S13–S22.

Chez MG, Bourgeois BF, Pippenger CE, Knowles WD. Pharmacodynamic interactions between phenytoin and valproate: individual and combined antiepileptic and neurotoxic actions in mice. *Clin Pharmacol* 1994;**17**:32–7.

Datta PK, Crawford PM. Refractory epilepsy: Treatment with new antiepileptic drugs. *Seizure* 2000;**9**:51–7.

Gatti G, Bonomi I, Jannuzzi G, Perucca E. The new antiepileptic drugs: pharmacological and clinical aspects. *Curr Pharm Des* 2000;**6**:839–60.

Ketter TA, Post RM, Theodore WH. Positive and negative psychiatric effects of antiepileptic drugs in patients with seizure disorders. *Neurology* 1999;**53(suppl 2)**:S53–S67.

Case 107

UNEXPECTED BENEFIT FROM AN OLD ANTIEPILEPTIC DRUG

Matti Sillanpää

History

A 30-year-old man had an uneventful previous history, except for moderate head trauma at the age of 3 years. Four years later, he started to have generalized convulsive seizures with abrupt loss of consciousness and some concomitant absence seizures. Most of the convulsions occurred on awakening; those few that did not occurred at random. There was no family history of epilepsy or febrile convulsions. At this time, the patient's sleep rhythm was irregular. He was awake late in the evenings and got up late in the mornings. According to his mother, he suffered from sleep deprivation. He was active in youth athletics but was somewhat hyperactive and restless. Antiepileptic drug therapy was initially unsuccessful but, at the age of 10, he was seizure-free.

After this, despite frequent discussions and advice, he continued his lifestyle with irregular and apparently inadequate nocturnal sleep. As an adult, he was well motivated to take his medication because of the risk of having his driving licence revoked. He did not use alcohol.

Examinations and investigations

Neurological examination was normal. His IQ was 80. The initial EEG showed massive 3–4 Hz bilateral symmetric spike-and-wave discharges, easily provocable by flicker light and hyperventilation. Eight years later, during a seizure-free period, EEG was normal in the waking state but during sleep there were a few right-sided spikes and spike-and-wave complexes, and flicker light and hyperventilation sensitivity had disappeared. Clinically, the patient's seizures were obviously primarily generalized without any warning, but the assymmetric spike-and-wave complexes on the EEG were interpreted by a neurophysiologist as a sign of a focal origin of the seizures. Not unexpectedly, however, a magnetic resonance imaging (MRI) scan of the brain was normal. A recent repeat MRI scan was also normal.

421

Diagnosis

Generalized tonic–clonic seizures on awakening, and absence seizures.

Treatment and outcome

The patient was initially administered phenytoin but without success. Valproate up to 30 mg/kg per day replaced the phenytoin. Because of continued seizures, a daily dose of 50 mg phenobarbital was combined with the valproate and the seizures disappeared. After 3 years, phenobarbital was tapered off, and as a result of a complete seizure-free period of a further 4 years, valproate was slowly decreased to 25 mg/kg per day. However, a relapse occurred 6 months later. The dosage of valproate was increased to 40 mg/kg per day and later combined individually or in combination with phenobarbital, primidone, carbamazepine, phenytoin and lamotrigine, but without success. More than 1 year later, as a last resort, ethosuximide 750 mg/day in two divided doses was combined with valproate. Since the first dose of ethosuximide over 5 years ago, no seizures have occurred.

Commentary

The early age of this awakening epilepsy and subnormal intelligence of the child initially did not lead initially to the correct epilepsy diagnosis. This case again shows the importance of an accurate and careful previous history in recognizing different types of epilepsy syndromes. The head trauma in the past history might argue for the Janz's hypothesis that the onset of this genetic epilepsy is precipitated by or predisposed to by traumatic or ictogenic brain lesion.[1] Despite an asymmetric EEG, no abnormality was found on MRI.

Valproate is the first drug of choice in awakening epilepsy, but if it or lamotrigine do not work, one cannot reject the diagnosis *ex juvantibus*. The high frequency of relapses after reduction in dose or withdrawal of medication is well known, but the drug resistance in this case was embarrassing.

Still more striking was the beneficial effect of ethosuximide. It is still unclear why ethosuximide was beneficial. Its effect in both experimental and human studies has proved to be very selective against typical absences in young subjects. Ethosuximide might actually exacerbate, rather than prevent, generalized tonic–clonic seizures, even though this has not been proved. The clinical diagnosis of seizure was definitely ascertained by EEG in this case, so the diagnosis of seizures or epilepsy syndrome cannot be wrong. The mode of action of ethosuximide is still largely unknown. Although I cannot explain the effect, this case shows that one must never lose hope but must try even 'impossible' antiepileptic medications in apparently hopeless cases.

What did I learn from this case?

I learnt several things from this case. Even very young children may have generalized tonic–clonic seizures on awakening. One must be able to differentiate between functional and lesional focal findings on the EEG to avoid misclassification of the origin of seizures. The medication should not be changed if seizures stop. If the patient has drug-resistant seizures, one should not lose hope but should try drugs that are not supposed to work.

To my mind, this case again shows that whatever you say in medicine is correct in no higher than 90 % of cases. The importance of life habits and personal responsibility for one's health should be emphasized to children. One should make them realize that everyone is the moulder of his or her own fortune and is also personally responsible for his or her own health.

Reference

1. Janz D. The grand mal epilepsies and sleep–waking cycle. *Epilepsie* 1962;3:69–109.

Further reading

Janz D, Kern A, Mössinger HJ, Puhlmann HU. Rückfallprognose während und nach Reduktion der Medikamente bei Epilepsiebehandlung. In: Remschmidt H, Rentz R, Jungmann J, eds. *Epilepsi 1981, Verlauf und Prognose, neuropsychologische und psychologische Aspekte*. Stuttgart: Thieme Verlag;1983:17–24.

Wolf P. Epilepsy with grand mal on awakening. In: Roger J, Bureau M, Dravet C, Dreifuss FE, Perret A, Wolf P, eds. *Epileptic syndromes in infancy, childhood and adolescence*. London: John Libbey;1992:329–41.

Case 108

STATUS EPILEPTICUS RESPONSIVE TO INTRAVENOUS IMMUNOGLOBULIN

Joseph I Sirven and Hoan Linh Banh

History

One week before admission, a healthy 30-year-old man developed flu-like symptoms. Four days later, he had three generalized tonic–clonic seizures, which began with focal left facial twitching. He had recovery of consciousness between the seizures. However, the night of seizure onset, he developed a cluster of generalized seizures with no recovery of consciousness.

He was admitted to an intensive care unit at a local community hospital. He was initially treated with phenytoin and phenobarbital, but his seizures failed to respond despite a phenytoin level of 20 µg ml and phenobarbital level of 45 µg ml. A magnetic resonance imaging (MRI) scan of the brain with gadolinium enhancement, a lumbar puncture, blood cultures and cerebrospinal fluid cultures for fungal, bacterial and viral organisms, and polymerase chain reaction for herpes virus were all normal. The patient was then given a continuous infusion of pentobarbital. Generalized tonic–clonic seizures were successfully terminated with phenytoin 300 mg intravenously every 6 hours, valproate 750 mg intravenously every 6 hours and phenobarbital 90 mg intravenously every 8 hours. When the pentobarbital was tapered, generalized tonic–clonic and myoclonic seizures returned, and these correlated with generalized polyspike–wave formations on the EEG. The patient subsequently relapsed into status epilepticus, both clinically and on EEG. He was then transferred to our institution for management of refractory status epilepticus.

Examination and investigations

Upon arrival, continuous pentobarbital infusion was continued, and phenytoin and phenobarbital were restarted to control his seizures. A brain MRI scan with gadolinium enhancement, a lumbar puncture, serum pyruvate and lactate levels, serum electrolytes, liver enzymes, and blood and cerebrospinal fluid cultures were all normal. Despite titration of the pentobarbital infusion to suppress all

424

electrographic activity completely, generalized convulsive and myoclonic seizures persisted. The myoclonic seizures became a prominent feature of the status epilepticus at this time in the clinical course. The myoclonus was both spontaneous and induced by tactile stimulation. The entire body was involved, but particularly the proximal muscles of the body and trunk. The EEG revealed generalized polyspike–wave activity during the myoclonic seizures.

Diagnosis

Generalized tonic–clonic status epilepticus with myoclonic seizures secondary to an unidentified postinfectious etiology.

Treatment and outcome

Table 108.1 lists the antiepileptic drugs that were unsuccessfully tried as adjunctive therapy to the pentobarbital infusion.

Forty-five days after the initiation of pentobarbital, the infusion was terminated. The patient was not responsive to verbal stimuli and he developed both generalized myoclonus and occasional generalized tonic–clonic seizures. Cisatracurium (neuromuscular blockade) continuous infusion was used to control his severe generalized myoclonic twitching and to protect renal function against myoglobinuria.

Since the patient's myoclonus and seizures were not responding to antiepileptic drugs and his level of consciousness did not improve despite termination of pentobarbital, high-dose methylprednisolone was tried for 1 week. The patient awoke, but the myoclonus persisted. Because of the response to methylprednisolone, consideration of a potential underlying immune mechanism responsible for the status epilepticus was given. Thus, a decision was made to initiate intravenous immunoglobulin (IVIG) 30 g/day (0.4 g/kg per day) for 7 days. Initially, no dramatic improvement in myoclonus was observed. However, on day 4 of IVIG therapy, the patient's myoclonic activity stopped and he was able to communicate with hand gestures. Four days after the completion of IVIG therapy, the patient became completely alert, awake and verbally communicative.

Because of some breakthrough myoclonic jerking of the face, 5-hydroxytryptophan and carbidopa were initiated. The patient was transferred back to his local community hospital 2 weeks later on 5-hydroxy-L-tryptophan 200 mg every 8 hours, phenobarbital 90 mg every 6 hours and lamotrigine 100 mg every 6 hours. He was eventually transferred to a rehabilitation hospital and no further seizures were reported.

425

Table 108.1 The antiepileptic drugs that were unsuccessfully tried in this patient as adjunctive therapy to pentobarbital infusion.

Start (day number)	Stop (day number)	Drug	Dose	Comment
1	45	Pentobarbital	[1]infusion	
52	59	Methylprednisolone	500 mg intravenously every 12 hours	
0	59	Phenobarbital	90 mg intravenously every 8 hours	
0	2	Valproate	750 mg/day intravenously	
0	60	Phenytoin	300 mg intravenously every 6 hours	Drug fever developed secondary to phenytoin
1	6	Carbamazepine	200 mg by mouth every 6 hours	
6	12	Carbamazepine	2000 mg by mouth every 6 hours	Suspected to be the cause of pancreatitis
12		Topiramate	Titrate to 100 mg by mouth every 12 hours	
25		Lamotrigine	Titrate to 100 mg every 6 hours (delivered per PEG tube)	
28	68	Clonazepam	3 mg by mouth every 8 hours	
30	68	Cisatracurium	[2]infusion	
59	63	Intravenous immunoglobulin	30 g/day	
68		5-hydroxy-ʟ-tryptophan	200 mg by mouth every 8 hours	Given to control myoclonic seizures

[1] 10 mg/kg load followed by 1.5 μg/kg/hr

He has been subsequently discharged to home with minimal neurological deficits. All blood and cerebrospinal fluid cultures have remained negative for all organisms. No specific antibodies for herpes virus, western equine encephalitis, eastern equine encephalitis or St. Louis encephalitis were detected.

Commentary

Our patient had a severe refractory myoclonic status epilepticus clinical syndrome that failed to respond to conventional management and management for refractory status epilepticus. IVIG has been used for intractable seizures in children at a dose 2 g/kg given over 5 days. The specific mechanism of action of IVIG in epilepsy is unclear, but it is clearly immunomodulatory. IVIG has many potential ways of modulating humoral and cellular immune responses. Anti-idiotype antibodies within IVIG could neutralize or counteract with particular seizure-inducing antibodies. Perhaps IVIG has antibodies that down-regulate the production of epileptogenic antibodies. Additionally, IVIG may alter complement-mediated neuronal damage. Uncontrolled clinical observations suggest that IVIG may be effective in some patients with intractable epilepsy, especially children, and may be considered as a safe adjunctive therapy. Our patient clinically improved with IVIG and it was well tolerated.

The major limitations to this treatment are the severe national shortage of IVIG, its cost and the risk of transmission of infectious diseases associated with blood derivatives.

What did we learn from this case?

We learned two major points from this case. In the absence of an etiology for refractory status epilepticus and no overt structural lesion on imaging, immune therapies such as corticosteroids and IVIG should be considered in the management of refractory status epilepticus and residual myoclonic activity. Although these are not clearly the treatments of choice for status epilepticus, one should at least consider their use when status epilepticus has persisted despite prolonged treatment with pentobarbital. The second major lesson was that patients can make a meaningful recovery despite prolonged duration of a protracted and serious status epilepticus.

How did this case alter our approach to the care and treatment of our epilepsy patients?

Because of this case, we are more optimistic about recovery from generalized status epilepticus in the absence of a clear catastrophic etiology. We are

427

also willing to initiate corticosteroids in status epilepticus without a clear etiology.

We now know that one can never give up when treating status epilepticus regardless of its duration, criticisms from colleagues who advise discontinuing therapy, and the absence of the medical literature to guide treatment.

Further reading

Ariizumi M, Shiihara H, Hibio S, *et al*. High dose gammaglobulin for intractable childhood epilepsy. *Lancet* 1998;2:162–3.

Baziel GM, van Engelen BG, Renier WO, *et al*. Immunoglobulin treatment in epilepsy: a review of the literature. *Epilepsy Res* 1994;19:181–90.

Duse M, Notarangelo, D, Tiberti E, Menegati S, Plebani A, Ugazio AG. Intravenous immune globulin in the treatment of intractable childhood epilepsy. *Clin Exp Immunol* 1996;104(suppl 1):71–6.

Etzioni A, Jaffe M, Pollack S, *et al*. High dose intravenous gamma-globulin in intractable epilepsy. *Eur J Pediatr* 1991;150:681–3.

Fayed MN, Choueiri R, Mikati M. Landau–Kleffner syndrome: consistent response to repeated intravenous γ-globulin doses: a case report. *Epilepsia* 1997;38:489–94.

Imbach P, d'Appuzo V, Hirt A, *et al*. High dose intravenous gammaglobulin for idiopathic thrombocytopenic purpura in childhood. *Lancet* 1998;1:1228–31.

Lagae LG, Silberstein J, Gillis L, Casaer PJ. Successful use of intravenous immunoglobulins in Landau–Kleffner syndrome. *Pediatr Neurol* 1998;8:165–8.

Van Engelen BG, Renier WO, Weemaes CM. Immunoglobulin treatment in human and experimental epilepsy. *J Neurol Neurosurg Psychiatry* 1995;57(suppl):72–5.

Case 109

SURGICAL SUCCESS IN A PATIENT WITH DIFFUSE BRAIN TRAUMA

Brien J Smith

History

The patient is a 26-year-old right-handed man who sustained a severe closed head injury 8 years before presentation. He was in a comatose state for 23 days and, on regaining consciousness, was severely impaired. He required retraining of language (speaking and writing), simple motor tasks (tieing shoes, eating) and other basic skills during an 18-month inpatient rehabilitation. Residual deficits included a left hemiparesis, bilateral fourth nerve palsies, impaired reading comprehension, and difficulty in processing short-term memory.

During his rehabilitation, the patient began experiencing episodes of a 'rising sensation' similar to a 'rapid unexpected descent in an elevator'. Initially these events were brief and infrequent. Subsequently, he began experiencing multiple events a day, with progression of symptoms to include difficulty swallowing, gagging, drooling and regurgitation. With most of these episodes he did not report an alteration in consciousness, but with longer events (duration 30–40 seconds) he reported 'phasing out'.

He was subsequently diagnosed with partial seizures and placed on carbamazepine. Despite treatment with various antiepileptic drugs, including valproate, phenytoin, gabapentin and clonazepam in monotherapy and polytherapy, he continued to have daily seizures and significant side effects from medical therapy.

There was no history of birth complications, febrile seizures, meningitis, encephalitis or other head trauma and there was no family history of seizure disorders.

Previous EEG studies reported sharp wave discharges over the left frontotemporal and left central head regions with intermixed slowing. A magnetic resonance imaging (MRI) scan of the brain 2 years earlier showed encephalomalacia of both frontal lobes and evidence of a remote parenchymal hemorrhage in the left frontal lobe (Fig. 109.1). There was also evidence of progressive degenerative changes involving the body and splenium of the corpus callosum.

429

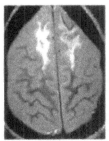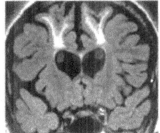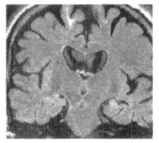

Figure 109.1: MRI scan of the brain (axial and coronal images) demonstrating atrophy, encephalomalacia, and bifrontal signal changes consistent with gliosis.

Examination and investigations

Neurological examination revealed dysconjugate eye position, mild left hemiparesis, hyperreflexia and a positive Babinski sign on the left.

After an extensive discussion explaining the limitations and risks of surgical intervention, the patient wished to pursue the presurgical evaluation. Baseline EEG continued to show epileptiform discharges in the left frontotemporal and central head regions and bursts of delta-wave slowing. A repeat MRI scan showed no significant interval change with the exception of right ventral tegmental atrophy, suggestive of wallerian degeneration.

Inpatient monitoring with scalp and sphenoidal electrodes captured multiple typical simple partial seizures and some complex partial seizures. EEG ictal changes suggested left hemisphere lateralization but no clear-cut focal or regional pattern was evident. Ictal single photon emission computed tomography (SPECT) was completed 17 seconds after clinical onset and demonstrated focal increased uptake in the left temporal, left parietal and left basal ganglia regions compared with the interictal study. The ictal and interictal SPECT studies both revealed hypoperfusion in both frontal lobes (concordant with the abnormalities on the MRI scan) and marked scattered heterogeneity in radiotracer distribution.

A battery of neuropsychological tests demonstrated short-term memory dysfunction and a full-scale IQ of 96 (verbal IQ 101, performance IQ 102). Language evaluation demonstrated anomia, and paraphasic and semantic errors. Intracarotid amobarbital procedure (Wada study) was suggestive of left hemisphere language dominance and showed borderline memory scores after injection on each side.

Owing to the evidence of bihemispheric injury, the limited localizing value of non-invasive testing and the need to limit a potential cortical resection to a small, well-defined ictogenic zone, intracranial implantation was suggested. Widespread bilateral subdural coverage, more comprehensively on the left, demonstrated multiple seizures with a focal ictal pattern over the left anterior and mid-parahippocampal gyrus.

Diagnosis

Medically refractory partial seizures arising from the left anterior and mid-parahippocampal gyrus secondary to head injury.

Treatment and outcome

Focal resection included the anterior temporal pole (2 cm), uncus, and parahippocampal gyrus (including the hippocampus up to 3 cm from the pes). The patient has had only seven simple partial seizures in more than 1-year's follow-up, compared with at least three to five seizures a week before surgery. No significant change in language or memory function was noted in early post-operative testing.

Commentary

Head trauma is a common risk factor for the development of partial epilepsy.[1,2] The option of epilepsy surgery for patients with refractory partial epilepsy secondary to a severe head injury is frequently pursued with reservation. This is, in part, because literature analyzing surgical outcome in post-traumatic epilepsy is limited[3 9] and also because the outcomes have been considered suboptimal[3,4] compared with the outcomes from surgery for other etiologies.

The approach to post-traumatic epilepsy is complicated by the variability of the clinical picture. Considerations include:

* the type of injury (penetrating or closed);
* the severity of the injury (mild, moderate or severe);
* the mechanisms of neuronal injury (primary or secondary);[10]
* the potential sites of epileptogenicity (diffuse bilateral, unilateral, multilobar, hippocampal or neocortical); and
* the age of the patient (pediatric or adult).

Moreover, the functional neurological reserve of a patient with previous severe brain injury is difficult to estimate when surgical resection is being considered.

Marks et al.[3] noted an association between head injury at an early age (less than 5 years) and mesial temporal sclerosis. Some patients with hippocampal atrophy on MRI scan, which was helpful in localization, had seizure-free outcomes. Other studies[4,5] have not found that the age at the time of the injury is a significant factor in determining outcome. The seizures of patients without clear-cut focal lesions on MRI and of those with evidence of diffuse brain injury were difficult to localize and the patients had poor outcomes. In smaller series of patients with a focal or regional destructive lesion from penetrating injuries, patients have typically done better when complete resection of the site has been undertaken.[7–10]

Patients are often excluded from surgical consideration based on the presumption of a coup–countercoup injury or bilateral frontotemporal polar injuries. These injuries have been demonstrated in neuropathology and imaging studies,[11] but they have never been clearly demonstrated to result in multifocal sites of epileptogenicity. At my center, we recognize that these patients may have multiple epileptogenic sites, but we do not routinely exclude them from surgical evaluation.

What did I learn from this case?

I learned that even in a patient with a severe closed head injury and diffuse changes on MRI, a small epileptogenic zone may be localized and successfully resected. The mechanisms of injury and subsequent development of epileptogenesis in post-traumatic brain injury is a complex process that has not been fully elucidated. MRI scanning may not have the same localizing value in these patients as it does in other patients because it may show no abnormalities or only diffuse changes. This case demonstrated atrophy that was more prominent on the right side, which was consistent with the acute neurological manifestations of the brain injury (left hemiparesis) but falsely localizing with regard to the seizures.

How did this case alter my approach to the care and treatment of my epilepsy patients?

I am now less likely to form a premature impression about surgical candidacy on the basis of a clinical history of severe head trauma or when viewing an MRI scan with diffuse bilateral changes. This case also reinforces the importance of obtaining a detailed history of the clinical semiology of seizures and of the frequency and severity of each seizure type, including the propensity to secondary generalization. In my experience with such patients, the history of frequent simple partial seizures or limited complex partial seizures with the same clinical semiology and no secondary generalization may actually be a positive prognostic factor.

432

References

1. Annegers JF, Grabow JD, Grover RV, *et al*. Seizures after head trauma: a population study. *Neurology* 1980;**30**:683–9.

2. Rocca WA, Sharbrough FW, Hauser WA, *et al*. Risk factors for complex partial seizures: a population-based case-control study. *Ann Neurol* 1987;**21**:22–31.

3. Marks DA, Kim J, Spencer DD, Spencer SS. Seizure localization and pathology following head injury in patients with uncontrolled epilepsy. *Neurology* 1995;**45**:2051–7.

4. Schuh LA, Henry TR, Fromes G, *et al*. Influence of head trauma on outcome following temporal lobectomy. *Arch Neurol* 1998;**55**:1325–8.

5. Mathern GW, Pretorius JK, Babb TL. Influence of the type of initial precipitating injury and at what age it occurs on course and outcome in patients with temporal lobe seizures. *J Neurosurg* 1995;**82**:220–7.

6. Foerster O, Penfield W. The structural basis of traumatic epilepsy and results of radical operation. *Brain* 1930;**53**:99–119.

7. Kazemi NJ, So EL, Mosewich RK, *et al*. Resection of frontal encephalomalacias for intractable epilepsy: outcome and prognostic factors. *Epilepsia* 1997;**38**:670–7.

8. Cukiert A, Olivier A, Andermann F. Posttraumatic frontal lobe epilepsy with structural changes: excellent results after cortical resection. *Can J Neurol Sci* 1996;**23**:114–7.

9. Mathern GW, Babb TL, Vickrey BG, *et al*. Traumatic compared to non-traumatic clinical–pathologic associations in temporal lobe epilepsy. *Epilepsy Res* 1994;**19**:129–39.

10. Miller DJ, Piper IR, Jones PA. Pathophysiology of head injury. In: Narayan RK, Wilberger JE Jr, Povlishock JT, eds. *Neurotrauma*. New York: McGraw–Hill; 1996:61–70.

11. Clifton GL, McCormick WF, Grossman RG. Neuropathology of early and late deaths after head injury. *Neurosurgery* 1981;**8**:309–14.

433

Case 110

DIETARY TREATMENT OF SEIZURES FROM A HYPOTHALAMIC HAMARTOMA

Vijay Maggio and James Wheless

History

The patient is a 16-year-old male with a history of seizure onset at the age of 2 years. Initially, the seizures were brief and consisted of staring spells, occurring mainly at night during the transition from waking to sleep. They were refractory to medical treatment and increased in frequency with time. Neuroimaging studies revealed a hypothalamic hamartoma.

The patient was evaluated at our institution at the age of 6½ years. During a typical event he would get a frightened look and complain of hearing or seeing scary things. He also perceived the room getting dark and fading away. These events were sometimes accompanied by facial grimacing (a smiling appearance). The events lasted for 15–20 seconds. There was no history of secondarily generalized tonic–clonic seizures except for one event that occurred after missing a medication dose. His longest seizure-free interval was 2 weeks. His partial seizure count was as high as 753 seizures in 1 month and 96 in 1 day; he typically averaged between three and five seizures a day.

His birth history was unremarkable. His medical history was significant for behavioral problems consisting of obsessive–compulsive traits, attentional deficits and perseveration. In addition, consecutive neuropsychological evaluations revealed progressive decline in intelligence and verbal memory skills and the development of a psychosis (Table 110.1).

Medications tried alone or in combination included acetazolamide, carbamazepine, valproate, felbamate, gabapentin, phenytoin, phenobarbital and lamotrigine. He had been treated with methylphenidate, amoxapine and thioridazine for behavioral modification.

Examination and investigations

The patient's general examination was unremarkable. His neurological examination showed evidence of cognitive slowing, dysarthria, slowing of speech

434

Table 110.1 Neuropsychological profile of the patient on assessment (WISC-R, Wechsler intelligence scale for children – revised; PPVT-R, Peabody picture vocabulary test – revised.)

Age (years)	IQ test	Full-scale IQ	Verbal IQ	Performance IQ	Other diagnoses
7.25	WISC-R	116	110	120	Attention disorder, poor right hand dexterity
8.80	WISC-R	98	92	105	Attention disorder, poor right hand dexterity, impaired expressive language, reduction in affective tone
9.40	WISC-R	74	75	78	Attention disorder, poor right hand dexterity, impaired expressive language, reduction in affective tone, marked disruption of memory abilities, worsening of fine motor skills
11.5–14.2					Attention disorder, poor right hand dexterity, impaired expressive language, reduction in affective tone, marked disruption of memory abilities, worsening of fine motor skills
13.4 (began the ketogenic diet)					
15	PPVT-R	105	Average		

and perseveration. His cranial nerve and motor examination revealed no focal deficits.

Multiple routine EEGs were normal. Magnetic resonance imaging of the brain revealed a hypothalamic mass 10–12 mm in diameter from the center of the hypothalamus, consistent with a hypothalamic hamartoma.

Video-EEG monitoring at the age of 13 revealed a diffusely slow background (4.5–5 Hz with admixed delta activity in the waking state) without epileptiform discharges. Over 2 days he had 150 partial seizures. Most were simple partial seizures without EEG change; some were complex partial seizures with diffuse EEG attenuation.

Diagnosis

Refractory seizures in a patient with hypothalamic hamartoma.

Treatment and outcome

All treatment options were discussed with the family, including surgical removal of the hamartoma, which was believed to be the only curative treatment for his condition. However, our patient did not want to risk the endocrine complications. He therefore agreed to a trial of the ketogenic diet, and then surgery if necessary.

The patient was initiated on the ketogenic diet and within days showed remarkable improvement. Within 1 year his antiepileptic drugs and the drugs used for behavioral therapy were withdrawn.

He has now been on the 4:1 ketogenic diet for 2 years and his urinary ketones are consistently 160 mg/dl. He is off all medications and only has one or two brief (5-second) simple sensory partial seizures a day. These are very mild and no one but the patient can tell when he has one.

The patient's neuropsychological examination was repeated 21 months after initiation of the ketogenic diet. There was improvement in his intelligence, which was now estimated to be in the average range with potential for further improvement. He was also found to be capable of making rapid academic progress. His executive functions were well developed.

He tolerates the ketogenic diet wonderfully and has had no complications. His lipid profile is normal. His dysarthria has showed significant improvement.

Commentary

Hypothalamic hamartomas are congenital malformations that consist of masses of neuronal tissue in ectopic locations. They typically originate from one of the mamillary bodies and extend into the interpeduncular cistern.[1] The histological structure most often resembles that of normal posterior hypothalamus, containing neurosecretory granules. Extralesional abnormalities of cerebral structure may also be present.[2]

These malformations may be asymptomatic or they may cause cognitive decline, a seizure disorder, behavioral problems or precocious puberty. The wide seizure spectrum associated with this condition is characterized by gelastic seizures, which are usually brief, repetitive, stereotyped attacks of laughter that begin in early childhood. Later, there may be complex partial seizures and a pattern of symptomatic generalized epilepsy with tonic, atonic and other seizure types in association with slow spike–wave discharges.[3] Hypothalamic hamartomas are intrinsically epileptogenic.[2] There may be other epileptic foci in the presence of dysplastic cortex.

Seizures are often refractory to medical management. Abatement of seizures has been reported after surgical removal, but larger series imply that patients are unlikely to become seizure-free and extirpation of the hamartoma may be associated with significant morbidity, including diabetes insipidus and panhypopituitarism.[4] For patients with a midline hamartoma, surgery may mean a lifetime of endocrine replacement therapy. In a cognitively impaired child this can be difficult and, during acute illnesses, potentially life-threatening.

Other operative procedures include resection of epileptogenic cortex[5] and corpus callosotomy.[6] These surgical approaches have not been shown to have a favorable outcome in reducing seizures. Recently, we have seen seizure improvement with vagus nerve stimulation in some patients.[7]

What did we learn from this case?

We learned that the ketogenic diet might be efficacious in the management of refractory seizures in a patient with hypothalamic hamartoma. Additionally, this patient's progressive cognitive decline and psychosis were reversed.

How did this case alter our approach to the care and treatment of our epilepsy patients?

This case suggested that earlier institution of the ketogenic diet might have prevented the cognitive decline and the development of behavioral problems. As a result, we now offer the ketogenic diet early for seizures associated with hypothalamic hamartoma. We also offer vagus nerve stimulation as a treatment

437

option. If these therapies are not successful we recommend direct surgical removal or gamma knife treatment.

References

1. Diebler C, Ponsot G. Hamartomas of the tuber cinereum. *Neuroradiology* 1983;**25**:93–101.

2. Berkovic SF, Kuzniecky RI, Andermann F. Human epileptogenesis and hypothalmic hamartomas: new lessons from an experiment of nature. *Epilepsia* 1997;**38**:1–3.

3. Tasch E, Cendes F, Dubea F, *et al*. Hypothalamic hamartomas and gelastic epilepsy: a spectroscopic study. *Neurology* 1998;**51**:1046–50.

4. Breningstall GN. Gelastic seizures, precocious puberty and hypothalamic hamartoma. *Neurology* 1985;**26**:509–27.

5. Cascino GD, Andermann F, Berkovic SF, *et al*. Gelastic seizures and hypothalamic hamartomas: Evaluation of patients undergoing chronic intracranial EEG monitoring and outcome of surgical treatment. *Neurology* 1993;**43**:747–50.

6. Pallini R, Bozzini V, Coliccho G, *et al*. Callosotomy for generalized seizures associated with hypothalamic hamartoma. *Neurol Res* 1993;**15**:139–41.

7. Murphy JV, Wheless JW, Schmoll CM. Left vagal nerve stimulation in six patients with hypothalamic hamartoma. *Pediatr Neurol* 2000;**23**:167–8.

VI

CONCLUSION

We are now in the era of evidence-based medicine. Medical books and the peer-reviewed literature frown on case reports in favor of patient series, cohort studies and multi-center trials. As technology advances, patients are increasingly screened, diagnosed and treated based on computerized protocols and algorithms – all derived from homogenized population-based data.

Yet, clinicians know that there is no *average* patient. There is no patient who perfectly fits the textbook description of a condition or who can be fully characterized by means, medians and chi square statistics. We recognize the importance of treating each patient uniquely, of bringing our knowledge and experience to the specific details of their individual situations and life histories. Knowledge comes from textbooks and the literature, but experience is still derived from listening to and caring for patients, one at a time, and being prepared to recognize the unexpected.

This book reminds us of the importance of the doctor-patient relationship because it shows that epileptologists, no matter how seasoned or experienced, learn powerful lessons from their patients. It further demonstrates that there is no substitute, no matter how hi-tech, for spending adequate time with patients.

We are grateful to the clinicians who shared their memorable cases with us, and to their patients. The readers of this book and their future patients are the beneficiaries.

Steven C Schachter, Boston
Dieter Schmidt, Berlin

CASE INDEX

Index

443

445

451

For Product Safety Concerns and Information please contact our EU
representative GPSR@taylorandfrancis.com
Taylor & Francis Verlag GmbH, Kaufingerstraße 24, 80331 München, Germany

www.ingramcontent.com/pod-product-compliance
Ingram Content Group UK Ltd.
Pitfield, Milton Keynes, MK11 3LW, UK
UKHW021445080625
459435UK00011B/373